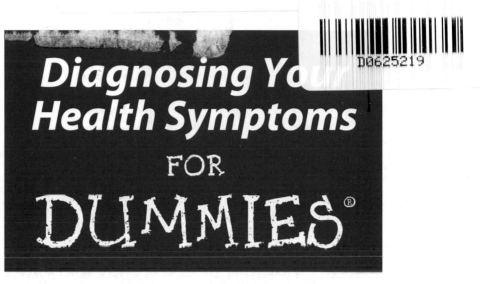

Diagnosing Your Health Symptoms

FOR DUMMIES®

by Dr Knut Schroeder
MD MSc PhD MRCP FRCGP CertMedEd

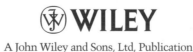

WILEY

A John Wiley and Sons, Ltd, Publication

Diagnosing Your Health Symptoms For Dummies®

Published by
John Wiley & Sons, Ltd
The Atrium
Southern Gate
Chichester
West Sussex
PO19 8SQ
England

E-mail (for orders and customer service enquires): cs-books@w

Visit our Home Page on www.wiley.com

Copyright © 2010 John Wiley & Sons, Ltd, Chichester, West Susse

Published by John Wiley & Sons, Ltd, Chichester, West Sussex

For general information on our other products and services, please contact our Customer Care Department within the U.S. at 877-762-2974, outside the U.S. at 317-572-3993, or fax 317-572-4002.

For technical support, please visit www.wiley.com/techsupport.

Wiley also publishes its books in a variety of electronic formats. Some content that appears in print may not be available in electronic books.

British Library Cataloguing in Publication Data: A catalogue record for this book is available from the British Library

ISBN 978-0-470-66096-6 (paperback), ISBN 978-0-470-66469-8 (ebk), ISBN 978-0-470-66470-4 (ebk), ISBN 978-0-470-66498-8 (ebk)

Printed and bound in Great Britain by Bell and Bain Ltd., Glasgow

10 9 8 7 6 5 4 3 2 1

WILEY

About the Author

Dr Knut Schroeder is a practising General Practitioner in Bristol, Honorary Senior Clinical Lecturer at the University of Bristol, a Fellow of the Royal College of General Practitioners and a GP trainer. His main interests (as far as work is concerned) include medical education and clinical diagnosis, and to these ends he has co-developed and taught courses on clinical diagnosis and evidence-based medicine to undergraduate students and postgraduate medical doctors.

Knut has written two previous books – *Top Tips for GPs - A Beginner's Guide to General Practice* and the best-selling *The 10-Minute Clinical Assessment* – and is guest author on the third edition of the *Oxford Handbook of General Practice*. He co-wrote two chapters for the *Oxford Textbook of Primary Medical Care* and had articles and research papers published in major peer-reviewed international medical journals, including the *British Medical Journal*, *The British Journal of General Practice*, *Family Practice* and *Archives of Internal Medicine*. Knut's passion is spending time with his wife and their two young boys and being outdoors running or cycling.

Dedication

Firstly, this book is dedicated to all the patients who trust their GPs with their worries and health concerns, particularly those whom I had the honour to know quite closely over the years and who've inspired me to write this book. I also dedicate it to all the caring, hardworking and enthusiastic nurses, doctors and other people working in the NHS – particularly my colleagues and the staff at The Stokes Medical Centre, who work so tirelessly at the 'frontline' (and behind the scenes!) towards better patient care.

Author's Acknowledgements

I owe much gratitude to a number of people who stimulated and encouraged me to write this book – in particular Mary Banks, Rosie Gilmour and Stewart Redpath, who helped so much with 'sowing the seeds'. Various people commented on earlier versions of the manuscript, and I'm very grateful to the staff and colleagues at the Stokes Medical Centre in Bristol for their inspiration, advice and constructive criticism, with special thanks to Tracey Frost, Sharlene Hodson, Lou Simeone, Wendie Smith and Mandy Stewart.

A big thank you also to Monisha Choudhury, James Dron, Clive Haddrell (from *First Response*) and Hauke Jörgensen who commented on parts of the book, came up with some great ideas and made a number of excellent suggestions! I would also like to thank the wonderful editorial and production team at Wiley – in particular Nicole Hermitage and Steve Edwards – along with the copy editor, Andy Finch, the technical reviewer, Dr Rodger Charlton, and the proofreader, Dawn Bates, for all their kind support, gentle advice, patience, inspiration, enthusiasm and hard work throughout.

Finally, I thank my wife Sharmila and my fantastic sons, Kiran and Rohan, for being so supportive and tolerant throughout.

Publisher's Acknowledgements

We're proud of this book; please send us your comments through our Dummies online registration form located at www.dummies.com/register/.

Some of the people who helped bring this book to market include the following:

Commissioning, Editorial, and Media Development

Development Editor: Steve Edwards

Commissioning Editor: Nicole Hermitage

Assistant Editor: Ben Kemble

Copy Editor: Andy Finch

Technical Editor: Dr Rodger Charlton

Proofreader: Dawn Bates

Production Manager: Daniel Mersey

Cover Photos: © Jeffrey Coolidge

Cartoons: Ed McLachlan

Composition Services

Project Coordinator: Lynsey Stanford

Layout and Graphics: Ashley Chamberlain

Proofreader: Melissa Cossell

Indexer: Ty Koontz

Special Help:

Brand Reviewer: Carrie Burchfield

Contents at a Glance

Table of Contents

Introduction

· ·

*E*verybody develops new health problems sometimes. Often, these prob-lems are familiar and not especially worrying. When you wake up with a slightly sore throat or get a mild headache after a long, busy day, for exam-ple, the chances are that you've already had this kind of thing before and you know instinctively what to do about it. You probably wait for a few days to see what happens, and in the meantime you might take some painkillers to help ease your symptoms.

But what if your sore throat doesn't settle? What if your headache gets worse rather than better? And what if you develop other additional symptoms such as vomiting or a fever? At some stage, you're likely to start worrying about your symptoms and start thinking what to do next, and whether you should seek medical advice.

Finding answers to these types of questions can be difficult. Your nan may have given you answers and advice on home remedies in the past, and yes, one of your friends might have spoken about a particular 'catch-all cure' for headaches. But then you remember that a distant relative of yours became seriously ill once because he ignored his health symptoms for too long, and so you begin to wonder whether it's safe to ignore your own symptoms. That's where this book comes in.

About This Book

This book tries to answer these types of questions. Think of it as an expe-rienced friend, whom you can rely on when you're dealing with a medical symptom and just don't know what to do about it. This book (like a well-trusted and experienced granny) does the following:

- ↙ Explains in plain language what your symptom may mean, and what a sensible course of action may be.

- ↙ Gives you straight-talking information and advice before you call the doctor or go on the Internet to look up health information.

- ↙ Makes clear to you when you're safe to wait and see what happens – and when you're better off seeking professional, medical advice.

- ↙ Points you in the right direction of where to look or go next, because no book or friend can possibly give you the answers to every question about your health.

As the last point implies, you need to be aware of any book's limitations as regards dealing with health symptoms, which are often straightforward but can sometimes be difficult to interpret. I do all I can to enable you to 'read' your symptoms, but if in doubt, always seek medical help and advice.

I based my decisions on what to include in this book largely on my own experience as a General Practitioner, and so I cover the topics that many patients tell me are important to them. The information and advice I give about symptoms and what to do about them is wherever possible based on good research evidence and current accepted medical guidelines in the UK.

I designed the book to be a health reference that you can dip in and out of as you like without the need to read from cover to cover, but if you want to read it all, to discover more about health symptoms and what they may mean, jump right in here!

Conventions Used in This Book

I use a few conventions in this book to help you navigate the text:

- ✔ *Italics* highlight new words – particularly medical terms. Usually I give you lay terms in plain English, but mention and explain medical terms as well, so you can look these words up in medical dictionaries or on the Internet if you want to. This approach may also help you to better understand any medical language that you hear health professionals using.
- ✔ **Boldfaced font** highlights the key concepts in a list, or the action part of a numbered list.
- ✔ Monofont is used for website addresses.

For general examples, I use the male gender in odd-numbered chapters and female in even-numbered chapters.

Scattered throughout the book are shaded areas called *sidebars*. In these sidebars you can find information that's interesting but not essential – you can skip them if you want and still understand everything else.

What You Won't Find in This Book

This book is neither a medical textbook, nor a reference about every health problem that exists. Also, I don't provide detailed information about medication and other treatments, because they depend in many cases on the final diagnosis – which you always need to leave to a health professional if you're in any doubt.

Foolish Assumptions

In writing this book, I make the following assumptions about you:

- ✔ You want to enjoy your life to the full and stay healthy.

- ✔ You don't know the meaning of certain health symptoms and medical terms and although you don't want to become a medical expert, you do want to have the information on hand to help you deal with any health problems that you and your family may encounter.

- ✔ You don't want to waste your GP's or other health professionals' time unnecessarily, but you want to know under what circumstances you really need to take action about your health.

- ✔ You haven't had medical training in managing the types of symptoms that I cover in this book, but you want to be able to tackle minor health problems yourself and feel that you have the confidence to do so.

How This Book Is Organised

I divide this book into six parts to help you find the information and advice you need about your health problems. A photo section in the middle shows you what certain conditions can look like

Part I: Spotting and Assessing Illness: The Basics

Part I gives an introduction to the best ways to approach health symptoms. It guides you through sensible questions you can ask yourself when faced with a medical problem, ways to check your body for any signs of illness and where to find appropriate medical help.

Part II: Looking at Emergencies and 'All-Over' Symptoms

This part provides the essentials about assessing and managing common emergencies and more on general health symptoms.

Part III: Going From Top to Toe: Looking at Specific Areas of the Body

Part III devotes individual chapters to various parts of the human body, looking at health symptoms that affect particular areas.

Part IV: Dealing With Health Problems in Specific Groups

Part IV takes a different approach and looks at common and important health problems in different age groups – babies, children, teenagers and older people – as well as problems specific to women and men, and those more common in later life.

Part V: Approaching Mental Health Problems and Addictive Behaviour

Here you find out how to spot and deal with symptoms surrounding your mental health, such as stress, anxiety or depression. This part also looks at unusual thoughts and behaviour as well as alcohol and drug problems.

Part VI: The Part of Tens

No *For Dummies* book is complete without a Part of Tens. Here I present some key suggestions – the stuff you most need to know, but perhaps least want to know. You get an introduction to providing first aid and basic life support and find out about some common medical tests in case you ever need them. This part also gives you details of ten reliable websites you can trust, pointing you in the right direction when you want to look up medical information on the Internet.

Icons Used in This Book

Every *For Dummies* book contains a selection of icons to highlight information that may be of particular interest to you, that make important points you don't want to miss or even indicate what you can safely miss when you're short of time.

Here's an explanation of each icon:

Getting scared or even panicky when you're faced with certain medical symptoms is all too easy. This icon tells you when a health problem is unlikely to be serious and highlights information that I hope reassures you.

This icon acts as a warning. It draws your attention to issues and symptoms that suggest a health problem may be due to a serious underlying cause. This situation may not always be the case, but if you see this icon you need to be alert and seek medical advice if you're unsure of what to do.

When you see this icon, you need to act quickly – for example, consult a doctor or even call for an ambulance in the case of a true emergency.

Many health symptoms and illnesses have myths attached to them – through word of mouth or unfortunate reports in the media, or even just common fears about a particular condition. This icon dispels one or more myths around certain health symptoms or their management.

This icon means that the information is essential and worth bearing in mind.

When you see this icon, the text next to it contains advice that may be particularly useful to you, or save you time and effort.

This icon gives you some deeper background that you can skip if you prefer, although the information may increase your knowledge about a particular topic.

Where to Go from Here

I've written this book so you can approach each chapter individually without having to read from cover to cover. The Table of Contents can help you to jump straight into any chapter or section that you think may be relevant, and the Index allows you to locate any particular symptoms or illnesses.

But if you want to get a good basic knowledge of how to assess and manage health problems, you may enjoy reading the whole book from start to finish. The choice is yours! Where information is relevant to more than one topic, I provide cross-references to other chapters.

I sincerely hope that you enjoy reading this book and that you gain increased confidence to deal with your health symptoms. I hope that it gives you plenty of reassurance and puts your mind at rest when you're faced with a minor medical problem. After all, the vast majority of health complaints are minor and nothing to worry about in the long term.

I also hope that this book kick-starts you into action if you ever have a symptom that indicates a potentially serious health problem . . . which does at times happen – though rarely.

Part I
Spotting and Assessing Illness: The Basics

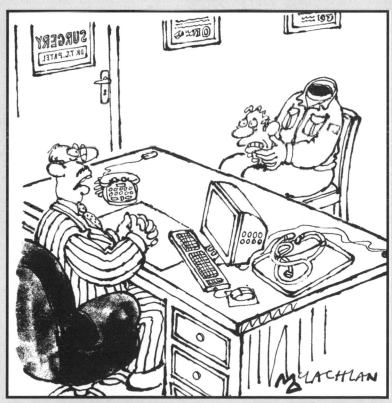

'I wish you'd come to me earlier when you realised self-harming was becoming a habit and getting worse.'

In this part . . .

Dealing with medical problems doesn't come naturally to many people and can be quite scary if you're not used to it. The good news is that things can be different, and armed with a bit of basic knowledge you can identify and assess many illnesses yourself.

Part I is all about basic strategies for approaching and managing almost any health problem sensibly. This part gives you an overview and insight into how your body works, and you can find guidance on where to get further help and information when you need it as well as advice on how to access the right health services for you.

Chapter 1

Understanding Your Health Problems

In This Chapter

▶ Recognising and approaching health problems in yourself

▶ Discovering more about your body

*H*ealth problems are part of life. The fact is that everyone gets ill sometimes – though hopefully not too often – and when you develop a
medical symptom you need to decide what to do about it. For example, you
may choose to see your pharmacist, consult your doctor, go to the nearest
Accident & Emergency (A&E) department – or, in the worst case, phone for
an ambulance. You may even choose to do nothing at all.

So that you stay healthy and get the best available health advice and treatment when you fall ill, you need to be able to make sensible decisions about
your health. Doing so can be tricky and occasionally a bit scary. Not surprisingly, you can feel out of your depth all too easily. Most people successfully
make decisions about their healthcare just by using common sense, but
instances do occur when you're not quite sure what to do or your health
problems develop gradually and you start to think about getting medical help.

These situations are where *Diagnosing Your Health Symptoms For Dummies*
can help. In the same way that you don't have to be a professional mechanic
or engineer to identify and deal with simple problems relating to your car or
dishwasher, you don't have to be a doctor to be able to recognise common or
potentially serious health problems or to have the confidence to decide what
to do about them. You do have to be a health professional, though, to deal
with and treat a great many conditions, and so knowing when you can treat an
illness yourself and when to seek medical advice is an essential skill.

In this chapter I introduce you to ways in which you can approach your
health symptoms sensibly (I cover some useful tips, tricks, tools and strategies in more detail in Chapters 2 to 4). I provide a brief overview of your
body's anatomy and how certain parts of it work, so you can more easily
understand the health problems that I cover elsewhere in this book.

Thinking Like a Medic: You Can Do It!

Medical problems come in all shapes and sizes. Some are easy to recognise, simple or harmless, whereas others may not be so obvious, are complex, or even dangerous. Telling the difference between them can be quite tricky, and making a formal medical diagnosis is best left to the professionals.

Whenever you develop a health problem, you automatically make a diagnosis yourself – whether you know it or not. If you develop a headache, for example, you may decide to ignore it for a few days and see what happens, or take some simple painkillers to relieve your symptoms. But what if the headache gets worse, or if it's very severe? When – and how – can you tell whether you should seek medical advice? This section aims to help you make these types of decisions by thinking like a medic – so that you can approach a variety of common or potentially serious problems appropriately. I give you some tools to help you make more informed decisions about your health and decide when to seek help, explaining the symptoms of common conditions and how to spot signs of serious illness.

Reacting to medical problems sensibly

Everyone reacts to medical problems differently, but broadly speaking, people often behave in one of the following three ways. Think whether any of these approaches sounds like the way you usually deal with health concerns:

- **Dealing with a medical problem appropriately:** Most people first have a quick think about possible causes of their health problem and then deal with the problem themselves, seeking advice or treatment from a health professional such as a pharmacist, nurse or doctor when necessary.

- **Having a 'stiff-upper-lip' attitude:** Other people are stoical, thinking that they know what's going on and that nothing needs to be done, or can be done. Stoics tend to 'wait and see' for a long time even when they're quite unwell, their symptoms get worse rather than better and others tell them to call the doctor because they're worried about them – sometimes stoics behave this way with great detriment to their health.

- **Worrying far too much:** Some people are preoccupied with their body functions and tend to think that even minor problems must be due to a potentially serious medical condition, meaning that they continually feel anxious about their health. This worrying makes them 'trigger-happy' about approaching health professionals – mainly for reassurance.

Having to deal with medical problems in yourself and other people can feel quite scary, and you can be forgiven for panicking or calling a health professional straight away. However, to think like a medic, a better idea is to:

✔ **Stay calm:** Try not to get too anxious over a symptom – the vast majority of health problems aren't due to serious illness. Don't make things worse for you and other people by worrying unnecessarily, but don't delay seeking medical advice and reassurance when you need it.

✔ **Take your time:** Apart from acutely life-threatening emergency situations, such as bleeding profusely or having a major heart attack (see Chapter 5 for more info), you normally have a bit of time to assess your health problem yourself in a basic way. So try not to panic!

Throughout this book you can find situations where not worrying and waiting to see is appropriate and, in contrast, when getting medical help fast is best.

Acquiring basic skills in self-diagnosis

When you're in the right frame of mind, you can approach health problems in the same way that you tackle any other problem in your daily life, assessing your symptoms in the following way:

1. **Ask questions:** Asking yourself a number of questions relevant to your health problems can help you to narrow down the causes of your symptom and make an initial diagnosis. But more importantly, asking questions is really about *prognosis* – that is, whether your health problem is more likely to be benign or serious, and what this fact means for your future health. Chapter 2 looks at this process and gives you just enough information to ask yourself some key questions.

2. **Check your body:** Looking for physical signs can help you find out what may be going on. Chapter 3 looks at general physical pointers to illness, and how to spot them. After checking your body, use the contents pages to find the chapter relevant to your health problem for specific information. And don't worry, this process is all pretty straightforward.

You don't need any background knowledge or experience to use this book for diagnosing your health symptoms, although you may find that certain techniques get easier when you practise them a bit (such as checking your temperature or feeling for a pulse). This book gives you the basics – think of it as a starter kit that you can use quickly when health problems arise – and as much information as you need to decide what to do next. If you want to gain more confidence in dealing with emergencies, read Chapters 5 and 24. If you acquire a taste for self-diagnosis and want to discover more, flip to Chapter 25 where you can find a list of websites that you can trust.

Looking at health behaviour

Researchers have looked at people's health behaviour and tried to explain why different people deal with health problems in different ways. They uncovered various influencing factors, such as:

✔ **Feeling threatened by a health condition:** The bigger you think your risk is of suffering from a health problem (say, a heart attack or HIV infection), the more likely you are to seek help from a health professional. And vice versa – if you don't think you're at risk, you're more likely to wait and see. Generally speaking, the higher the threat, the more likely you are to try and do something about it, and if you feel that the consequences of ignoring your health condition are potentially serious, you're more likely to seek medical advice.

✔ **Getting 'cues to action':** This factor means that physical symptoms (such as a severe pain or feeling dizzy) or some other cue (such as watching a TV programme or reading a newspaper article about a health condition) may prompt you to go and see your doctor.

✔ **Having confidence in dealing with medical problems:** You may feel quite confident in dealing with a medical symptom, or you may always need or want reassurance.

✔ **Thinking about medical problems in a certain way:** The environment in which you live or work can affect how you approach health problems. You may belong to a family or group of friends who are always anxious about their health, or you may work in a hard-nosed business where succumbing to medical problems is frowned upon. Or the way in which you're brought up may influence how you respond to any health symptoms. For example, you may say things like 'my mum/dad always panicked when it came to health problems', which now makes you anxious about your health. Or you remember that 'I was always told not to be a crybaby – to ignore the pain and just get on with it', which may lead you not to pay attention to your health symptoms – even when they're potentially serious.

Trying to figure out what influences your behaviour can be worthwhile when dealing with health symptoms. Becoming more self-aware and being able to 'step back' can be very useful when assessing and managing your medical problems.

Discovering How Your Body Works

In this section I give you a short guided tour through your anatomy, so you can understand the symptoms that I cover in this book. You don't need to become an expert, but having a rough idea about where the major structures in your body are located and how they work goes a long way towards making sense of medical symptoms. And don't worry, you're safe to read on – I haven't included any gory pictures or overly detailed descriptions here!

Getting around with cells

At the root of everything are the tiny *cells* that make up your body. You can't see cells because they're very, very small – smaller than the sharp end of a pin. Cells can divide and develop into different types such as, for example, nerve cells, muscle cells, or skin cells – and loads of others. Many cells don't live as long as you do – they die off after a certain amount of time and are replaced by new ones, which explains why your body can grow, your wounds heal and your bones join back together again.

When cells multiply at a higher rate than they die, the process is called *cancer*. Because the body contains so many different types of cells, numerous types of cancer exist that produce many different symptoms. Cancer treatment has vastly improved in recent years and helps people with cancer to live longer and lead a better life, but the condition is still a huge problem worldwide and a major cause of illness and death. (You can read more about cancer in Chapter 6 and in chapters relating to specific areas of the body.)

Knocking about with the bare bones

Just over 200 bones support your body and protect some of your organs – your brain, lungs and heart in particular. But your bones have other functions, too: some of them – for example, the long bones in your legs and arms – provide levers for your muscles, which can contract and relax, ensuring that you can walk around and carry out actions with your hands. Your bones also contain *bone marrow*, which produces your blood cells (see 'Pumping blood around your body' later in this chapter).

More than 24 separate bones (called *vertebrae*) form your spine and connect at the top to the base of your skull. Your spine holds your *spinal cord*, which contains *nerve fibres* that convey messages from your brain to your arms, legs and other organs (you can find more info in the 'Checking in with your brain and nerves' section later in this chapter). The ends of your bones in particular are often covered by a strong and smooth material called *cartilage* – usually in spaces where two or more bones move against each other. These places are called *joints*, which come in various forms and sizes, such as:

- **Ball and socket joints:** In joints that you need to be able to move within a wider range (such as your shoulder and hip joints), you can find ball and socket joints, which enable you to move in various directions.

- **Hinge joints:** These joints allow movement in only one direction – your fingers, toes, knees and elbows are good examples. To make these joints more stable, strong fibrous tissues called *ligaments* are attached to both bones that form a joint and hold them nicely together.

- **Saddle joints:** You can find saddle joints, for example, in your thumbs, which can move sideways as well as back and forth.

A thin membrane covers your joints so they can contain a small amount of fluid for lubrication.

Muscles are attached to your bones through *tendons* and exert their force onto your bones by becoming shorter (they *contract*). Most joints have at least one pair of muscles attached to them to pull the joint in opposite directions.

Common symptoms when something isn't quite right with your bones, joints, or muscles may be due to inflammation. *Inflammation* is your body's response to injury or irritation and shows itself through swelling, pain, redness and heat. When one or more of your joints shows these signs, the cause can sometimes be overuse or – on rare occasions – infection, in which case you may have a fever, too (see Chapter 7 for more info on fever).

Common medical conditions that can affect your joints are inflammation due to overuse, breakage of a bone (called *fracture*), 'wear and tear' (known as *osteoarthritis*) or ongoing joint inflammation (such as *rheumatoid arthritis*). Arthritis may in the long run lead to joint stiffness and distortion. You can read more about bone and joint problems in Chapter 13.

Because bone cells continuously replace old bone with new bone, following a healthy diet that contains vitamins (Vitamin D in particular), protein, and calcium is important.

Pumping blood around your body

Your *blood* is a fluid that consists of red blood cells (or *erythrocytes*), which transport oxygen to your cells, white blood cells (or *leucocytes*), which are responsible for, among other things, fighting infections, and blood platelets (known as *thrombocytes*), which help to stop any bleeding. These cells are suspended in a clear yellowish fluid called *plasma*, which also contains proteins, salts and other chemicals. All your tissues need blood like a plant needs water, and blood vessels help with the 'irrigation'.

Mapping out your heart

Your *heart* pumps blood around your body. Think of it as a hollow muscular pump made up of four separate chambers, to which are attached large blood vessels that carry blood around your body and to and from your lungs.

The two main types of blood vessels attached to your heart are:

 ✔ **Arteries:** Arteries are thick-walled blood vessels that can tolerate higher pressures and contain the blood that's being pumped out of your heart. Arteries run from your heart to your lungs and from your heart to other areas of your body such as your brain, limbs and internal organs.

✔ **Veins:** Veins have thinner walls and generally carry blood to your heart from other parts of your body. Most veins run close to the surface of your body before they link up to the deeper veins, and you may be able to see them on the back of your hand, your forearm or your lower legs.

When your heart muscle contracts at (usually) a regular rate, the pressure inside your heart increases, so that blood flows out of your heart into the arteries to your body or your lungs, where it picks up _oxygen_ (one of the most important nutrients for your tissues). When your heart muscle relaxes, the heart expands, allowing blood to return to your heart through major veins. _Heart valves_ prevent the blood from flowing back, so your blood always only flows in one direction – called _circulation_ – and your heart then pumps it on to other areas of your body.

Understanding the importance of good circulation

Like the flow of water in the plumbing of your house or in your washing machine, blood flows properly only when your blood vessels are open and not obstructed by clots or fatty deposits (which can occur in what's known as _cardiovascular disease_). Your blood pressure also needs not to be too high, because persistently raised blood pressure (known as _hypertension_) causes a strain to your heart and can lead to damage of your blood vessels.

When you have your blood pressure checked, you may hear your GP or nurse mumble something like '. . .your blood pressure is 140 over 80', or you may see it written down as '140/80 mmHg'. Here's what these terms mean:

✔ **Systolic blood pressure** is the maximum pressure in your arm artery at the time when your heart contracts.

✔ **Diastolic blood pressure** is the resting blood pressure at the time when your heart fills up again and relaxes between beats.

✔ **mmHg** is the unit in which your blood pressure is measured. mmHg is the pressure needed to push a column of mercury (the chemical symbol for mercury is _Hg_) within a cylindrical vial up a certain distance (measured in millimetres), hence mmHg. Traditional blood pressure machines have now largely been replaced with newer electronic ones, but the same units of measurement are still being used.

Your blood pressure is said to be too high if it's above 140/90 mmHg each time you have a reading taken. You can have:

✔ **High systolic blood pressure:** For example, a blood pressure of 170/84 mmHg.

✔ **High diastolic blood pressure:** For example, a blood pressure of 132/98 mmHg.

✔ **Combined systolic and diastolic high blood pressure:** For example, a blood pressure of 184/114 mmHg.

Treating raised blood pressure reduces your risk of suffering a heart attack or stroke, but in deciding whether you need to receive treatment your doctors consider various factors in addition to the actual level of your blood pressure. 'Acceptable' blood pressures can therefore vary from person to person.

If your blood vessels are too narrow or blocked, or your blood pressure is too high or too low, you may develop health problems. Depending on which area of your body isn't receiving enough blood (or enough of the oxygen and other nutrients that your blood transports), you may notice:

- **Brain symptoms:** If the blood supply to your brain is impaired you may feel dizzy, faint, confused or develop sudden limb weakness in the case of a complete blockage (for example, because of a stroke).

- **Heart symptoms:** When the blood supply to and from your heart is compromised, you may feel breathless, develop chest pain or suffer from palpitations.

- **Leg symptoms:** A blood clot in your *veins* (which carry the blood back to your heart) can cause pain and swelling in one of your legs (known as *deep venous thrombosis*, or *DVT*). This condition is dangerous because the clot can dislodge and travel to your lungs, where it can block a blood vessel. This can be dangerous and requires urgent treatment (see *pulmonary embolism* under 'Lung symptoms' in this list).

- **Limb symptoms:** Lack of blood supply to one or both of your legs can lead to intermittent pain on walking (called *intermittent claudication*) or leg sores (called *ulcers*).

- **Lung symptoms:** A blood clot in the artery leading from your heart to your lungs (known as a *pulmonary embolism* causing symptoms such as chest pain, shortness of breath, coughing up blood and collapse) may develop from DVT and can be life-threatening.

To find out more about circulation problems, check out Chapters 5, 10 and 20.

Filling up on oxygen

Imagine your *lungs* to be like two big sponges inside your chest, which expand when you breathe in (*inhaling*) and contract when you breathe out (*exhaling*). Air flows from your nose or your mouth through your throat (called the *pharynx*), voice box (known as *larynx*) and windpipe (or *trachea*) into your lungs, where the air gets into the lung tissue through branching tubes (called *bronchi* and *bronchioles*). The passages through which the air travels to your lungs are called *respiratory tract* or *airways*.

A thin lining covers your airways from the inside to help keep the air warm and moist. The most common problem affecting the respiratory tract is an inflammation of this lining caused by an infection such as a cold, but many conditions can affect your airways and lungs. Common symptoms include:

- ✔ **Cough:** Coughs can be *acute* (in other words, they come on suddenly and last no longer than three to four weeks) or *chronic* (ongoing).

- ✔ **Shortness of breath:** Breathing difficulties may be due to respiratory problems, but can also be brought on by heart problems or other medical conditions (you can find more on breathing problems in Chapter 10).

- ✔ **Wheezing:** Wheezing is the noise you make when you breathe through narrowed airways and is common in asthma or chronic obstructive pulmonary disease (see Chapter 10 for details on these conditions).

Smoking dramatically increases your risk of developing problems with your airways. (For information on respiratory symptoms, see Chapters 5, 9 and 10.)

Travelling down to your intestines

Your *digestive system* stretches from your mouth to your back passage – with the bit containing your stomach and your bowels called your *gastrointestinal tract*. The main function of your digestive system is to break down food and drink that you take in, so your body gets the protein, carbohydrates, fats, minerals and vitamins it needs.

After chewing food in your mouth, a mixture of food and saliva travels down your gullet (or the *oesophagus*) into your stomach, where it gets broken down by acidic digestive juices. When the stomach contents have become a bit more liquid, they move into the *duodenum* (the first part of your *small bowel*), where more digestive juices from organs called your *pancreas* and *liver* break down the liquid further to enable your body to extract the necessary nutrients in the *small intestine*. Everything that's left over flows as a thin fluid into your large bowel (known as the *colon*), which absorbs most of the water contained in the fluid back into your body. After this process you're left with 'poo' (or *stool*), which is stored in the last bit of your large bowel (your *rectum*) which tells you to go to the toilet to open your bowels when it becomes full.

Your *liver* is a large and important sponge-like organ located in the right upper part of your abdomen and has many functions. It 'cleans' your blood from toxins, recycles ageing blood cells and helps regulate the breakdown of waste products in your blood. Drinking too much alcohol – a widespread problem around the world – can cause liver problems.

If you have liver problems, or other issues with your gastrointestinal tract, you may develop one or more of the following symptoms:

- ✔ **Abdominal pain:** Tummy pain can occur for many reasons and is one of the most important indicators that something may be going on inside your abdomen.

- ✔ **Constipation:** Hard stools or problems with opening your bowels is a common symptom.

- ✔ **Diarrhoea:** Runny stools are common with bowel infections but may also occur for many other reasons.

- ✔ **Jaundice:** If you have severe liver damage or blocked digestive tubes running from your liver to your intestines, you may develop a yellow tinge in the whites of your eyes and your skin known as *jaundice*.

- ✔ **Nausea and vomiting:** Feeling and being sick are common with stomach infections and liver problems, but many other causes may be responsible.

These symptoms are just a few that can indicate gastrointestinal problems. For more information, flip to Chapter 11.

Checking in with your brain and nerves

Your *brain* is the 'control centre' for your activities, both conscious (such as moving about, talking and thinking) and unconscious (digesting food, breathing or doing things automatically). Your *nerves* pass on 'commands' from your brain to other parts of your body by means of small electrical impulses and act as messengers for sensations such as temperature or pain. Many nerves are bundled together in your *spinal cord*, which acts as your 'information highway', collecting and passing on messages from the brain and your peripheries and running through the bones in your spine.

Your brain needs oxygen and a good blood supply, and your brain cells are in serious trouble if they don't get enough oxygen for more than a couple of minutes. If the blood supply to your brain is completely interrupted (for example, due to a stroke), you may suffer irreversible damage to your brain with potentially severe consequences. Symptoms arising from your brain and nerves can come in various forms and include the following:

- ✔ **Difficulty speaking or understanding:** These symptoms may be due to a brain problem and are common in stroke.

- ✔ **Pain:** Pressure on a nerve often causes pain and can be one of the reasons for back pain (for example, sciatica – see Chapter 13).

- ✔ **Tingling or numbness:** Also referred to by doctors as *paraesthesiae*, these symptoms commonly affect the hands or feet and can be due to a variety of different conditions.

- ✔ **Weakness:** Weakness in a limb or other part of your body may be due to a nerve or brain problem (such as a stroke).

This list contains only a selection of problems that can affect your nervous system – for additional details check the table of contents or the index for problems in specific body areas.

Accepting that it may be your hormones!

Hormones are chemicals produced by organs called *glands*. They facilitate various body functions, but in a different way to nerves (described in the preceding section). Whereas nerves convey 'messages' through electrical impulses, think of hormones as 'chemical messengers'.

Here's a quick low-down on some of the important glands:

- **Adrenal glands:** These glands sit on top of your kidneys and produce hormones (known as *steroid hormones*) to help maintain the right levels of fluid, salts and sugar in your body. They also produce another hormone called adrenaline, a stress hormone that helps to 'get you going' when you're faced with physical or emotional stress.

- **Ovaries:** The ovaries are two olive-size organs deep inside the pelvis of women that produce eggs as well as sex hormones, which are important for sexual and reproductive function. (You can find more information on women's health issues in Chapter 18.)

- **Pancreas:** The pancreas gland is an organ that lies behind your stomach in the back of your abdomen. It helps to make digestive juices that break down your food and produces hormones called insulin and glucagon that are important for keeping your blood sugar levels stable. Insulin acts like a 'key' for getting glucose from your blood into your cells. If you suffer from diabetes mellitus (which I discuss in detail in Chapter 20), you have a lack of insulin in your blood, and your blood sugar levels rise.

- **Pituitary gland:** This gland sits on the base of your skull and, in a nutshell, controls the function of some other hormone- producing glands in your body (including your thyroid gland and your sex hormones).

- **Testes:** Testes are the 'balls' inside the skinny bag between men's legs. These glands produce a hormone called testosterone, which starts off puberty and helps develop some typical male features such as hair growth, the shape of the body and a deeper voice.

- **Thyroid gland:** Your thyroid gland lies in front of your throat and produces a hormone that helps to maintain an even body temperature and keep a check on the way your body converts food into energy.

In essence, hormone problems can be two-fold: the levels may be too high or too low, and the subsequent problems very much depend on the role of the particular hormone. A lack of the hormone insulin, for example, causes diabetes – which is very common. If you lack the thyroid hormone, you may, for example, feel tired and cold. And if you're a man and don't have enough testosterone floating around your body (which is in fact less common than many men think), you may have a reduced sex drive and lack of energy.

Checking out your plumbing

Various organs and structures make up your *urinary system* or *tract*, which is responsible for filtering your blood and getting rid of waste chemicals and excess fluid from your body. These organs include two *kidneys* and two tubes known as *ureters* that drain urine from your kidneys into your *bladder*, which is a hollow organ in your lower abdomen. When your bladder is full, urine passes through another tube (called the *urethra*) and out of your body.

Various symptoms can arise from your urinary tract, which may include:

- ✔ **Pain:** Sudden pain in your *loin* (the area on either side of your backbone, between your ribs and hips) may be due to a small stone (which can form within your urinary system) getting stuck in one of your ureters, or to urinary tract infection.

- ✔ **Urinary symptoms:** Such symptoms are common in urinary tract disorders and include passing urine frequently, painful urination, and blood in your urine. The most common problem affecting the urinary system is bladder infection (or *cystitis*).

You can read more about urinary problems in Chapter 12 and problems with women's and men's sexual functions in Chapters 18 and 19, respectively.

Chapter 2

Conducting a Symptom Check

. . . .

In This Chapter

▶ Establishing the story of your health problem

▶ Considering timing

▶ Narrowing down your problem

▶ Looking out for additional clues

▶ Thinking about other relevant issues

. . . .

Developing a medical symptom is very much like a story: it contains a beginning, a middle and an end. You can usually tell the story of a medical symptom by describing what happened and when, and what the particular circumstances were when everything started. Going through these different story elements can help you make sense of your problem and decide what to do about it.

This chapter is about the different elements of the 'story' of your medical symptoms; it looks at the 'ingredients' of a medical history. I give you an overview of ways to look at your medical problem in more detail and I cover the issues to consider, using a similar structure to the one doctors learn in medical school. This process enables you to get a better idea of what may be going on with your body, to know the important signs to look out for (also check out Chapter 3) and to manage your symptoms confidently (you can find out more about this aspect in Chapter 4). It's all about deciding when a symptom is mild and is something you can deal with yourself, and when to seek professional medical help. The more you know about medical symptoms and conditions, the easier it is for you to make appropriate decisions when you're faced with them – and the more confident you'll be.

Getting the Story Clear

The more you can find out about any new health symptom you develop, the easier you'll reach the right conclusion in terms of what to do next. Like a detective, the best way to gather information is to ask yourself questions. In this section I give you tips on how to spot medical clues and ask the types of questions that can help you get to the bottom of what's going on.

Asking yourself the right questions

Broadly speaking, gathering further information – pulling all the relevant facts and details together to get a clearer picture about what may be happening to you – is a useful first step in conducting a symptom check. For example, with a minor health problem such as a sore throat, you know that the problem's likely to go away on its own and you need only treat your symptoms until the problem disappears within a week or two. But establishing the facts is still useful to identify whether you may be faced with a more complex health problem than you first thought.

Which questions are relevant and important depends on the medical problem facing you. The following sections give you a general overview of the types of questions to ask and why. You can then consult Parts II to V to find out more about the key questions for individual medical problems.

Up to now, maybe you've left this fact-finding mission – called *taking the history* – largely to a health professional. And rightly so: taking an effective history is a complex task and helps medical professionals to gather all the information they need to reach a working diagnosis, order further tests and agree the best plan of action with you – it takes many years of training to do this well.

But you can also do a bit of detective work yourself. Armed with a bit of basic knowledge, which I try to provide in this book, doing this helps you to consider possible underlying causes of your health problems. And knowing what's happened and when – and under which circumstances – can give you and your doctor some important clues. But don't worry – this is really only about becoming better at deciding when to seek medical help. In the same way that you can learn to sort out simple computer problems without being a software engineer – while knowing your limits – you can become better at managing your health symptoms yourself and knowing at what stage to ask for help.

Deciding what you think is wrong

Without much consideration, people often come to their own conclusions about a health problem. Even when you're unsure precisely what's going on, you may often have a feeling about whether your problem's likely to be serious or not. This process is often almost automatic and subconscious, and so try consciously to work out what your instinct is telling you – and why. You may in fact already have an idea of what's causing your symptom(s).

Establishing the Timing of Your Health Problem

When you develop a health problem such as a headache, tiredness or shoulder pain, mapping out a timeline of your symptoms can be extremely useful for identifying the underlying cause and helping you – as well as health professionals – with assessing your symptoms.

Try to remember when the problem started and how it developed. Consider the following factors:

✔ **Onset:** Ask yourself:

- What date and time did you first notice your health problem?

- Did the problem come on suddenly or develop gradually over time?

To give you an example of why establishing this information is important, a sudden severe pain in your knee that starts while you're playing football and that doesn't get better suggests a *ligament injury*, whereas a gradual onset of knee pain over months or years is more likely to be due to something such as *arthritis*. (Turn to Chapter 13 for information on bone and joint troubles.)

✔ **Circumstances:** Ask yourself:

- What were you doing and where were you when the problem started?

    For example, diarrhoea and vomiting a few hours after a 'dodgy' meal suggests food poisoning, or a pain in your foot that comes on after playing sports is likely to be due to an injury or overuse.

- If your problem is due to a particular activity, did you do anything differently to what you normally do?

    Sometimes your activities in the hours or day before the problem started are relevant.

After establishing when the problem started and under which circumstances, look in more detail into what happened. In particular, try to figure out the following:

✔ **Frequency:** Ask yourself:

- If you don't have the symptom all the time, how often do you get it?

To give you an example, an intermittent headache that you have for a while up to a few times every month, lasts for a few days and completely disappears between episodes, is probably more likely due to migraine than to anything else (you can find more on headaches and migraine in Chapter 9).

✔ **Duration:** Ask yourself:

- How long do your symptoms last, and for how long have you had them altogether?

- How long are the periods when you don't have any symptoms?

- When you don't have the symptom, are you completely well between episodes, or does the problem never go away completely?

For example, diarrhoea for only a day or so is likely to be due to an infection, whereas if you have loose stools for weeks, months or even years, other causes are much more likely (see Chapter 11).

✔ **Progression:** Ask yourself:

- How have your symptoms developed over time?

- Are they getting worse? If so, how quickly?

To give you an example, a tummy pain that you've had for only a few hours that gets worse very quickly is likely to be more serious than one that you've had occasionally for years that only very gradually gets worse. Generally speaking, you can be a bit more relaxed about health problems that get better by themselves.

Mapping Out Your Problem

After establishing the timing of your medical symptom, the next essential step to take in working towards a solution is defining the problem, and the clearer you are about what's going on the better.

Identifying and describing your health problem

You can experience medical symptoms in various ways, and the differences between them can sometimes be quite subtle. Thinking about what your main symptom is and describing it to yourself can be very useful for deciding what may be going on. In addition, if you need to see a doctor about your symptoms, being able to paint a picture of your problem and what it means to you can go a long way towards making sure that you get the most from the consultation.

Here is a list of some common medical symptoms and ways to describe them:

- ✔ **General symptoms:** 'General' body symptoms are common and include feeling tired or dizzy. Tiredness, for example, can mean different things: not getting enough sleep, being physically exhausted or lacking in energy because of stress. (To find out more about the causes of tiredness, check out Chapter 6, and read about stress in Chapter 21.)

- ✔ **Pain:** Pain can show up in very different ways. Yours may be stabbing, burning, sharp or dull in nature – you may have another description that fits even better. Being able to describe the type of pain that you experience can sometimes help you identify possible underlying causes.

- ✔ **Sensations:** As well as pain, you may notice other sensations such as tingling, burning, pins and needles or a loss of sensation anywhere on your body. Such symptoms can sometimes indicate that a disturbance to one or more nerves is causing the sensation. For example, nerve problems are fairly common in long-standing diabetes, but may also have other causes such as pressure on a nerve (for example, in *sciatica* – described in Chapter 13). The presence of additional symptoms can sometimes help to identify certain patterns of disease.

Locating your symptoms

The next step in describing your symptoms is to identify exactly where you notice the problem – which is particularly relevant when you have pain. Usually – though not always – the location of your pain gives helpful clues as to what may be wrong.

Here are some examples: the cause of stomach pain often depends on where in your abdomen you notice the pain, or whether it moves about. A gradually worsening pain in the centre of your stomach near your belly button, which moves into the right lower area, for example, is typical of appendicitis – although stomach upsets due to tummy bugs are much more common. Pain in the upper right-hand corner of your stomach, which comes and goes and is quite severe, may be due to gallstones. Pain in one of your loins, which comes on suddenly, may suggest a kidney stone – among many other causes. (You can find more information about these conditions and others in Chapter 11.)

The other important issue is whether a pain spreads (or *radiates*) to other areas. In chest pain, for example, any pain or heaviness in the centre of your chest, which spreads to your jaw, neck, back, shoulders or arms, may suggest heart problems such as angina or a heart attack. (You can read up about these conditions in Chapters 5 and 10.)

Conveying the severity of your symptoms

Rating your symptoms according to their severity is useful. Try using a scale from zero to ten to estimate the severity of your symptom (such as pain), with zero being no symptoms at all and ten being the worst possible symptom you can imagine. A 'ten out of ten' pain would be really, really bad and prevent you from doing almost anything: generally speaking, the more severe your symptom, the more urgent your need to do something about it.

If you have symptoms that fluctuate over time, consider keeping a diary with your symptom scores, to give you an idea whether your underlying condition is improving or getting worse. The information you collect can also help your doctor or another health professional decide on the best type of treatment and assess your response to pain relief.

Always be honest with yourself and health professionals – don't underplay or exaggerate your health problem.

Assessing the impact on your life

One of the most important aspects of a symptom is the impact it has on your quality of life. The same health problem can affect people in very different ways. For example, if playing the piano is an important part of your life, suffering an injury to your little finger may feel catastrophic to you – whereas you may not be as bothered about a stiff knee. However, the situation would be the other way round if you're a professional football player.

You can see, therefore, that assessing the impact a symptom has on your daily life, work or hobbies is important in helping you decide what to do about the problem and how quickly you need to get help. Using the same examples, if you're the piano player you'll be more inclined to undergo an operation on your little finger than if you're the footballer. Assessing the impact of a health problem on your life also helps health professionals to estimate the potential risks and benefits of any treatment that they want to discuss with you.

Noting things that make a difference

The next step to take in making a diagnosis is to think whether you've noticed anything that makes your symptom better or worse. For example, if you have stomach or loin pain that only laying very still improves, you may possibly be suffering from an inflammation or infection of your abdominal lining known as *peritonitis*. However, if you find yourself pacing around the room with pain, you're more likely to have a kidney stone wedged in the tube running from your kidneys to your bladder (called *renal colic*). (You can read more about stomach and urinary symptoms in Chapters 11 and 12 respectively.)

If you have tried anything to ease your symptom, make a list of what worked (particularly any medication) and what didn't. Your list is sure to be useful for yourself and for medical professionals when considering the treatment options. Also make a note of anything that you notice improves your health problem – some people get better after eating or drinking, with rest or when moving around – as well as anything that brings on your symptoms.

Listing other signs

Many symptoms don't appear on their own but instead show up at the same time (or earlier/later) as other symptoms. A combination or set of symptoms occurring together is called a *syndrome*. An example of a syndrome is a *stroke*, which brings on sudden loss of speech, loss of vision and weakness in a limb (you can read more on stroke in Chapter 5). Another example is bowel cancer, when you may notice bleeding from the back passage, a change in bowel habit and weight loss occurring together. (Chapter 11 contains more details on bowel cancer.)

Individual syndrome symptoms don't always occur at the same time and aren't always obvious, and so making a diagnosis can sometimes be quite tricky – including for experienced medical practitioners. Even if you can't make a connection, do mention to your doctor any other symptoms or events that happen at the same time as your health problem. Things that seem minor to you can give your doctor important clues – especially so for 'red flag' symptoms, which need to prompt you to see your GP to rule out any underlying medical conditions.

Here are some examples of important red flag symptoms:

- ✔ Constant and gradually worsening pain.
- ✔ Loss of appetite over weeks and months for no apparent reason.
- ✔ Lumps or bumps anywhere on your body that are new and persistent (that is, for more than two weeks).
- ✔ Sweating (particularly at night).
- ✔ Unexplained fever.
- ✔ Unintentional weight loss.

These symptoms don't mean that something serious is definitely going on, but acting on them and seeking medical advice is important.

Things that health professionals want to know

As well as the other details I cover in this chapter, doctors and nurses are often keen to find out about your particular concerns, expectations and ideas:

✔ **Your concerns:** Say when you're worried that something serious may be going on, you're concerned about receiving a particular diagnosis or you think that you're going to die/lose your job/suffer for the rest of your life.

✔ **Your expectations:** Make clear early on what you want to get out of the consultation, because this information is useful for doctors. Let your doctor know when you think that you need painkillers or antibiotics, you just want reassurance, you need a

sick note or you feel you need a referral to a specialist. Not all your expectations may be realistic and appropriate, but stating them to your doctor can help to ensure that the outcome of the consultation is satisfactory for you both.

✔ **Your ideas:** Let your health professional know what you think's going on and what you know about your symptom and its management.

Try to think through and be clear about these details in advance of a consultation with a health professional so you get a better idea about what to focus on.

Looking for Clues in Your Medical Background

Past and current health problems can be linked to new symptoms, and so be sure to think about and consider any other medical issues that you may have when conducting a symptom check. Certain conditions that you've had in the past may sometimes recur (such as thrombosis or migraine), and new problems may be a complication of a current medical problem that you suffer from. The link isn't always obvious, though, so this section aims to give you some ideas about how you can spot such connections.

Considering past health problems

If you've had any significant illnesses, operations or accidents in the past, consider whether any of these incidents may be connected with your new symptom. For example, a previous bone fracture involving a joint can potentially lead to arthritis later on, which may be the cause of gradually developing joint pain and swelling. Likewise, if you were diagnosed with cancer in the past, your symptoms may be due to a recurrence (you can read about the symptoms of cancer in Chapter 6).

Make a list of all the medical tests that you've undergone – such as blood tests, X-rays, electrocardiograms or any scans or endoscopic investigations – together with the dates and results of what they showed. If you can't remember them, ask your doctor for a copy of your test results – but try to limit this only to any apparently relevant ones. (You can find more information on medical tests in Chapter 26.)

Listing current health problems

Any current medical problems that you have may give important clues as to the cause of any new symptom that you develop. For example, if you already suffer from diabetes, you're more likely to develop infections – which may explain recurrent bladder or skin infections (you can find more on diabetes in Chapter 20). Likewise, existing asthma can explain an episode of shortness of breath and wheezing (for more on asthma, take a look in Chapter 10).

In addition, think about whether your new symptom has any effect on other health problems that you have. For example, stress, anxiety and depression (check out Chapter 21) can get worse if you develop problems with alcohol (which I discuss in Chapter 23) or you get frustrated because of ongoing pain in your hip (Chapter 13 contains much more on joint pain).

Knowing about your current health problems also helps your doctor or medical practitioner to make decisions about treatment. For example, asthma or indigestion limit the medication options that your doctor can prescribe to you.

Finding out about medication

Drugs form an important part of modern medicine. Many drugs are effective in relieving symptoms and preventing death and can literally be life-changing; without them doctors just can't treat many diseases. Most people tolerate most drugs well, and so when your doctor prescribes a new medicine, don't get put off by long lists of possible side effects. You can find relevant side effects on the information sheet that comes with the drug (or ask your pharmacist or GP if you're not sure), but many of these side effects are rare – so the chances are that you're going to be fine.

Almost any medicine can cause side effects, though, and so when you take medicines regularly, or have just started taking a new drug, the drug may be causing your new symptom. Here are some examples of side effects for a selection of commonly prescribed drugs:

Keeping notes

Although your medical notes usually get passed on from one surgery to another when you move house, this process can sometimes take a while. So, keeping an up-to-date summary of your medical history just in case you need to see a doctor – and particularly if you're about to register with a new one – is a good idea. You don't necessarily have to refer to it, but having your summary to hand is useful when any questions about your medical history arise. Doing so saves time for health professionals and gives you more opportunity to talk about your current health problem. Include details about any past and present medical problems, when they started and how they've been managed so far. Also make a list of all hospital admissions or surgery in the past, including dates and reasons.

✔ **Antidepressants:** Many of the newer antidepressants known as *selective serotonin reuptake inhibitors (SSRIs)* can give you a number of side effects, particularly when you first start taking them. These symptoms include light-headedness, feeling a little 'spaced out', headaches, tummy symptoms and problems with sleeping. However, these side effects usually settle after a week or two, and persevering with the medication is usually worthwhile.

✔ **Aspirin-type medicines such as ibuprofen or diclofenac:** These medicines can be a bit tough on your stomach; taking them with food helps.

✔ **Blood pressure lowering medication:** Tiredness and problems with erections in men may happen with some blood pressure medicines.

✔ **Painkillers:** Some codeine-containing drugs commonly cause problems with constipation, and so if you need to take these drugs at higher doses or longer-term and you have trouble opening your bowels, speak to your pharmacist or GP about using additional laxatives.

Knowing about your regular medication is also important for any health professional who needs to treat you for a new problem, because certain medications may interact with each other and bring additional side effects that you could really do without. Here are some examples:

✔ **Combined oral contraceptive pill and antibiotics:** If you're a woman taking the combined oral contraceptive pill, also starting to take certain antibiotics (such as some forms of penicillin or other preparations that you may need for chest or urine infections) can make the pill less effective and put you at higher risk of becoming pregnant. Doctors and pharmacists therefore advise that you take extra contraceptive precautions (such as avoiding sex or using condoms) while you're taking the antibiotics and for another week thereafter (called the *seven-day rule*). The seven-day rule is only valid for new prescriptions of antibiotics and not necessarily when you've been taking antibiotics in the long-term – ask your doctor or pharmacist for further details.

✔ **Statins and macrolide antibiotics:** If you take a cholesterol-lowering drug belonging to a group of drugs called *statins*, also taking a type of antibiotic of the *macrolide* group (such as erythromycin or clarithromycin) increases the risk of muscle aches. This interaction means that when you have to take one of these antibiotics (which may be the preferred alternative when you have an allergy to penicillin), your doctor usually advises you to stop the statin while you're taking the antibiotics.

Many more other drug interactions exist. If you think that your problem may be due to a drug interaction, speak to your pharmacist or GP.

As a rule, never use any prescription-only medicine from someone else. If in doubt, always seek further advice from your pharmacist or GP.

Over-the-counter medication

Although you can get over-the-counter preparations without a prescription, they can still cause adverse effects and/or interact with other over-the-counter or prescription-only medicines. Be aware of this fact when you're tempted to take any over-the-counter medicines from other people. Your pharmacist can advise you on any likely problems when you purchase the medication.

Situations in which not to take certain medicines

If you suffer from certain health conditions, you may need to avoid particular medications altogether, or at least take them with caution. Such circumstances are known as *contraindications*. In most cases, your doctor and pharmacist check whether any drugs may be 'contraindicated' for you before you receive a particular prescription or drug. However, if you forget to mention such circumstances, if you've forgotten about them or if you develop a new medical problem while you're already taking medication, starting contraindicated drugs can cause potentially serious – and sometimes fatal – health problems. Consider contraindications if you develop symptoms after taking a drug and you can't think why you suddenly feel unwell.

Two main types of contraindication exist:

✔ **Absolute contraindication:** Taking two drugs together, or taking a new drug while you suffer from a particular health condition, which creates a potentially life-threatening situation for you is called an *absolute contraindication*. Your doctor or pharmacist can advise.

✔ **Relative contraindication:** Taking two particular drugs together, or at the same time as suffering from a certain health condition, and having detrimental side effects on you – though not too serious or life-threatening – as a result is called a *relative contraindication*. The benefits of taking the new drug may outweigh the risk of developing problems. Again, ask your doctor or pharmacist.

Taking stock of your drugs

If you take medicines regularly, keep a list that contains the drug name, current doses and frequency at which you take them. Note down the dates of any dose changes and any side effects that you experienced. Some drugs need regular blood tests for monitoring. For example, if you take certain blood pressure lowering medications, you need to have blood tests to check your kidney function at certain intervals. Therefore, make a note of when you last had a blood test, and whether the results were normal. Also make a list of any over-the-counter or herbal medication that you're taking.

Here are some examples of contraindications – but remember that many more exist:

- ✔ **Asthma:** If you suffer from asthma, taking aspirin-type medicines such as ibuprofen or diclofenac (often used for pain relief or to treat inflammation) or beta-blockers (sometimes used for treating high blood pressure or preventing migraine), can potentially make your breathing worse.

- ✔ **Bacterial skin infections:** If you suffer from an untreated bacterial, fungal or viral skin infection, avoid using topical steroids (which are commonly used for the treatment of eczema).

- ✔ **Combined oral contraceptive pill:** Although the combined oral contraceptive pill is commonly prescribed and perfectly safe for most women, you must not take it when, for example, you're pregnant, you suffer from severe migraines, you've had a thrombosis or stroke, or you have certain liver problems. For this reason, be sure to mention any health problems to the medical professional prescribing the pill – particularly if you have a new health problem you haven't mentioned before.

- ✔ **Pregnancy:** Many drugs are contraindicated in pregnancy or during breastfeeding.

Allergic reactions to medicines

If you suddenly develop a new symptom such as a rash, itching or difficulty breathing after taking a new medicine, or you become otherwise unwell, you may be suffering from an allergic reaction to the medication. You can have an allergy to certain medicines just as some people are allergic to certain foods or insect bites. For example, allergies to antibiotics such as penicillin are fairly common. (For more information on allergy and anaphylaxis, check out Chapter 5.)

If you know or suspect that you suffer from an allergy, make sure that your doctor's surgery and other people close to you know about the condition. In addition, at home keep a supply of drugs called *antihistamines*, which can help relieve the symptoms of minor allergic reactions. Your pharmacist or doctor can advise you.

Taking a Look at Other Issues

Your new health symptom may be caused by other aspects of your life, some of which are more obvious than others. In this section I run through some factors that are worth bearing in mind when conducting a symptom check.

Running in the family: Inheriting illnesses

When conducting a symptom check, consider whether you may be at a higher risk of suffering from certain medical conditions that are common (or 'run') in your closer family members. Some conditions (known as *genetic* or *inherited* disorders) are passed on directly from parents to their children, whereas with other conditions you may only be at higher risk of developing the condition. Broadly speaking, the more direct family members are affected by a particular condition, the higher your own risk of developing it. An example of a fairly common and serious inherited disease in humans is cystic fibrosis, which affects over 8,500 people in the UK.

The following conditions commonly run in families, which means that you're likely to develop them; they're not infectious or genetic diseases that are directly passed on from one person to another:

- ✔ Autoimmune conditions (such as an underactive thyroid gland).
- ✔ Certain cancers.
- ✔ Cardiovascular disease (causing heart attack and stroke).
- ✔ Diabetes.
- ✔ Mental disorders (such as depression).

If you're concerned that you may suffer from an inherited condition or one that runs in your family, or you worry that you're at higher risk of a disease because some family members are affected, speak to your GP about it.

Sussing out the impact of your symptom on your quality of life

Whenever you develop a new symptom or suffer from a longer-term health condition, consider its impact on your life in general – the same symptom may affect different people's quality of life in various ways. In general, the more a health problem affects your day-to-day life, the more important getting help is early on. In particular, think about the following areas:

- **Driving and other activities:** Driving can be affected through ill health. A number of medical conditions (such as a recent fit or problems with your vision) may render you temporarily or permanently unfit to drive, and so you need to inform the Driver and Vehicle Licensing Agency (DVLA). Any medical information that you pass on to the DVLA is always treated in the strictest confidence. (For further details check out the DVLA website at www.dft.gov.uk/dvla.)

- **Exercise:** As well as being fun, exercising is also important for keeping your muscles and general health in good shape. Not being able to exercise because of a health problem can make you feel miserable, and you may put on weight. On the other hand, if exercise caused your health problem (such as through overuse, injuries in your legs or a neck sprain from playing rugby), or exacerbates your symptoms, you need to reduce your activities until your symptom settles down, and work out ways in which you can continue your interests without incurring health problems in the future (perhaps by warming up properly, stretching or buying better equipment such as good running shoes).

- **Family issues:** An illness affects not only you, but also the people around you. Small children, for example, may depend on you and your illness can make you unable to look after them. This problem can mean that you need to get medical help more quickly than someone whose role as a parent isn't affected. If you're older and already find coping difficult, support from family members makes dealing with your illness easier than when you have to struggle by yourself.

- **Friends and socialising:** Many medical problems can affect your social life, which may be very important for your general wellbeing. For example, a foot injury may prevent you from taking part in group activities, and if you're anxious or depressed, you may not feel like seeing anyone at all – which in turn can make your symptoms even worse.

- **Hobbies:** For many people, hobbies are a large, important part of their lives. Not being able to play football on a Saturday, do needlework or play an instrument because of physical problems can reduce the quality of your life considerably.

- **Home life:** Some medical problems (such as a bad knee) can cause major disruption to your daily routine, causing problems with cooking, shopping, washing, getting dressed and many other activities.

✔ **Relationships:** Illnesses – particularly chronic ones – can cause you to be more irritable, which can considerably affect your relationship and sex life.

✔ **Work:** Maybe you just need a sick note, but some illnesses can stop you getting to work and doing your job properly. Not being able to work through illness, and the subsequent financial implications, can cause you stress and create problems for your employer, and so don't wait too long before consulting a health professional when you need support.

Taking account of alcohol and other drugs

When a doctor takes a medical history, the use of alcohol and drugs is sure to be a major aspect. Therefore, you also need to consider these issues when conducting your symptom check because of their potential impact on your health. Alcohol and drugs are frequently responsible for symptoms that you might never suspect can be connected.

Although drinking small amounts of alcohol may be good for some aspects of your health, remember that no such thing as a safe limit for alcohol exists – whenever you drink alcohol you may put your health at risk, particularly in regard to driving and accidents. Drinking alcohol can affect your health in a number of ways (turn to Chapter 23 for more details). Whenever you drink – and particularly if you drink larger amounts of alcohol regularly – you increase the risk of developing any of the following:

✔ **Accidents:** Many accidents (particularly related to driving) are alcohol related. Even drinking small amounts of alcohol reduces your ability to react quickly – which can make the difference between life and death when you're the driver.

✔ **Chest pain and stroke symptoms:** Drinking alcohol can directly increase your risk of suffering a heart attack or stroke. So if you drink regularly and heavily, any chest pain that you develop is more likely to be due to heart disease compared to someone who doesn't drink. For more info on heart attack and stroke, turn to Chapter 5.

✔ **Liver problems:** The *liver* is an organ in your abdomen that helps break down alcohol in your bloodstream. If you drink too much alcohol for too long, your liver can't cope, and you may develop problems such as liver failure or liver cancer. Should you suffer from abdominal pain, tiredness or yellow skin (called *jaundice*), be aware that your symptoms could be due to liver problems.

✔ **Mental health problems:** Alcohol often causes mental health problems such as depression, anxiety and difficulty concentrating or sleeping. And if you keep drinking too much, you also increase the chances of developing dementia or brain damage.

✔ **Poisoning:** Drinking too much at a time puts you at risk of developing potentially fatal alcohol poisoning.

✔ **Stomach problems:** Problems such as stomach pains or persistent diarrhoea are common and can sometimes be severe. If you drink regularly or heavily, this may well be the main cause of your symptoms.

Alcohol can interact with certain medicines (both prescription-only and over-the-counter ones), and so make sure that you ask your pharmacist or GP for advice if you're worried. The take home message is: consider whether your symptoms may be due to alcohol consumption, particularly if you drink regularly over the recommended limits.

Smoking

If you smoke, this fact needs to form part of your symptom check. Most people know that smoking can cause lung cancer, but you may be surprised to hear that ciggies can cause a lot of other trouble, too. Smoking can lead to the following minor problems:

✔ Bad breath.

✔ Coughs, colds and flu-like illnesses.

✔ Gum problems and mouth ulcers.

But the real issues come with the bigger diseases that can potentially cause serious health problems:

✔ **Chest symptoms:** Chest symptoms like cough, shortness of breath or chest pain may be directly related to smoking. Smoking can directly cause asthma attacks, or make your asthma worse if you've already been diagnosed with it, and is a common cause of other chronic lung problems (turn to Chapter 10 for more info on lung problems). Smoking also increases your risk of developing lung cancer.

✔ **Fertility problems:** If you're a man, smoking can directly affect your fertility.

✔ **Leg problems:** Leg pain can be due to clogged-up blood vessels which can fur up because of smoking. Eventually, this may lead to gangrene and even amputation, in severe cases.

✔ **Urinary symptoms:** Blood in your urine can sometimes be a symptom of bladder cancer – and smoking increases the risk of developing this condition (turn to Chapter 12 for more info on bladder cancer).

✔ **Vision problems:** Certain eye conditions such as cataracts become more common if you smoke.

Because smoking can cause or contribute to many symptoms, trying to give up cigarettes if you possibly can is a great idea. Stopping smoking can be very difficult – but the good news is that lots of help is available to you. You can find more information on ways to stop smoking at http://smokefree.nhs.uk, or contact your GP surgery. Stopping is worthwhile – both for your health and your wallet!

Increasing health risks through poor diet and lack of exercise

A large number of health symptoms such as shortness of breath, joint problems and tiredness can stem from an unhealthy diet and lack of exercise. Consider whether you eat too much and mostly the wrong stuff (find out more at http://www.nhs.uk/livewell). If so, you're more likely to develop potentially serious health problems such as clogged-up blood vessels, heart disease, stroke or obesity.

Being a couch potato makes you more prone not only to an increased risk of heart attack and stroke, and therefore to symptoms like chest pain or sudden weakness (flip to Chapter 5 for how to spot these conditions), but also muscle and bone problems such as back ache, knee pain or neck problems.

Taking the fast track to your symptoms

To remind yourself quickly of the things to consider when approaching a health problem, here's a brief summary:

✔ **Develop your story:** How did the symptom start? What happened then? How often and for how long do you experience your symptom?

✔ **Describe your problem:** What's wrong? How bad is it? How badly does it affect you? What makes it better or worse?

✔ **Look for other clues:** Do you have (or have you had) other health problems that may be responsible? Do you take any medication that may have something to do with your symptoms?

✔ **Consider further issues:** Do any illnesses run in your family? May your problem be due to alcohol or drugs? Also, consider stress, diet and exercise.

Writing down your symptoms can help to make things clearer for you and any health professionals you consult.

Chapter 3

Looking Out for Signs of Illness

. . . .

In This Chapter

▶ Checking for visual pointers to ill health

▶ Feeling your way around your body

▶ Moving about and checking that your body still works

▶ Using medical equipment

. . . .

A detective trying to solve a crime usually asks questions to find out what's happened and gathers evidence before checking out the crime scene for clues. Likewise, your dentist first asks you where the pain is and what's happened before having a detailed look at your teeth. Medical professionals do the same – they conduct a kind of interview before moving on to a physical examination. If necessary, they then arrange further medical tests.

When you're not sure if a medical symptom is serious and whether you need to do something about it, you can follow the same course of action: ask yourself some questions (you can read up on this process in Chapter 2) and then have a closer look and feel. Being able to perform a basic physical examination enables you to make a straightforward diagnosis yourself. Also, you can use various medical gadgets at home, which are tremendously useful for helping you to make decisions about your health.

In this chapter I look at ways in which you can examine your body. I show you what to do (for example, look, feel and move) and how to spot the difference between normal and abnormal. I also tell you about some useful gadgets and pieces of equipment that you may want to keep at home and how you can use them to their best effect. And don't worry – none of this process is as scary as it may sound: everything that I cover in this chapter is fairly straightforward. But as I say throughout this book, do seek medical advice whenever you're unsure about the significance of your finding.

Spotting Abnormalities: This Doesn't Look Right

One of the main skills you need for carrying out a basic physical assessment is the ability to make careful observations. You may think that doing so without medical training must be an impossible task, particularly where serious illnesses are concerned. Well, in the same way that you can tell that your toaster isn't in brilliant shape when it starts going up in flames or that engine trouble is likely if your car starts to splutter and smoke, you can spot certain signs of serious disease even with little medical knowledge.

Bear in mind that you almost certainly know your body quite well already and therefore can normally spot any part that suddenly looks or feels different. (If you develop symptoms in a certain area of your body, check out the relevant chapter that tells you what particular signs to look out for. For more details on dealing with emergencies and giving first aid, turn to Chapters 5 and 24.)

Looking for trouble

If you suspect that you or someone else may be seriously ill, start by looking for clues. Here are some examples:

- **Airways and breathing:** Not being able to breathe properly is often a sign that something more serious may be going on. Although shortness of breath or breathing much faster than usual can occur in anxiety and panic (and of course during exercise), it may also indicate a potentially serious chest or heart problem. Consider the possibility of choking or an inhaled object in other people if difficulty breathing comes on very quickly and without much warning.

- **Bleeding:** Take any bleeding seriously, particularly if it's profuse and doesn't stop. Bleeding is commonly the result of major injuries but can also occur from the mouth or the back passage, or from the vagina in women. After an injury (such as a fall) always check for any evidence of bleeding, but take care in the case of head and neck injuries (you can find further information on first aid essentials in Chapter 24).

- **Confusion:** Not knowing who and where you are, and why, or the year, season and month, can be a sign of impaired brain function (perhaps after a head injury or a stroke – check out Chapter 5) and needs urgent medical attention.

- **Deformities:** If your body looks deformed after an injury and the affected body part is painful, an underlying fracture is likely.

✔ **Drowsiness:** Becoming very drowsy and less responsive is a sign of a potentially serious illness and can develop into unconsciousness and coma.

✔ **Eye opening:** Not opening the eye in response to speech or pain may indicate a serious underlying illness.

✔ **Looking pale or blue in the face:** Anyone who's seriously unwell usually also looks unwell. If you're very pale or blue in the face you may be suffering from a potentially serious underlying condition. Being pale is normal after a simple faint, but your colour normally returns fairly quickly; remaining pale possibly indicates more serious problems.

✔ **Skin lesion:** Skin lesions are common and in most cases not serious. However, ruling out the possibility of skin cancer is important, particularly in lesions that get bigger, bleed, are very dark or don't heal. (You can read up about skin problems in Chapter 8.)

✔ **Speech:** Being unable to talk and/or get words out properly can be a sign of serious illness.

✔ **Swelling, redness and tenderness:** These signs can indicate tissue inflammation due to, for example, a skin infection or an *abscess* (a collection of pus), or an inflammatory condition like arthritis. An abscess usually causes a red and hot swelling within or under your skin, and tends to be painful and tender to the touch. Most abscesses need a small incision to drain the pus and/or a course of antibiotics, and so seeking medical advice is best – particularly if you feel unwell. Severe infections or abscesses can also cause a fever. (For more information on fever and its causes, flip to Chapter 7.)

Searching for trouble in children

Fortunately, the vast majority of children who fall ill don't have a serious underlying illness. But because small children in particular can't often tell you what's wrong with them, you have to rely more heavily on a physical assessment when deciding whether your child may be suffering from a potentially more serious illness. Reassuringly, though, this is far less common than many people think.

In a nutshell, here are a few things to look out for in children that – on rare occasions – need to prompt you to seek medical advice immediately (you can find more on recognising illness in children in Chapters 14 to 17):

✔ **Alertness:** If your child appears sleepy or drowsy or doesn't respond to you, a serious injury or illness may be present.

✔ **Difficulty breathing:** If your child's breathing is faster than usual, more laboured or you can hear new sounds (for example, wheezing or grunting), or your child's chest looks abnormal during breathing – the skin between your child's ribs is likely to get 'sucked in' with each breath when breathing is difficult – he may have a serious underlying illness such as a chest infection. (You can find more information on breathing problems in children in Chapter 15.)

✔ **Fever:** Fever – a feeling of being hot and cold or sweaty, and when the body temperature rises above 38 degrees Celsius (100.4 degrees Fahrenheit) – in children is extremely common and in most cases not due to any serious underlying illness. Chapters 14 and 15 tell you more about danger signs to check for when your child has a fever – and when you don't have to worry.

✔ **Head injury:** Always take head injury in children seriously, particularly if your child is drowsy, has lost consciousness, has a severe headache or vomits (you can read more about head injuries in children in Chapter 15). Look out for any open head wound and whether you can see any blood or clear fluid coming out of your child's nose or ears, which suggests a more serious head injury.

✔ **Persistent vomiting/diarrhoea:** Your child may lose too much fluid and be dehydrated through persistent vomiting or diarrhoea. (Check out Chapter 14, which tells you what to look out for specifically.)

✔ **Rashes:** Rashes are common in children and can have various causes – most are benign, but some may be due to serious underlying illness, particularly if your child also has a fever. Chapter 15 tells you the signs to watch out for.

✔ **Stomach pain:** Most children have occasional tummy aches, which by themselves aren't much to worry about when they're not severe, your child is otherwise well and the aches go away by themselves. However, if your child's tummy seems bloated or he doesn't let you touch it, the problem may be a more serious one, such as appendicitis. (Chapter 16 contains more information on tummy pain in children.)

Many parents start to worry or panic when their child falls ill and they don't know whether something serious may be going on. The good news is that the vast majority of children don't fall severely ill, even when they appear miserable or cry a lot. Conditions that parents often worry about – such as meningitis or cancer – are fortunately very rare. In most cases your child will be suffering from an illness that gets better by itself, such as a viral infection, and treating the symptoms, and making your child feel better until the illness has passed, is the most important thing to do.

Nevertheless, even though they're rare, serious illnesses do occur in children. If you're worried or unsure what's wrong with your child, seek medical help, particularly in the case of babies and children under one year of age. (For more information about childhood illnesses see Chapters 14–17.)

Spot the difference: Viral and bacterial infections

Infections caused by small microbes (or 'bugs') are very common, and they usually belong to one of two types: viruses or bacteria. The main difference between them is that you can destroy *bacteria* with drugs called antibiotics, but these drugs have no effect on *viruses*. Generally speaking, you can catch bacterial infections again and again, but you can have many virus infections (like chickenpox or mumps) only once because your body develops immunity against them after infection. Sadly, this fact isn't true for cold and flu viruses, and many other ones as well. Because viruses cause most colds and coughs, you don't normally take antibiotics for them.

Inspecting yourself

Whenever you develop a new symptom, expose the affected body part (and perhaps other areas as well) to check whether you can see anything that looks abnormal to you. Take a very close look, and for areas that you can't see properly these tips may help:

✔ **Employ mirrors:** Using one mirror in front of you and one held with your hand behind you enables you to look at areas on the back of your head or neck, or on your back. By laying a mirror on the floor, you can inspect around your bottom or genitals, which you can't normally see.

✔ **Take a photo:** If you find using mirrors a bit tricky, perhaps because you have joint problems or can't move very well for other reasons, ask someone with a digital camera or camera-phone – someone you don't mind looking at you – to take a photo of the affected area.

Even if you can't make out what's going on, if you keep inspecting yourself over a period of time you can often see whether a rash or any other skin problem changes – many conditions get better by themselves.

Knowing Your Body Through Touch

After inspecting your body visually (as I describe in the preceding section), the next step is to feel your way around to get clues as to what may be wrong.

Knowing how to check your pulse and becoming familiar with how your body normally feels is worthwhile so that you can easily notice significant abnormalities when you fall ill.

Testing for tenderness

If you have pain anywhere on your body, checking for *tenderness* – an unusual sensitivity or pain in an area when you touch or press it – can give you additional clues. Here's a guide to what tenderness in certain body areas may mean:

- ✓ **Bones and joints:** If your bones or joints are very tender and sensitive to touch (particularly after an injury and when the bone also appears deformed), visit your GP or – in the event of an injury – your local Accident & Emergency (A&E) department for further assessment. (Turn to Chapter 13 for more info.)

- ✓ **Skin:** A tender swelling in your skin that's also red and feels hot may be due to a skin infection. See your GP or practice nurse for further assessment: you may need any pus draining and/or a course of antibiotics. (For more on skin conditions turn to Chapter 8.)

- ✓ **Tummy:** If you have tummy (also known as *abdominal*) pain, press it gently. If doing so makes your pain worse and you don't like this pressure, you may rarely have a more serious underlying problem (such as *appendicitis*, where the tenderness is usually in the centre of the tummy to start with before it moves to the right lower part). You can find more on tummy pain in Chapter 11.

Checking your pulse

Your *pulse* is the throbbing of blood vessels (called *arteries*) produced by the regular contractions of your heart. You can feel your pulse at various places on your body, but the easiest and most practical place for checking your pulse is your wrist. Being able to check your pulse is a useful skill because it can tell you how fast and regular your heart is beating. Changes in heart rate – particularly if it becomes irregular, very fast or very slow – can be important indicators when assessing illness.

Heart rates vary between people, but normal ranges at rest are as follows:

- ✓ 60–90 beats per minutes in adults.
- ✓ 90–110 beats per minute in children.
- ✓ 110–140 beats per minute in babies.

To check your heart rate, and to see whether your pulse is regular, follow the steps below. Get a feel for what your normal pulse is by checking your pulse at rest, but also find out how your pulse changes during or after exercise.

1. **Put out one hand in front of you, with the palm facing upwards.**

2. **Place the pads of your first/index finger and your middle finger of your other hand on the inside of your wrist. Put them near the base of your thumb – roughly where the strap of a watch would be.**

3. **Press gently and feel for the pulse. If you can't feel it, press a little harder or move your fingers around slightly.**

4. **Feel your pulse. The pulse is measured in beats per minute, so count your pulse for a minute, checking for:**

- **Heart rate:** Your heart rate can go up for various reasons – for example, when you're excited, during exercise or a fever, when you're angry or when you're in pain. If your pulse is going too fast even at complete rest, particularly if you have other symptoms such as chest pain or shortness of breath (find out more about these in Chapters 5 and 10), seek medical advice.

- **Irregular heartbeat:** Normally, your pulse has a regular rhythm – like a clock or a metronome – so that you can predict the next beat. But when your pulse is irregular, you may not be able to predict the next beat – such as in the case of a common rhythm abnormality called *atrial fibrillation*. If you notice that your heartbeat is irregular, see your GP for further assessment. If you suddenly develop shortness of breath or chest pain (or if you've had these repeatedly over time), consult your GP more urgently or dial '999' in an emergency. (You can find more detail on how to deal with heart and lung problems in Chapters 5 and 10.)

- **Occasional missed beats:** Missed beats are common and if you're otherwise well you don't usually have to worry about them.

For more information on taking your pulse, look at the British Heart Foundation website at www.bhf.org.uk.

Assessing lumps

If you develop somewhere on your body a new lump that persists for two weeks or more, getting it checked out by your GP is usually best, unless for some reason you know that the lump is due to an entirely benign reason.

Here I give you some hints as to when you need to make an appointment with your GP sooner rather than later:

- ✔ **Attachment to underlying structures:** A lump that you can move a bit within the tissues is less worrying than one that seems fixed to the underlying tissues (which is relevant for breast lumps, for example).

- ✔ **Consistency:** A lump that feels soft (like the muscular bit at the base of your thumb) is much more likely to be benign than a lump that feels rather hard (a bit like one of your knuckles).

- ✔ **Pain and tenderness:** Lumps that are painful and tender are more likely to be benign than those that are painless. A painful soft swelling that comes on fairly quickly is often due to a collection of pus (check out the 'Looking for trouble' section earlier in this chapter).

- ✔ **Shape:** Most benign lumps are round, whereas lumps due to cancer for example sometimes have an irregular shape.

- ✔ **Size:** Any new lump more than 2 centimetres (just under an inch) in size and growing needs checking out.

- ✔ **Surface:** Check whether the surface of the lump feels smooth or more irregular or 'craggy' – the latter is more suspicious.

Even a lump that has some of these worrying features doesn't mean that you have something nasty such as cancer – but it needs to prompt you to get it checked out by your GP. In particular, don't delay making an appointment when you notice a lump in the following areas:

- ✔ **Breast:** Breast cancer is a common cancer in women. Most breast lumps aren't due to breast cancer, but do get any new and persistent lump checked by your GP. (Chapter 18 has more details on breast issues.) Remember that you can also get breast cancer if you're a man. Breast cancer in men is very rare (about 100 times rarer than in women), but if you notice a lump, see your GP. Saying that, breast lumps behind the nipple area are common in teenage boys and are due to hormonal reasons. These settle by themselves and are completely harmless.

- ✔ **Neck lumps:** Any lumps in your neck that appear for no apparent reason, get bigger and last for two weeks or more are suspicious, particularly if they have further 'red flag' features such as the ones that I mention in the preceding list (turn to Chapter 9 for more on neck problems).

- ✔ **Testicle:** If you're a man, go and see your GP if you notice a lump that seems attached to one of your testicles to rule out testicular cancer. (Chapter 19 contains more details on testicular problems.)

Again, the vast majority of lumps aren't due to cancer – but getting them checked by a medical professional if you're worried is important. If you're concerned that you may suffer from cancer, you can find more information about spotting the symptoms and signs in Chapter 6.

Checking Function: In-out, in-out – Shake It All About!

Bone, muscle and joint problems can be disabling, and so if you develop pain or stiffness in any part of your body, check how far it affects your normal movements. Particularly after sustaining an injury or being involved in an accident, or when more than one area is affected, doing a systematic body movement check can be a good move. Here's a quick checklist:

- **Arms and hands:** Check for any problems with movements in your elbows, wrists and hands. Difficulties with moving these joints freely can have a severe impact on your life.

- **Hips, knees and feet:** Problems in these joints may have an effect on getting around and can greatly reduce your mobility.

- **Neck:** You should be able to bend your neck forward and sideways and rotate it to both sides as well. Being able to rotate your neck freely is important when you drive a car, and problems with looking up or down can cause problems when trying to reach items higher up (for example, shelves at home or when out shopping).

- **Shoulders:** Check whether you can move your arms freely or whether any movements are restricted. Shoulder problems may cause considerable problems with day-to-day activities at home or at work.

You can read more about bone and joint problems in Chapter 13.

Using Medical Gadgets and Other Tests

Being able to perform basic medical tests is a great help when you assess your health symptoms. In particular, using a thermometer to identify a fever or checking your blood sugar levels when you're diabetic can be very useful.

Using a thermometer to check for fever

Your normal body temperature is between 36.5 and 37.2 degrees Celsius (97.7–99 degrees Fahrenheit). Your temperature is high if it rises above 38 degrees Celsius (100.4 degrees Fahrenheit), which means that you have a *fever*. Typical symptoms of fever are feeling flushed, sweaty and hot (or cold). You can read more about fever and what it means in Chapter 7.

Having a thermometer enables you to check your temperature quickly and easily. Make sure that your thermometer is always clean and take care reading the instructions for use beforehand. If you get a raised temperature reading, confirm your reading by checking again 15–20 minutes later.

You can buy different types of thermometers from pharmacies, including:

- **Digital ear thermometers** are expensive, but easy and quick to use, and accurate when you use them correctly. Be aware that readings may not be accurate when you've just returned from outside and have cold ears, or if you've been lying on a pillow. In these instances, wait for 10–15 minutes before taking a reading. In any case, ear thermometers aren't always entirely accurate and may not be suitable for use with smaller babies; be sure to check the instructions prior to use.

- **Digital thermometers** check your temperature from your mouth or armpit. If you take a reading from your armpit, remember that the measured temperature is about 0.5 degrees Celsius (0.9 degrees Fahrenheit) lower than your actual body temperature – so you need to add this amount to the reading. Although armpit measurements aren't the most reliable way of measuring your temperature, they come in handy and are safe when measuring the temperature of babies and small children (check out Chapter 14 for more details on doing so).

- **Mercury thermometers** are more old-fashioned and contain mercury, which is poisonous when you swallow it or it comes into contact with your skin. Other types of thermometer are easily available now, so mercury thermometers are being phased out. If you've still got an old mercury thermometer at home, avoid using it to take a child's temperature. To take your temperature with one, place the tip in your armpit or mouth, but make sure that you don't bite on it accidentally.

- **Thermometer strips** go directly onto your forehead skin, and are popular because they're easy to use. However, thermometer strips give you only an approximate reading and aren't very accurate.

Home monitoring in chronic disease

If you suffer from chronic conditions like diabetes or raised blood pressure, your GP or diabetic nurse can advise you whether you may benefit from measuring your blood sugar (or *glucose*) or blood pressure at home. Doing so can be useful while you're getting started on medication, or when you suddenly become unwell and want to know whether your illness is affecting your blood sugar levels or blood pressure – or whether these factors may even be responsible for your condition. Various gadgets are available to you to measure your blood sugar or blood pressure – ask your practice nurse, pharmacist or GP for advice on when and how to use them.

Chapter 4

Managing Your Health Problems

In This Chapter

▶ Gaining confidence for dealing with medical problems

▶ Using simple self-help strategies

▶ Getting help from the professionals

*E*veryone falls ill at some stage – and knowing what to do can sometimes be difficult. Even just thinking straight can be hard when you're in pain or worried that you may have a serious illness, which doesn't help when you need to make a decision about managing your health problem or don't feel confident about taking matters into your own hands.

As a rule, if you're seriously worried about your health or you're quite unwell, the best thing to do is seek advice from a health professional. However, many health problems are minor and benign, and armed with a bit of knowledge and confidence you can often manage most of these issues yourself.

In Chapters 1–3 you can find more information on health symptoms and how to distinguish between minor problems and the ones that may indicate a more serious underlying illness. In this chapter I let you know what you can do to manage your health symptoms yourself – and how to seek help from health professionals. For more information on getting the right help first time and to ensure that you're approaching the most appropriate service for your health problem, remember to check out the NHS websites and helplines I look at in Chapter 25.

Self-Managing Your Health Problem

You can manage a large number of health problems yourself. In this section, I advise you on ways to treat and relieve your symptoms such as pain, fever and many others – and how to access additional help and advice. If you're not sure what's going on, or you want guidance on how to check over your body, refer to Chapters 2 and 3.

Making use of time as a healer

The old saying 'time's a good healer' contains a lot of truth. However, time itself isn't what does the healing – getting better is all thanks to the capabilities of your body and mind for self-repair. Health professionals often talk about *self-limiting illnesses*, which are those that sort themselves out and go away without the need to do anything. In these cases, waiting and seeing is usually fine, but the 'seeing' means that, although the illness may be self-limiting, you still need to remain alert to the possibility of complications. However, you can do a lot to relieve your symptoms and make yourself feel better 'while-you-wait'.

Here are some examples of common conditions for which you don't usually need any specific treatment, other than relieving your symptoms with painkillers such as paracetamol or ibuprofen:

- **Coughs and colds:** Most coughs and colds are due to virus infections that stay with you for around ten days. Some people say that they 'come over three days, stay with you for three days and go over three days' – which in many cases is exactly what happens, give or take the odd day or two. Sometimes coughs and colds linger on for a bit longer (say for three to four weeks), but that's the limit in the vast majority of cases.

  Apart from taking painkillers and drinking plenty of fluids to make you feel better, you don't need to do much else because you're likely to feel better again soon. You can also try over-the-counter cough medications, but little scientific evidence exists about how effective these preparations are, and so unless danger symptoms are present (check out Chapters 9 and 10 for more details), let your body get on with fighting the infection itself.

- **Earache in children:** Many children get earache – particularly in the first few years of life. Unless you see any danger signs (turn to Chapter 15 for more information), you don't need to do much apart from giving fluids and painkillers to keep your child comfortable. In most cases, earache settles by itself and doesn't need treatment with antibiotics.

- **Gastroenteritis:** If you suddenly get very loose and frequent stools (also called *diarrhoea*), perhaps together with feeling sick and vomiting, you're likely to be suffering from *acute viral gastroenteritis* – particularly if other people in your household or workplace are also affected. A serious potential complication of gastroenteritis is dehydration, but otherwise these infections are usually not dangerous, get better without any complications and don't need any treatment apart from keeping up your fluid intake. Read Chapter 11 for more about gastroenteritis.

✔ **Sleeping problems:** Problems with sleeping are common – and can be very annoying. However, if you normally sleep well, your sleep problems are likely to be short-lived and get better by themselves. Even though not sleeping well for a few nights makes you feel tired, it doesn't harm your body. Chapter 6 gives you some ideas for tackling sleeping problems. If your lack of sleep is due to stress, you can find some stress-busting strategies in Chapter 21.

✔ **Viral warts:** Viral warts are common: they're round and up to 1 centimetre (about ½ inch) in diameter, with a cauliflower-like surface and pinkish in colour. Most warts don't cause any problems and usually go away within two years, and so if they don't bother you, leaving them alone is perfectly safe. You can read more about skin problems in Chapter 8.

Using RICE for an injury

If you injure or strain any of your soft tissues (such as muscles or ligaments) through sports or an accident, you can shorten your recovery time and reduce pain by using a treatment method called *RICE*, which stands for rest, ice, compression and elevation:

✔ **Rest:** Resting is very important if you want to get better quickly after a soft tissue injury. Without rest, your injury takes longer to get better, and your tissues may not heal properly. If you keep going regardless, you continue to strain the affected area, which results in ongoing inflammation and pain – and you even run the risk of making your injury worse because the tissues are already damaged.

As a rule, try to rest until you can use your affected body part again without any major problems and the pain is more or less gone. How long this process takes can vary and depends on the location and severity of your injury. Many sports medicine doctors and physiotherapists advise *relative rest*, which means that you can keep exercising as long as you rest the injured limb and avoid activities that make the pain worse.

✔ **Ice:** Cooling down the affected area can help reduce inflammation and pain – particularly in the initial phase after the injury. To make sure that you don't damage your skin, wrap ice inside a towel before wrapping it around the painful area. Leave the ice on for about 20 minutes or so and then take it off for 40 minutes. Usually, just employ this approach for no more than 24 to 48 hours – continuing for longer may even be harmful and lead to a delay in your recovery.

✔ **Compression:** Inflammation is usually accompanied by a swelling of the affected tissues. To reduce this swelling – which can affect how your limb works and delay your recovery – you can wear an elastic bandage (your pharmacist can advise you about which type is suitable) over the affected area. The bandage needs to be a snug fit – but make sure that it isn't too tight or you may impair blood flow to the injured area.

✔ **Elevation:** An injury is a great excuse for putting your feet up! By elevating your limb you help drain blood and fluid from the injured tissues, which reduces swelling. Obviously, you can't always keep your limb elevated – you've probably got other things to do – but in a leg injury, for example, try to raise your limb whenever you sit down. Remember to keep a balance between rest and keeping mobile.

RICE isn't a cure as such, but it can help speed up your recovery in minor injuries or sprains where you feel seeking medical advice isn't necessary. Also, if you suspect that you have a more serious injury (flip to Chapter 13 for more details), RICE is a good first aid method to use before you attend an Accident & Emergency (A&E) department.

Taking things easy

Many illnesses are caused or made worse simply by doing too much. Resting is just as important for dealing with these problems as for injuries and physical strains (which I discuss in the preceding section). If you're suffering from a viral infection such as a sore throat or cough, for example, try not to overdo things and cut down on unnecessary activities until you feel better. If you suffer from depression or a stress-related problem (which you can read up about in Chapter 21), having too much on your plate can prevent you from getting better – or even make things worse.

When you take things easy while you're sick, you're much more likely to recover quickly. This advice doesn't, of course, mean that you don't do anything – you still have to do the dishes! But simply taking a gentler pace until you feel better can make all the difference.

Employing home remedies

Your mum or granny may swear by certain home remedies, but for many of them little evidence exists to say that they're effective. However, this fact doesn't necessarily mean that these remedies don't work. Many people commonly use home remedies to treat minor medical conditions, believing that they work, so you too may try home remedies and if you find they work for you then that's great. The good thing is that they're usually as cheap as chips, and so you may want to give any of the home remedies listed below a go. Do check the relevant section in this book first, though, to make sure that you're dealing with a minor illness:

✔ **Cold sores:** Cold sores can be extremely irritating. You can try to relieve symptoms such as pain and stinging by dissolving an ice cube every hour for a few hours on the lesions around your mouth. Some people say that pressing a used tea bag on the lesions also helps to reduce symptoms.

✔ **Common cold:** Lemon and honey is a cheap and commonly used home remedy for the common cold. Add the juice of a whole lemon with a teaspoon of honey to a glass of warm or hot water and drink slowly. For more information on cold symptoms and coughing, turn to Chapters 9 and 10.

✔ **Constipation:** If you suffer from hard or 'difficult-to-get-out' stools, eat more fruit, vegetables and wholemeal products to add fibre to your diet, together with drinking plenty of water. For more information on constipation and other tummy symptoms, check out Chapter 11.

✔ **Cystitis:** If you suffer from or are prone to bladder infections (known as *cystitis* – discussed in Chapter 12), drinking lots of fluids can help with treating and preventing problems. Drinking two glasses of cranberry juice a day also can reduce your chances of getting a urine infection. If you're a woman and you get urine symptoms frequently after having sex, make sure that you empty your bladder before and just after having intercourse.

✔ **Ear wax:** If you suffer from a build-up of excessive ear wax, try putting a couple of drops of olive oil into the ear canal, tilting your head to the opposite side (or lying down with your affected ear facing upwards to ensure that the oil gets to the deeper areas in your ear canal) for about 5–10 minutes and gently pressing your finger on the cartilage-like bit near the opening of your ear canal. This process helps to dissolve the ear wax, which usually comes out naturally over the next week or two – but you need to use olive oil three to four times a day. To avoid any mess, buy some olive oil from your pharmacist – it's cheap and comes in a little bottle with a dropper to make putting it into your ear easier. After straightening or getting up again, mop up any oil that comes out of your ear with a soft tissue.

✔ **Headache:** Some people with tension headaches find that vigorous exercise relieves their symptoms. A hot or cold foot bath before going to sleep may also help.

✔ **Irritable bowel syndrome:** If you suffer from stomach or bowel problems such as *irritable bowel syndrome* (or *IBS* for short), try drinking peppermint or camomile tea instead of ordinary tea or coffee to relieve your symptoms. In addition, a fibre-rich diet and plenty of exercise may also help.

Generally speaking, one of the most effective home remedies can be simply to adopt a healthier lifestyle: exercising more, eating a healthier diet, drinking alcohol only in moderation, not smoking, reducing stress and getting enough sleep can sometimes improve symptoms dramatically – without the need for any additional treatment. However, seeking medical advice is best when you're not sure whether your symptom is benign or potentially serious, or you're not getting better as quickly as you expect.

Taking over-the-counter medicines – sensibly

When you're unwell, remember that you can head for your local pharmacy, where you can get a variety of over-the-counter medicines for treating minor medical conditions. Even if you're not sure whether a treatment for your condition is available, your clued-up local pharmacist can offer you advice on suitable preparations that may help.

Here I give you an overview of some symptoms and conditions for which you can buy medicines without prescription:

- **Children's problems:** If your child suffers from a minor medical problem such as colic, some common childhood rashes, head lice, teething problems, nappy rash, oral thrush or threadworms, you can buy a variety of preparations from your pharmacy.

- **Coughs and colds:** Various cough, cold and sore throat preparations are widely available, as are medicines for allergic symptoms in hay fever and other related conditions.

- **Ear and eye problems:** Many medicines are available from your pharmacy for common ear and eye symptoms and conditions.

- **Mental health issues:** If you suffer from stress or problems with sleeping, talk to your pharmacist who may be able to recommend suitable preparations for you.

- **Pain:** Your pharmacist can advise you about relief for headaches and musculoskeletal problems.

- **Preventative treatment:** You can buy preparations from your pharmacy that aim to prevent conditions such as heart disease or brittle bones (known as *osteoporosis*).

- **Skin problems:** If you suffer from eczema, acne, cold sores, athlete's foot, scabies, warts, psoriasis, hair loss or dandruff, your pharmacist can advise you on suitable preparations for self-treatment.

- **Stomach and bowel problems:** Treatments are available for symptoms such as heartburn, nausea and vomiting, indigestion, motion sickness, diarrhoea and constipation. You can also find preparations for mouth ulcers, haemorrhoids and irritable bowel syndrome.

- **Women's health:** Consider talking to your pharmacist if you're a woman and suffer from bladder infection, vaginal thrush, painful periods or you're pregnant and suffer from one of the common pregnancy symptoms, such as heartburn. You can also get emergency hormonal contraception without prescription.

Stocking your home medicine cupboard

Even minor ailments can significantly impair your quality of life, and so be prepared! Keeping a basic stock of medicines and other equipment at home ensures that you're ready when illness strikes suddenly – particularly in the middle of the night.

Here's a list of medicines that you may want to consider keeping at home. These items are only my suggestions and not an exhaustive list – talk to your pharmacist about any particularly personal requirements that you may have:

✔ **Anti-diarrhoea tablets:** These tablets can improve the unpleasant effects of diarrhoea from food poisoning or a viral infection. However, don't give them to children under 12 years of age and seek medical advice if the diarrhoea is severe or doesn't start to improve after a few days (you can read more about diarrhoea and other bowel problems in Chapter 11).

✔ **Antihistamines:** These medicines help with relieving symptoms of hay fever, allergies and insect bites and can soothe some itchy skin rashes.

✔ **First aid equipment:** Keep a basic stock and range of plasters, bandages, medical tape and sterile dressings for those minor bruises, sprains and cuts. A thermometer is also useful (you can read more about using these instruments in Chapter 3). Other items worth having handy include antiseptic solution, eyewash solution (although fresh tap water usually works just as well) and a pair of tweezers for pulling out splinters.

✔ **Indigestion relief:** Simple drugs such as antacids can help relieve symptoms such as 'trapped wind', heartburn or stomach aches. Having them to hand can be useful if you've been partying a bit too hard!

✔ **Painkillers:** Paracetamol, ibuprofen and aspirin are effective for many minor aches and pains as well as reducing fever and inflammation. Remember not to give aspirin to children under 16 years of age.

✔ **Sunscreen:** Choose sunscreen with a high factor (at least 15) that provides UVA as well as UVB protection for those sudden unexpected outbursts of sunny weather, when all you want to do is be outside.

Always keep your medicines out of the reach of children and store them (the medicines, not your kids!) in a cool, dry place. Whenever you use over-the-counter medicines from the supermarket or pharmacy, never take more than the recommended dose and make sure that you read the label and instructions. Take care to check the expiry dates on the packets regularly; when a medicine is past its use-by-date take it back to the pharmacy for safe disposal instead of throwing it away. Your pharmacist can advise you whether you need to avoid taking particular medicines because of medicines you already take or pre-existing medical conditions (turn to Chapter 2 for more info on this).

Accessing and Using Health Services Appropriately

If you decide that you can't deal with a particular health problem yourself, or the treatments you try fail to work, you're likely to need further advice and help from a health professional.

Many different professions form part of the wider health community, and in the NHS you can choose which services to approach. Identifying the most appropriate service for your individual problem – and knowing how and when to access it – can be a tricky business. Helping people to access the right health services and get the most out of them is a big priority for the NHS, and so I devote this section to the topic and look at a selection of the main ports of call that are open to you.

Finding and using NHS services

Medical treatment is more effective when you can choose, understand and control your care. The NHS therefore regards you as a partner and aims to assist you in looking after your own health and making the right choices when it comes to lifestyle decisions, staying healthy and accessing health services appropriately.

To enable you to do this, the NHS provides comprehensive information services that aim to put you in the driving seat when it comes to your healthcare. Depending on where you live in the UK, you can access a huge amount of up-to-date and authoritative information on the Internet (for individual NHS website addresses, turn to Chapter 25).

Check out the NHS websites for information in the following areas – and much more:

- **Answers to your health questions:** Get answers to common health questions such as Can I get pregnant just after my period has finished? or Which vaccinations do I need to travel abroad?

- **Caring:** Get advice and support when you are the carer for another person.

- **General health information:** Obtain information on current and important health topics, such as swine flu, accidents and first aid, current health scares or health-related headlines, information about drugs and medication, and how to stay healthy in winter.

- **Healthcare services:** Locate healthcare services close to you, such as GP surgeries, emergency and urgent care services, hospitals, pharmacies, dentists, opticians and other additional services.

✔ **Healthy living:** Check out tips and advice on how to keep yourself and your family healthy.

✔ **Initial assessment:** Get an initial online assessment of your health problem, for example if you have symptoms that concern you, a dental health issue or a question about your medicines.

✔ **Medical conditions:** Check the latest information about symptoms, causes, diagnosis and management of over 800 medical conditions and treatments.

✔ **Self-help:** Find symptom checkers and self-help guides.

✔ **Useful telephone numbers and links:** Obtain telephone numbers and web links for useful contacts that may be able to help you, like The Samaritans, Alcoholics Anonymous, Child Line, MacMillan Cancer Line, and many more.

NHS Direct (England), NHS 24 (Scotland) and NHS Wales (turn to Chapter 25 for contact details) are the services for you if you have health worries and need personalised health advice rather than general health information. If you suffer from a health problem, they enable you to answer many of your questions about medical symptoms, dental health issues and medicines with an online initial assessment, or ask questions via email.

In addition, well-trained call handlers can help you with your health problem, reassure you when necessary and point you in the right direction if you need further medical assessment and treatment, particularly in the following areas:

✔ **Health advice:** Providing general health or dental advice out of hours, supporting GPs and dental services.

✔ **Health scares:** Giving you advice and reassurance in response to health scares.

✔ **Operations:** Providing you with support before and after any surgical operations.

✔ **Remote clinics:** Running remote clinics over the telephone.

✔ **Telephone support:** Offering telephone support when you suffer from a long-term medical condition.

Getting help from your pharmacy

Pharmacists (sometimes also called *chemists*) have special expertise in medicines and how they work. They work in pharmacies, which you can find on almost any high street, and play a major role in providing healthcare in the community.

Here are some examples of what the pharmacist's role includes:

- Advising on drug side effects and checking that taking certain medicines is safe for you.
- Advising on healthy living and treating minor health problems.
- Dispensing medicines prescribed by your doctor.
- Giving advice on using over-the-counter medicines and dispensing them.
- Providing various services related to specific conditions, for example, checking your blood pressure, doing routine blood checks such as sugar or cholesterol, or performing a medication review.
- Supplying items such as emergency contraception, incontinence supplies, oxygen or needle exchange.

Visiting minor injuries units

If you suffer a minor injury, you can go to a *minor injuries unit* for assessment and treatment instead of attending your GP surgery or an A&E department. Among other things, minor injuries units can treat:

- Broken bones.
- Minor animal and insect bites.
- Minor burns and scalds.
- Minor chest, shoulder or back injuries.
- Minor eye injuries.
- Minor head injuries.
- Minor wound infections.
- Muscle or joint sprains and strains.

Attending a minor injuries unit for conditions such as the ones above means that you get the help you need while freeing up A&E staff to concentrate on serious cases with life-threatening or severe medical problems. You're also likely to be seen and attended to much quicker. Nurses lead minor injuries units, and you can just turn up without the need for an appointment.

Minor injuries units can't treat serious conditions such as chest pain, breathing difficulties, stomach pains or alcohol-related problems, or indeed any condition that may require admission to hospital. They also can't treat very young children (the under-3s).

To find your nearest minor injuries unit, look on the NHS Choices website at www.nhs.uk.

Strolling into walk-in centres

At NHS walk-in centres you can conveniently and without the need to make an appointment see an experienced nurse or doctor (though a doctor may not always be available), who can assess and treat minor ailments and injuries such as:

- ✔ Common skin problems.
- ✔ Emergency contraception.
- ✔ Minor cuts, bruises and burns.
- ✔ Minor infections.
- ✔ Muscle or joint sprains and strains.
- ✔ Stomach upsets.

Walk-in centres are open to everyone and are usually managed by a nurse. Most centres are open every day all year round, and also outside office hours. They provide a complementary service to the more traditional A&E and GP services for the management of minor complaints – but aren't equipped to manage immediately life-threatening conditions or longer-term health problems.

The medical staff at walk-in centres won't usually have access to your medical record, and so if you need to seek medical help and advice for what appears to be a more complex health problem, you're probably better off booking an appointment to see your GP.

Making best use of your GP surgery

Your GP surgery (also called *GP practice*) is often your first point of contact if you're an NHS patient. Think of it as the 'hub' for your medical care, where a team of various health professionals look after you.

Many important people are beavering away, working 'behind the scenes' in your GP practice, providing a number of services (these vary slightly between practices). Specialist nurses run many of these services, and examples include the following:

- ✔ Asthma clinic.
- ✔ Baby clinic.
- ✔ Blood tests.
- ✔ Coil and contraception clinic.
- ✔ Diabetes clinic.

✔ Health prevention clinic.

✔ Hypertension clinic.

✔ Insurance medicals.

✔ Minor illness clinic.

✔ Minor surgery.

✔ Occupational health services.

✔ Smoking cessation advice.

✔ Travel and immunisation clinic.

You can freely choose your GP practice, but if you need to visit your GP frequently because of an ongoing health problem, or you're likely to require home visits, you may prefer to choose a GP surgery close to where you live. Most practices have a website nowadays, on which you can find details about the ethos of a practice, available appointment times, and the experience and special interests of individual GPs and other staff members.

Most GP surgeries are open from around 8.30a.m. to 6.30p.m. – and often longer – although opening times vary between surgeries and areas. If you need to access GP services between 6.30pm and 8.30am, an out-of-hours doctor is always available to you – on every day of the year including bank holidays and weekends. The provision of services and ways of accessing them can vary between regions, so check with your local surgery. Additionally, some under-doctored areas have created GP-led health centres, which are open between 8a.m. and 8p.m. every day of the week – you can usually book an appointment or walk straight in.

Introducing Your Wider Primary Healthcare Team

You probably already know your hard-working local GP, and you may have said hello to her friendly receptionist a few times when booking or attending your appointments, but you may not be aware of just how many other professionals are working away to deliver healthcare. In fact, many professionals work together in the community to try and keep people healthy and manage medical conditions.

In this section I look at the main roles of key individual team members within a GP surgery.

Getting more out of your GP appointment

Most GPs book their patients in at an average of ten-minute intervals. Here are some tips to help you make the most of the time available:

✔ **Prepare:** Make a list of symptoms, problems or questions that you have before seeing your GP. Be aware, though, that if you have a list of different problems, your GP may not be able to deal with them all during a single appointment, so decide which one or two problems are the most important ones for you to discuss. Also take a pen and paper with you to note down any points that you want to remember from the consultation – they're easy to forget!

✔ **Wear suitable clothes:** If a good chance exists that your GP may need to examine you, wear loose clothing and few layers.

✔ **Remember your medication:** Be prepared to tell your GP about any supplements or non-prescription drugs that you take – make a list if you find remembering them difficult.

✔ **Bring some support:** Your GP doesn't mind if you're anxious and want to bring someone else along for support. Another person can also be useful for discussing with you anything that was said during the consultation afterwards.

✔ **Ask questions if you don't understand something:** Your doctor also doesn't mind repeating or writing down things for you. Also, make sure that you know why you're being prescribed any drugs and how to take them correctly – and for how long.

Your practice receptionist

Receptionists are usually your first point of contact when you get in touch with your GP surgery. They meet and greet people and direct you to the most appropriate professional within or outside the practice. Your receptionist can make an appointment for you with a doctor, nurse or other member of the primary healthcare team and plays a hugely important role in keeping these services running like clockwork. If you're unsure whom you should see for your health problem, don't hesitate to ask the receptionist.

Your GP

GPs are experts in family medicine and take a central role in preventing health problems, informing and educating patients and their families about their health and treating people with acute as well as complex and long-term medical conditions. GPs are able to assess any medical problem and then decide on the best and most appropriate way to deal with it.

Your GP works closely with a team of other health professionals and is usually based in your GP surgery, but can also visit you at home when you can't get to the surgery because you're too ill or frail to travel. However, if possible, do always try to see your GP at the surgery because of the better access to medical instruments and treatment room facilities should you need them in connection with your appointment.

GPs provide personalised care within your local community and deal with a wide range of medical problems – including physical, psychological and social issues. If appropriate, your GP can refer you to hospital specialists and other services for diagnosis, further tests or help and advice on the management of your health problem(s).

Your practice nurse

Practice nurses in GP surgeries have many roles and play a very important part in delivering high-quality primary care. Some example activities that practice nurses perform include:

- ✔ **Health promotion:** Your practice nurse can inform you about health issues, give lifestyle advice, run smoking cessation programmes, provide travel services and give immunisations.

- ✔ **Managing chronic illness:** Practice nurses play a major role in identifying, diagnosing, monitoring and managing patients with long-term conditions such as high blood pressure, diabetes, asthma, epilepsy or chronic lung conditions. They also support patients with self-care of acute and chronic conditions, undertake health screening and conduct medication reviews, as well as prescribing medication.

- ✔ **Initial management and minor illness clinics:** With support and backup from the GP, practice nurses sometimes provide first-contact services and diagnose and manage your minor illness.

- ✔ **Women's health services:** Practice nurses provide services such as smear tests and vaginal swabs.

Your practice manager

GP practice managers oversee the business aspects of your GP surgery and make sure that the service runs smoothly and effectively for patients. They lead the administrative team and closely work with all the healthcare professionals within the surgery as well as with outside NHS and other teams. Among their roles, practice managers keep an eye on the quality of patient services that the practice provides as well as the level of patient satisfaction. So if you have a specific question or complaint, you may well find yourself being directed to the practice manager.

Getting out and about with the community team

Some members of the primary healthcare team work mostly outside the GP practice setting, and can visit people in their homes. Don't worry if the range of services available to you seems at first confusing – familiarising yourself with them puts you in a much better position to choose confidently the appropriate service. You can access these services directly or via your GP surgery – check your surgery website or ask the receptionist at your GP surgery if you're unsure.

Your health visitor

Health visitors are qualified nurses or midwives who have undergone training in community health to take up a special role within the primary healthcare team. One of their remits is to promote health and prevent illness in all age groups, but particularly in the under-fives and older people.

Health visitors work with mothers of young babies and advise on feeding issues, emotional and physical development of children and many other areas relating to childcare and child health. They also contribute to the care of people with disabilities or people suffering from a chronic illness, helping them with any difficulties connected to coping with their condition.

Health visitors also provide help and support for women with postnatal depression, bereaved people and families in which violence is an issue. In addition, they co-ordinate child immunisation programmes and baby clinics.

Your community midwife

Community midwives provide personal care during your pregnancy, throughout and after the birth. They can help to answer any concerns or questions that you may have, provide psychological support throughout, arrange a home birth or support your delivery at the hospital, according to your wishes, and support you in the period after your baby is born. Community midwives liaise closely with other members of the primary healthcare team and can independently arrange tests and referral to hospital if necessary.

Your community or district nurse

Community nurses play a vital role within the primary healthcare team in delivering healthcare. They visit people at home, provide medical and nursing care, and support carers and other family members. Their aim is to avoid you having to go into hospital unless absolutely necessary and help to ensure that you can return home as soon and as safely as possible after any stay in hospital.

Community nurses may visit you every day – or even more than once a day – if needed. They collaborate closely with other teams such as voluntary agencies, social services and other NHS organisations to help co-ordinate and deliver various care packages.

Going to A&E

A&E departments provide urgent care for people with serious injuries or who have a serious illness that needs immediate treatment. Generally speaking, visit an A&E department only in a genuine emergency – going to A&E with a minor health problem is like calling the Fire Brigade for a leaking tap!

Here are some examples of emergency situations in which attending an A&E department is appropriate:

- Acute confusion.
- Persistent severe chest pain.
- Poisoning.
- Problems with breathing.
- Serious tissue, bone or joint injuries (particularly if you suspect a fracture or are likely to need stitches) or an inability to walk.
- Self-harm (including medication overdose, self-cutting and attempted suicide).
- Severe mental health and alcohol-related emergencies (including severe suicidal thoughts with immediate danger to a person's health, acute severe psychosis or delirium – check out Part V for more info on acute mental health problems).

When you attend A&E, a nurse or doctor assesses your condition before deciding on further tests or treatment. Prepare yourself for having to wait for a while, particularly around busy times such as weekend nights. However, all A&E departments try their best to assess, diagnose and manage 98 per cent of the people they see within an average of four hours of arrival.

Major A&E departments are open around the clock on every day of the year – but not all hospitals have an A&E department. Remember that alternatives to A&E departments are available, including walk-in centres and minor injuries units (flip to the earlier sections 'Strolling into walk-in centres' and 'Visiting minor injuries units', respectively). These centres can see you without an appointment – but they do deal only with minor illnesses and injuries.

Calling '999' in an emergency

Don't hesitate to call '999' for those emergencies when you can't get to A&E yourself quickly or safely (for example, if you're too unwell to sit in a car, if you need to get to hospital quickly during rush hour or if you're too unwell to get to hospital using your own transport). Symptoms or conditions that justify calling '999' in such circumstances include, for example, the following (you can read more about these instances in Chapter 5):

- ✔ Acute confusion.
- ✔ Central chest pain and suspected heart attack.
- ✔ Loss of consciousness.
- ✔ Major accidents and injuries.
- ✔ Severe allergic reactions (known as *anaphylactic shock*).
- ✔ Severe pregnancy-related emergencies.
- ✔ Severe shortness of breath.
- ✔ Sudden collapse and loss of consciousness.
- ✔ Suspected stroke.

When you phone '999' because of an emergency, your call gets prioritised to ensure that you get the quickest response, in case you're suffering from a life-threatening condition. The ambulance crews who respond to these calls usually consist of a paramedic and an emergency care assistant, who are highly trained in managing a whole range of emergencies – from serious heart problems such as cardiac arrest to major trauma. The ambulances themselves carry various pieces of equipment including oxygen, intravenous drips, various drugs, spinal and traction splints as well as a machine to restore your heartbeat if necessary (known as a *defibrillator*).

If necessary, an ambulance can take you to hospital – but ambulance crews can also perform certain diagnostic tests and procedures directly at the scene. They can also arrange for you to go directly to specialist medical units, refer you to social services and administer drugs used for the treatment of asthma, allergies, diabetes, overdoses and heart problems.

Call '999' only in a genuine emergency, so that you don't divert care from seriously ill or injured people. In many areas ambulance services struggle to keep up with the demand – mainly because many people call '999' inappropriately, putting lives at risk.

Also consider other options instead of calling '999', such as using self-care at home, speaking to your pharmacist, going to a local NHS walk-in centre or contacting your GP surgery. You can also make your own way to your local A&E department, bearing in mind that you aren't necessarily seen quicker just because you arrive by ambulance. And if you're not quite sure how urgently you need treatment, you can always call the relevant NHS services first (flip to Chapter 25 for contact details).

Part II
Looking at Emergencies and 'All-Over' Symptoms

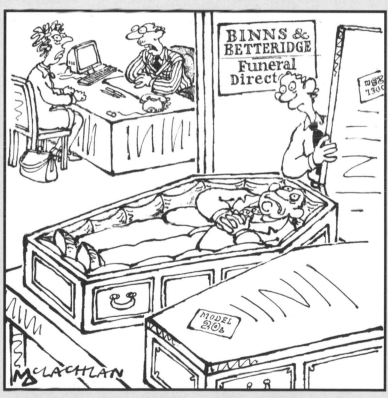

'Your husband must really think he's ill—
we don't get many customers coming in
for a fitting.'

In this part . . .

'Vague' health problems are relatively common, and feeling anxious about them is quite normal. To help, Part II gives you some straight-talking advice on assessing and managing a number of non-specific symptoms.

Also, you're introduced to ways of dealing with medical emergencies and of getting to grips with symptoms affecting your wider body.

Chapter 5

Coping With Medical Emergencies

- -

In This Chapter

▶ Discovering more about circulation and breathing emergencies

▶ Getting to grips with accidental injuries

▶ Looking at some other common emergencies

- -

Television medical dramas such as *Casualty*, *House* and *ER* are packed with scenarios in which people suffer sudden and often dramatic illness, but in fact relatively minor medical conditions are much more common. However, although you may only rarely have to deal with a true medical emergency in yourself or other people, by having some idea of what to do in such circumstances you can literally save your or someone else's life and prevent further damage to health. You're also likely to feel less scared and helpless if you ever find yourself in such a situation.

Medical emergencies can happen anywhere and at any time – in your home, when you're out shopping or on the road driving – and they can be due to all sorts of things. Head injuries, heart attacks, strokes, allergic reactions or problems due to diabetes are common and can be immediately life threatening. In many cases, you need to get help quickly and call '999'. In other cases, when perhaps things aren't that dramatic and symptoms develop more gradually, you usually have a bit more time to consider whether something more serious may be going on.

In this chapter I help you to recognise some important medical emergencies and give you some idea of how serious they may be. The emphasis here is on *recognising* – knowing *when* to seek help and *why* – but I also tell you what you need to do in particular emergency situations. You can find more on managing emergencies and providing first aid in Chapter 24, and if you can't find a particular emergency here, look up your symptom in the index and check the relevant chapters in this book.

 I can give you only some hints and basic guidance here. This chapter doesn't replace practical training in the management of emergencies and giving first aid. If you want to find out more and gain confidence in dealing with medical emergencies, I strongly recommend that you book onto a first aid course. You can find details about courses in your area and information on how to provide first aid on the St John Ambulance website at www.sja.org.uk. The British Red Cross (at www.redcrossfirstaidtraining.co.uk) also holds first aid and health and safety courses, and its website contains lots of useful tips and first aid advice.

Identifying Trouble With Vital Organs

You're unlikely to have any problems spotting a serious asthma attack, heart attack or stroke, particularly when you or the affected person develop symptoms quickly and are very unwell. Most people who are seriously ill usually also look seriously ill, and so when you're concerned that you or someone else is suffering from an acute and severe illness, speak to your GP immediately or call '999' straight away in an emergency.

In many cases, though, events may not appear quite as dramatic. For example, asthma can get worse gradually, and an asthma attack can sometimes look less severe than it actually is. Heart attacks and strokes may also present in quite a subtle way at times. Spotting the warning symptoms and signs of these conditions early allows you to do a lot of good by getting help quickly when appropriate.

Managing shock

People use the expressions 'I'm shocked' or 'to be in shock' to express surprise, horror or disgust. However, *shock* – in the medical sense – is a serious medical condition. Shock means that for some reason not enough blood is pumping through your body and your vital organs – such as your brain or your heart – therefore don't get enough oxygen.

Important causes of shock are as follows:

- **Burns:** Severe burns can cause shock, when fluid evaporates from the wounds.
- **Heart problems:** Suffering from an acute heart problem such as a heart attack can cause shock.
- **Losing blood:** You can develop shock if you, for example, lose large amounts of blood from your back passage or due to an injury.
- **Losing fluid:** People commonly lose too much fluid due to excessive sweating, severe vomiting or diarrhoea.
- **Poisoning:** Various poisons (such as a heroin overdose or a bite from a poisonous animal) can lead to severe problems with your circulation and can cause shock.

You may recognise the following features in yourself or someone else suffering from shock:

- **Breathing:** Breathing tends to be shallow and fast.

- **General wellbeing:** You or a person suffering from shock are likely to feel unwell, thirsty and sick – and vomiting is common. Weakness and dizziness are other important symptoms.

- **Mental state:** In more severe shock people become aggressive, restless and gasp for air. Eventually, they become drowsy and lose consciousness. Finally, the heart stops beating.

- **Pulse:** If you're able to feel your own or the casualty's pulse, it's usually quite fast in shock and may also be irregular, particularly if the underlying cause is a heart condition.

- **Skin:** The skin becomes clammy, cold and pale. If shock is severe, the lips may appear blue and skin can become grey or blue in colour. You may also notice excessive sweating.

If you suspect shock in a casualty, give first aid as I outline in Chapter 24. Shout for help and call '999' straight away. After you call for help, do the following:

1. **Lay the casualty down and raise and support the legs.**

2. **Try to keep the person warm – 'space blankets' are ideal (these are the 'foil' blankets that you see on marathon runners after they've crossed the finishing line).**

3. **Check breathing and pulse frequently (check out Chapter 3 on how to take a pulse).**

4. **Follow the resuscitation sequence described in Chapter 24 if breathing stops.**

5. **Give lots of reassurance and try to comfort the casualty – shock can be very frightening!**

Spotting a stroke

If the blood supply to your brain gets interrupted, you suffer a *stroke* – also sometimes called *brain attack*. If blood can't reach certain areas of your brain, the affected brain cells behind the blockage can die – and parts of your brain don't function properly afterwards.

The two main types of stroke are:

- ✔ **Ischaemic stroke:** In this common type of stroke, a clot narrows or blocks a blood vessel in your brain.

- ✔ **Haemorrhagic stroke:** This less common type of stroke happens when a blood vessel in your brain bursts, causing bleeding into your brain.

A 'mini-stroke' (also known as *transient ischaemic attack*, or *TIA*) is very similar to a stroke but does improve by itself within 24 hours – whereas damage from a full-blown stroke is more permanent (although symptoms may also improve after a while, but much slower and usually not fully). Sometimes, a TIA can be a warning sign that a more serious stroke may be imminent, which is why you need to take it just as seriously as a stroke.

You're at higher risk of suffering a stroke if you have underlying medical conditions such as diabetes, high blood pressure, raised cholesterol and/or an irregular heartbeat known as *atrial fibrillation*, or if strokes run in your family. Your lifestyle may also contribute, if you smoke, are obese or inactive, have a poor diet or drink too much alcohol.

You can recognise a stroke by any of the following features, which may appear alone or in any combination:

- ✔ You can see that your face has fallen to one side and you're unable to smile properly – your face may look contorted when you're trying to do so.

- ✔ You can't lift both arms in front of you (with the palms of your hands facing up) and keep them there. In the event of a stroke, one arm is usually noticeably weaker than the other and slowly drifts down and inwards (so that the palm starts to face down).

- ✔ You notice that your speech is slurred.

- ✔ You suddenly lose sight in one eye – partially or completely.

- ✔ You notice that one of your legs suddenly becomes weak or that you can't walk properly.

If you suspect that you or another person is suffering a stroke, call '999' immediately. The sooner you call for help, the better the chance of a good recovery.

Recognising a heart attack

In a *heart attack*, the blood vessels supplying your heart suddenly become blocked and your heart muscle doesn't get enough oxygen: the result is usually chest pain. The main danger of a heart attack is that your heart may stop beating, and so you need to treat a possible heart attack as a medical emergency – even if you still feel relatively well.

A number of factors can increase your risk of suffering a heart attack (called *cardiovascular risk*), some of which are preventable. See whether any of the following apply to you:

- You're a smoker.
- You suffer from high blood pressure, diabetes or raised cholesterol.
- You know that early heart attacks or strokes (suffered before the age of 60) run in your close family.
- You're overweight.
- You drink alcohol over and above the recommended limits.
- You lead an inactive lifestyle.

Heart attacks aren't always easy to spot, but call '999' if you recognise one or more of the following typical symptoms (which can occur alone or in any combination):

- You experience persistent central chest pain that feels like a 'tightness' or a heavy pressure, or like someone sitting on your chest.
- You have pain that spreads to your neck, jaw and/or down one or both of your arms. Sometimes the pain also spreads to your back, or you feel it in your upper abdomen rather than in your chest (a bit like indigestion).
- You have pain and in addition feel breathless, nauseous and sweaty, and your skin feels cold to touch. You may even be gasping for breath, or vomit.
- You have chest pain and collapse without much warning.
- You develop a pale appearance or blue lips.
- You have chest pain and notice that your heart is suddenly beating unusually fast, and your pulse may be irregular (refer to Chapter 3 for info on how to check your pulse). However, if you suffer from pre-existing conditions such as anxiety, a fast heart rate may be normal for you.

While you wait for the ambulance to arrive, take the following steps:

1. **Make sure that you're as comfortable as possible and try not to exert yourself.**

   Sit down in the 'W' position with your back at about 75 degrees to the ground (not completely upright but also not lying flat) with your knees bent if possible, while resting your back against the headboard of the bed or a wall (supported by a pillow) (see Figure 5-1). In this position, your heart finds pumping blood round your body easier.

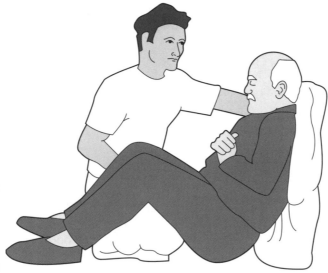

Figure 5-1:
Sitting down
in the 'W'
position.

2. **Take your medication.**

   If you have aspirin at home and you can't think of any reason why you shouldn't take it (for example, you're allergic to aspirin, or you have asthma and aspirin always makes your breathing worse) and assuming you're older than 16 years, take one 300-milligram tablet straight away. If you have medication for angina such as glyceryl-trinitrate (GTN) spray or tablets, also use these immediately.

Attacking asthma and other serious chest problems

If you suffer from *asthma* and have an asthma attack, the air passages in your lung narrow because they go into spasm and their lining swells. Therefore, air can't pass through your airways easily anymore, and you find breathing more difficult. (For more information on asthma, take a look at Chapter 10.)

If you suffer from asthma, certain situations (or triggers) may provoke an asthma attack. Common examples are:

✔ You suffer from a cough or cold.

✔ You have an allergic reaction.

✔ You smoke or are exposed to cigarette smoke.

✔ You exercise (in some circumstances, even mild exercise can cause an asthma attack).

✔ You go out in the cold, or the temperature is very hot outside.

An asthma attack occurs when your symptoms become suddenly more severe. Being able to recognise the danger symptoms and signs of severe asthma is important and may literally save your life. You can recognise an asthma attack by the following features:

✔ You have difficulty breathing, particularly breathing out.

✔ You notice an audible wheeze when you breathe out, and you breathe very fast.

✔ Your chest feels very tight.

✔ You can't complete a sentence without gasping for breath.

✔ You feel very short of breath or feel that you might suffocate.

✔ You feel anxious and distressed.

✔ You're also likely to have a cough.

If your doctor has already diagnosed asthma, you're likely to have been pre-scribed a blue *reliever* inhaler (usually containing a drug called *salbutamol*). Try the following:

✔ Using the blue inhaler straight away. If you don't notice an effect after three minutes or so, use the inhaler again.

✔ Staying calm, because doing so helps your breathing; and try to breathe calmly and deeply.

✔ Sitting up rather than laying down – take up the position that's most comfortable for you, which may be leaning forward with your arms rest-ing on a table, or sitting 'the wrong way round' on a chair and resting your arms and chest on the chair's back.

✔ If you're indoors, let some fresh air in, which can also help.

Don't delay calling '999' if this attack is your first ever, or if you think that your asthma attack is severe because:

✔ You're getting worse rather than better.

✔ You don't notice any effect within a few minutes from using your blue inhaler.

✔ You can't speak in full sentences without gasping for breath and may only whisper despite using your inhaler.

✔ You feel more and more tired and exhausted.

While waiting for the ambulance to arrive, use your inhaler every five to ten 10 minutes.

If you're dealing with an asthma attack in someone else and the person becomes very unwell or unconscious, you can find further advice on providing first aid in Chapter 24.

Dealing With Accidents

Some people are more accident-prone than others, but anyone can suffer an injury. Many injuries occur due to accidents in the house – falling while putting up curtains, suffering burns when cooking or tripping over carpets or things lying on the floor are common causes. And needless to say, roads are dangerous places, too. When you suffer an injury you may feel unsure whether it's likely to be serious or not, and so this section offers some tips that may help you decide what to do.

Handling head injuries

Take every head injury seriously because a possibility always exists that you may have suffered damage to the blood vessels inside your skull or sustained a skull fracture. (For head injury in children, check out Chapter 15.) A blow to your head that leads to you passing out – even if only briefly – is called *concussion*.

Seek medical advice immediately – and call '999' in an emergency – if you notice any of the following symptoms or signs in connection with a head injury, which can suggest a more serious underlying problem:

- ✔ You have an open head wound that bleeds profusely, or you can see the underlying bone.
- ✔ You feel increasingly drowsy or you may become unconscious.
- ✔ You have constant neck pain.
- ✔ You have problems speaking or understanding.
- ✔ You have a loss of balance and an inability to walk properly.
- ✔ You can't remember anything from before or after the injury.
- ✔ You have an ongoing headache, particularly if this pain gets worse rather than better.
- ✔ You're vomiting.

✔ You have clear or blood-stained fluid coming from your ears or nose.

✔ You suffer a fit following the head injury.

✔ You suffer a high-impact injury such as being hit by a car, a fall from a bike and landing on your head, or any fall onto your head from a height.

✔ You suffer a head injury in connection with drinking alcohol.

✔ You suffer from a blood-clotting disorder or take blood-thinning medication.

Always suspect an injury to the neck as well if you or someone else suffers a head injury. If you have any pain on moving your neck or at rest, keep as still as possible and ask someone to call for an ambulance. Avoid moving your head and neck until the ambulance arrives.

Similarly, seek medical advice immediately if you notice one or more of the following signs at any time in the days or weeks after a head injury:

✔ You become drowsy.

✔ You have a headache that persists or gets worse.

✔ You suffer from persistent vomiting.

✔ You can't see properly.

✔ You suffer a change in behaviour.

After a minor head injury, you may get mild headaches and feel a bit dizzy and tired for a few days, and you may also find concentrating or remembering things more difficult than usual, but these symptoms usually settle quickly. Rest and taking paracetamol for the headache are usually all that you need, but do contact your GP for advice if you can't make out what's going on or you're concerned.

Recognising fractures

Whenever you sustain an injury to a limb or other part of your body, one of the questions to ask yourself is whether you may have broken a bone (called a *fracture*).

Suspect a bone fracture when you notice:

✔ Abnormal mobility of the affected body part.

✔ A 'crunching' feeling (called *crepitus*) when you move the affected part.

✔ Bruising and swelling.

- Constant pain at the affected site, which is worse on movement.

- Deformity of the affected part of your body along with tenderness to touch.

- Inability to use the affected body part properly.

- Inability to weight-bear properly at the time of your injury and afterwards, when a lower limb is affected.

Many types of fractures exist, and so here's a selection of the more common ones:

- **Ankle:** Ankle injuries are common, especially due to sport. You may have suffered a *sprain* (a twisted, torn or partly torn ankle ligament – check out Chapter 13 for more on sprains and strains), but a fracture is more likely when you have the symptoms in the above list.

- **Collar bone:** Collar bone (or *clavicle*) fractures are usually caused by a fall onto your outstretched hands. If you feel a bit short of breath, you may have punctured the lining of your lung, causing your lung to partly or fully collapse (known as *pneumothorax* – this sometimes only causes mild symptoms. If your shortness of breath is very severe, call '999').

- **Hip:** Hip fractures are common in older people and are usually – but not always – due to a fall. Normally, you can't walk properly, but in some cases walking may not be severely affected. Suspect a hip fracture if you suffer constant pain around the hip joint or in your groin that's worse on walking and if you notice a shortening of your leg. Your affected leg may also turn outwards a little.

- **Scaphoid:** The *scaphoid* is a small bone inside your wrist, which can break from a fall onto your outstretched hand. You're likely to notice pain, swelling and tenderness over the back of the 'thumb' side of your wrist, which is worse when you press over the little dimple (also known as *anatomical snuffbox*) that forms when you move your thumb away from your fingers. This fracture is an easy one to miss, and you need to get this problem checked out because if you're not treated properly you run the risk of long-term wrist problems.

- **Wrist:** Wrist fractures are common in children and in older women suffering from brittle bones (known as *osteoporosis*). The wrist may be deformed – your wrist may take on a 'dinner fork' shape when you look at it from the side (called *Colles fracture*).

If you suspect that you may have fractured a bone, go to the nearest Accident & Emergency (A&E) department, because you may need an X-ray. In the meantime, keep the affected part as still as possible and take painkillers such as paracetamol, if you have them at hand. In an emergency – that is, if you're very unwell, are bleeding profusely or can't move – call '999'.

If, after being diagnosed with a fracture and getting discharged from hospital, you notice any of the following symptoms or signs, seek medical advice again to exclude potentially serious complications such as infection or a blood clot:

✔ Limb remains swollen or swells up later.

✔ New numb feeling in the affected limb.

✔ Offensive smell or discharge.

✔ Persistent severe pain (more than you'd expect).

✔ Red or mottled skin colour, or blisters, in your affected limb.

✔ Swelling and severe pain in the muscles around the injury, which gets worse when you stretch those muscles.

✔ The edges of your cast rub into your skin so that your skin gets damaged.

Experiencing eye injuries

Eye injuries are common, and in many instances visiting your GP or an Eye Hospital Emergency department (in case of more serious injuries) for further assessment is best.

Here's a quick summary of common eye injuries and advice on what to do:

✔ **Blunt injury:** You may suffer a blunt eye injury, for example from a squash or tennis ball, or from a fist. Depending on the force of impact, you may just get a 'black eye' – but you may also suffer a serious eye injury such as a *blow out fracture*.

Go to the nearest A&E if you notice one or more of these symptoms:

- You can't see properly from the injured eye.

- You develop double vision.

- You damage your eyelids or other parts of your eye.

- You notice, on close inspection, a blood level behind the clear front bit of your eye.

- You see that your pupil (the black central bit of your eye) is larger than in the other non-injured eye.

- You spot that your eye looks as if it's being pushed inside your skull (due to a blow out fracture – you also can't look upwards).

- You can't see your eye properly because of pain or swelling.

✔ **Chemical injuries:** Chemical burns (for example, from strong cleaning solutions, paint stripper or materials used by the building trade such as cement or hydrochloric acid) can cause serious damage to your eyes, particularly when the chemical involved is alkali based. The thing to do is to hold your eyelids apart and flush your eye with plenty of clear water immediately – you may use up to one or two litres – and then go to the nearest A&E immediately.

✔ **Damage to your cornea:** The *cornea* is the sensitive front-bit of your eye, and an injury to your cornea (called *corneal abrasion*) can be very painful. Corneal injuries are commonly caused by getting a twig in your eye when gardening or by children who reach out and accidentally scratch your eye. If the pain doesn't settle quickly, contact your GP.

Always seek medical advice when the pain in your eye is due to high-speed particles (for example, due to strimming or grinding), which can penetrate your eye and cause nasty injuries or infections if left untreated.

✔ **Foreign bodies:** Eyelashes often get into the eye and cause discomfort, but usually they come out again by themselves. Rolling your eyes while pulling gently on your eyelids may help.

Don't attempt to remove any larger foreign bodies by yourself – just use a bit of padding for support while you get medical help. Cover your other eye too, which makes you less likely to move your eyes, and take a friend or relative with you to help guide the way. Always see your GP or go to A&E when you have suffered an injury due to metal getting into your eye.

✔ **Penetrating wounds:** If a chance exists that your eye has suffered a penetrating wound – for example, you've been chiselling or working with a hammer and a small particle injures your eye – you need to visit your GP or go to your nearest A&E immediately, particularly if you notice any of the following:

• Your eye is painful and waters.

• Your eye can't tolerate the light.

• Your pupil is unusually wide or distorted.

Always try to prevent eye injuries by wearing protective goggles when you're doing activities that can damage your eyes, such as high-speed grinding or other do-it-yourself projects.

Getting the Low-down on Other Emergencies

In most emergencies you don't have any problem deciding what to do – either they're so minor that you're confident dealing with them yourself (such as a minor sprain or a graze to your skin), or you know immediately that you need to get medical help very quickly (for example, you're in fear of your life or have sustained a major life-threatening injury). In this section I cover a selection of emergencies where deciding what to do isn't so easy.

Suffering from allergies and anaphylaxis

When you suffer from an allergy, your body responds in an exaggerated way to an *allergen*. Various allergens exist, including: foods (for example, peanuts, fish, eggs), insect bites (for example, bee or wasp stings), drugs (for example, antibiotics such as penicillin or aspirin-type medicines) or exposure to a new drug (for example, you've been vaccinated). You may not always know, however, what's causing your allergy.

Allergies may produce symptoms such as tingling on your tongue, swollen lips or raised wheals on your skin (you can find more on this type of problem in Chapter 8, which covers skin problems). A severe allergic reaction, which can start suddenly and progress very fast, however, is called *anaphylaxis*.

After being exposed to something that you know – or may not know – you're allergic to, anaphylaxis can show itself with one or more of the following features:

- ✔ You notice skin changes such as itching, redness, flushing or swelling.
- ✔ You spot that your eyes, lips, tongue or other parts of your body have swollen up.
- ✔ You feel sick and develop a painful stomach.
- ✔ You have difficulty breathing and notice a wheeze.
- ✔ You feel that your heart is racing away.
- ✔ You faint or collapse – along with a feeling of impending doom.
- ✔ You can lose consciousness if the reaction is very severe.

If you're not sure whether you're suffering from an allergic reaction and you're not too unwell, phone your GP for advice. However, if you suspect a severe allergic reaction or anaphylaxis, call '999'. If you suspect anaphylaxis in someone else, check out Chapter 24 for some more first aid advice.

Soothing stings and bites

In the UK, you're unlikely to suffer any serious poisonous animal bites or stings – although you can suffer a severe allergic reaction to what appears to be a minor sting. Here's the low-down on some of the more common bites and injuries from animals:

- ✔ **Insects:** Stings from bees and wasps often cause some redness and swelling but usually aren't dangerous – unless you're stung by masses of them all at once (like in that Michael Caine film, *The Swarm*!). If you can see the sting, try to scrape it out gently if you can. Cooling the area with an ice cube can help prevent swelling.

✔ **Larger animals:** If you suffer a bite from a cat or dog where the teeth punctured your skin, seek medical advice because bite wounds can become septic if not treated adequately – even if the bite looks relatively minor to start with. Be aware that being bitten by a dog or fox when abroad poses additional dangers because of the risk of *rabies* – a serious infectious disease. Seek medical help immediately.

✔ **Snakes:** The only poisonous snake in the UK is the adder, but fortunately its bite is in most cases not dangerous (although children may become quite unwell). Seek medical attention when you receive an adder bite.

Evaluating burns and scalds

Getting burnt or scalded is easy, because most houses are full of heat sources. Burns due to steam, hot liquids, electricity or corrosive chemicals are therefore relatively common.

Most mild burns cause just a bit of redness. A burn is more likely to be more severe under these circumstances:

✔ You notice that your skin is broken as a result of the burn.

✔ You develop more than one or two smaller blisters.

✔ You see that your skin is charred.

✔ You suffer burns to a larger area.

Seek medical advice urgently, and take the following steps to prevent any further damage:

1. **Remove the cause of the burn (for example, put out the flames, switch off the electricity or remove clothes soaked in hot fluids).**

2. **Cool the affected area of your body with plenty of cold water, ideally under a running tap.**

Don't put any creams or ointment on your burnt skin, because you may do more harm than good. If you suffer severe burns that involve the insides of your hands, your head and neck, or the insides of your elbows and knees, or you inhale a lot of smoke, seek medical advice immediately or call '999'. Do so especially when you're short of breath, because your breathing may get worse. You can suffer cyanide poisoning from smouldering plastic, leading to headaches, dizziness or even seizures.

Hello, Sunshine!

Exposing your skin to a lot of sunshine – especially when the sun is hottest around the middle of the day – without adequate protection ages you and increases your risk of developing skin cancer. Take care not to burn in the sun by taking the following protective measures:

- Avoiding direct sunlight during the hottest part of the day.

- Covering your skin with sunscreen with a high sun-protection factor (25 or above) when you're in the sun.

- Wearing a hat and sunglasses and covering exposed skin with loose-fitting cool clothing.

- Wearing a UV-protective swimsuit when swimming outdoors or when you're on the beach.

You've had too much sun when you:

- Notice tingling of your skin, followed by reddening of your skin 2–12 hours later. Use calming lotions if needed – your pharmacist can advise you on suitable preparations.

- Develop skin blisters and painful skin, and your sunburn makes you feel unwell. These symptoms indicate more severe sunburn, and you need to seek medical advice.

Alleviating heat exhaustion

If you're not used to a hot environment, perhaps when you're on holiday, and you don't drink the extra fluids that you need, excessive sweating may lead to heat exhaustion. You're likely to notice the following symptoms:

- You feel tired and exhausted.

- You see that your skin looks pale and feels clammy.

- You feel dizzy, faint or nauseous, or you vomit.

- You notice your heart beating faster than usual, and/or your breathing becoming more rapid.

- You may suffer from headache.

- You can get muscle cramps.

If you think that you're suffering from heat exhaustion, follow this advice:

- Drink some cool water, to which add one teaspoon of salt per one litre (just over two pints) of water. If you have a special rehydration powder at hand, use that instead and according to the manufacturer's instructions. Cool sports drinks are another useful alternative.

- ✔ Lay down in a cool and quiet area and raise your feet a little (for example, under a rucksack or cushion).
- ✔ Loosen or remove any tight-fitting clothing.

If you don't start to feel better or your condition gets worse, seek medical assistance.

Chapter 6

Approaching Non-Specific Symptoms

*T*he phrase *non-specific symptoms* sounds a bit woolly, but sometimes that's the way things are. By 'non-specific symptoms', I mean those signals that you – as well as health professionals – can find 'vague' or difficult to get a handle on. This problem can arise when the symptom – such as being tired all the time, feeling generally unwell or feeling dizzy – doesn't point to any particular part of the body.

A variety of different conditions can cause non-specific symptoms – ranging from minor self-limiting illnesses, such as viral infections, to serious problems like cancer. Some people worry about such symptoms unnecessarily, whereas others don't consider seeking medical advice when this would be the right thing to do, not even when their problems persist for weeks or months or get worse gradually.

In this chapter I try to make sense of symptoms that seem strange to you, and help when you can't quite put your finger on what may be wrong. I cover some of the warning signs to look out for and provide general indications of when not to worry – and I tell you when consulting your doctor is best, to make sure that you don't have a more serious underlying health problem.

Looking at Ill-Defined Symptoms

In this section I cover the most common 'vague' symptoms, and those that many people have difficulty making head or tail of.

Experiencing constant tiredness

Feeling tired all the time is a common – no, make that a *very* common – problem, and a frequent reason why people visit their GP.

Feeling tired often means that you haven't had enough sleep or you've been doing too much – and by making you feel tired your body's telling you to slow down, rest and take it easy until your 'batteries are recharged' again. Usually, just feeling a bit tired without any other symptoms isn't a cause for concern, particularly if you're not too bothered by it and start to feel better after a while, rather than getting worse. However, sometimes you may feel that even when you do get plenty of rest, you still don't feel much better for it. If this situation sounds familiar, physical or psychological causes such as those in the following list may be responsible for your tiredness (I order them starting with the more common and/or harmless, moving on to relatively rare and/or more serious causes):

- ✔ **Lifestyle:** Having young children, lack of sleep and working long hours are common lifestyle reasons for feeling tired all the time. Try getting a break by, for example, organising additional childcare (perhaps a relative or friend can help) or changing your work patterns.

- ✔ **Medication:** Taking certain tablets regularly can make you feel tired. Common culprits are *beta-blockers* (which your doctor may have prescribed because you have high blood pressure or for preventing migraine or a heart condition), antidepressant medication or drugs used in the management of epilepsy. Check the information leaflet that comes with your drug to see whether tiredness is a common side effect and, if necessary, seek advice from your pharmacist or see your GP for a review of your medication.

- ✔ **Infections:** Colds and viral infections can make you feel tired, as can many other acute and chronic infections. If you're not sure what's going on, you feel quite unwell or your symptoms don't settle, consult your GP.

- ✔ **Mental health problems:** A number of mental health conditions such as stress, depression or anxiety, as well as alcohol and drugs, can lead to tiredness. Check out Part V on mental health problems and consult your GP for further assessment as appropriate.

- ✔ **Hormone problems:** Various hormone abnormalities can lead to tiredness. Hormonal changes in early pregnancy, for example, cause – sometimes excessive – tiredness. *Diabetes mellitus* is another cause, and is a condition in which you lack the hormone *insulin*. Diabetes may come on slowly and make you feel tired to begin with, but you may also show symptoms such as excessive thirst or passing urine frequently. You may be able to get a simple blood test for diabetes at your local pharmacy – otherwise contact your GP surgery. (You can read more about diabetes in Chapter 20.)

An underactive thyroid gland (called *hypothyroidism*) is another common hormone problem that causes tiredness. Other symptoms of hypothyroidism include constipation and heavy periods (in women), as well as feeling cold, developing a hoarse voice or generally lacking energy. See your GP, who can assess you further and diagnose this and other conditions with a simple blood test.

✔ **Chronic fatigue syndrome:** If you suffer from profound physical and mental tiredness – for example, you have difficulties concentrating, word-finding or multi-tasking – and exhaustion (particularly related to physical activity), you may have *chronic fatigue syndrome*. This condition is very different to the usual day-to-day tiredness. See your GP for further assessment, particularly if you've been feeling tired for weeks or even months without any obvious cause.

✔ **Anaemia:** In simplified terms, *anaemia* means 'lack of blood'. In women of childbearing age, anaemia is most commonly due to blood loss through heavy periods. Anaemia can also be due to insufficient iron intake, especially in unbalanced vegetarian diets. Even with good iron intake, however, if your stomach and bowels don't digest food properly you can have an insufficient uptake of iron and other vitamins, which can also lead to anaemia. Blood loss through a cause within your bowel, which may potentially be serious – particularly when you're older – can also lead to this condition (you can find more on bowel problems in Chapter 11).

If you're anaemic, in addition to tiredness you may also look pale and feel short of breath when you exert yourself. Always see your doctor for further assessment if you think you may be anaemic.

✔ **Chest problems:** Various chest problems, including weakness of your heart muscle (often referred to as *heart failure*), chronic lung conditions such as *chronic obstructive pulmonary disease (COPD)* and other medical problems, can cause persistent tiredness. Usually, you also notice other chest symptoms such as shortness of breath or coughing. Read Chapter 10 on heart and chest problems for further information and see your GP for further assessment as appropriate.

✔ **Cancer:** Tiredness is a common symptom of cancer – but of course this doesn't mean that you have cancer when you feel tired. Cancer can affect many parts of your body, and in addition to tiredness you're also likely to have symptoms related to the affected area of your body. You can find more information on how to spot the symptoms and signs of cancer later in this chapter, in the section 'Asking: Can This Be Cancer?'.

Many other causes can make you feel tired, and so if none of the above sound likely to you, consult your GP. Certainly don't wait to make an appointment if you notice any of the following:

✔ You've been losing weight for a while, don't have much appetite or suffer from fevers, night sweats and swollen lymph glands (some of these are located on your neck, in your armpits and in your groins).

✔ You suffer from symptoms of depression or anxiety (check out Chapter 21 for more information on these problems).

✔ You suffer from constant and persistent pain anywhere in your body.

✔ You pass a lot of urine frequently and drink much more than you used to (suggesting *diabetes mellitus*).

✔ Your tiredness is disabling and impacts on your day-to-day life.

Feeling faint

Feeling faint is quite a common problem, but passing out and losing consciousness even briefly can be very worrying. You can read more about collapse and more serious losses of consciousness in connection with a medical emergency in Chapter 5.

Consider the following causes when you feel faint, whether just once or more regularly (I list them starting with the more common/harmless causes, moving on to rarer/more serious ones):

✔ **Simple faint:** Fainting may occur when you've been exercising a lot or been out in the sun in hot weather without drinking enough fluids. It can also happen easily if you stand for too long in one spot, particularly if you're in a stuffy environment. You're likely to feel a bit light-headed before going pale and feeling cold and clammy, but you don't normally have any other significant symptoms. Sit or preferably lie down and drink some cool water, and you usually feel better soon.

✔ **Pregnancy:** If you're a woman of childbearing age, consider being pregnant as a possible cause for feeling faint, particularly if your period is late and you have other symptoms of pregnancy such as tender breasts, morning sickness and tiredness. Confirm or exclude being pregnant by doing a pregnancy test, which you can get from your pharmacy without prescription, or contact your GP surgery.

✔ **Low blood pressure:** Taking regular medication may cause your blood pressure to fall slightly when you get up too quickly from sitting, kneeling or lying (a condition called *postural hypotension*). See your pharmacist or GP for advice if you suspect that this problem causes you to feel faint.

✔ **Low blood sugar:** If you suffer from *diabetes mellitus* (which I describe in detail in Chapter 20) and haven't eaten for an unusually long time (or you've been exercising more than you normally do), low blood sugar can cause you to feel faint. Alternatively, taking too high a dose of insulin or medication for your diabetes can also make you feel faint. You usually feel better quickly when you drink a sugary drink or eat something containing sugar (such as a biscuit). Visit your GP or a nurse with special experience in diabetes if you suffer such episodes regularly.

✔ **Some other medical problems:** Occasionally, problems with your heart or blood vessels in general can cause fainting and episodes of passing out (which I cover in Chapter 5). Consult your GP for further assessment if you suspect an underlying condition or you're just not sure what's going on.

Always consult your GP in the first instance or even consider calling '999' when you're suddenly becoming very unwell or you don't get better quickly, particularly if you experience one or more of the following symptoms in addition to feeling faint:

✔ You get chest pain or feel short of breath, or your heart beats irregularly, very fast or very slow, during an episode (you can read more on heart and lung problems in Chapters 5 and 10).

✔ You suffer from confusion, blurred vision or numbness or weakness in one of your limbs, or you have difficulty speaking, which may indicate a *stroke* (Chapter 5 contains more on stroke).

✔ You notice blood in your stools, or your stools have become black lately (check out Chapter 11 for more information).

Chapter 24 tells you how to give first aid to another person who's fainted.

Delving into Functional Problems

Not being able to sleep or feeling dizzy are two very common problems. Worrying about them – because you're not sure whether you're suffering from a health condition or whether the problem isn't serious and you just have to put up with it – can make matters worse. In this section I give you some clues that help you to tell the difference.

Having difficulties sleeping

Sleep problems affect many people. Having the occasional bad night's sleep doesn't do any harm as long as you get a chance to catch up on your sleep over the following days. However, most people start to worry when their usual sleep pattern gets disrupted for more than a few nights. For example, you may have problems with getting to sleep, waking up after a couple of hours or so, getting up regularly during the night or waking up much earlier than you want.

Coping with sleeplessness

Not being able to sleep can be a real headache, and so try taking the following precautions (sometimes referred to as *sleep hygiene*) that many people find useful:

✔ Avoid exercising late in the evening, which can be counterproductive, and instead increase the amount of exercise you do during the day so that you feel more tired at bedtime.

✔ Avoid eating too much when you have your evening meal and ideally have it at least two to three hours before you go to bed. A light snack before bedtime is of course fine if you feel hungry.

✔ Avoid drinking too much alcohol both during the day and in the evening.

✔ Avoid trying too hard to get to sleep. If you haven't fallen asleep after 30 minutes or so,

get up instead of tossing and turning, do something 'boring' and not too stimulating (in other words, don't start reading an exciting thriller or watch an action movie), and try again as soon as you feel sleepy.

✔ Avoid working too late into the evening if doing so prevents you from sleeping.

✔ Avoid using sleeping pills – although they can sometimes be useful short-term. Always see your GP or pharmacist to discuss the pros and cons of sleeping pills, as well as the use of alternative medications or strategies. Additional help may be available, particularly if your problem is severe.

✔ Some people find that having a hot bath in the evening, or taking a well-padded hot water bottle to bed with them in colder weather, helps them get to sleep better.

Consider the following causes if you suffer from sleep problems:

✔ **Alcohol:** Alcohol can affect your sleep pattern – sometimes quite considerably. In fact, many people with sleeping problems drink alcohol to help them get to sleep without realising that this may only make things worse in the longer term. (Turn to Chapter 23 to find out more about alcohol-related problems.)

✔ **Anxiety, depression and stress:** These problems are very common reasons for lack of sleep. You can read more about them in Chapter 21.

✔ **Environment:** To improve your chances of getting a good night's sleep, make sure that your bedroom is the right temperature for you, that you make your bed as comfortable as possible and that you don't watch too much TV late at night before going to bed. You may perhaps have a snoring partner who prevents you from sleeping, in which case consider sleeping in separate rooms for a while, or ask your partner to seek medical advice for his or her snoring – help may be available.

✔ **Life events:** Acute life events, such as an upcoming exam or interview, marriage problems or the death of someone close to you, can all cause sleep problems. If your sleep doesn't improve, consult your GP.

- ✔ **Medication and other substances:** Drinking a lot of coffee or tea during the day or late in the evening may adversely affect your sleep. Prescribed drugs such as asthma inhalers or steroids, which may be given for asthma and a number of other medical conditions, can also make you feel more awake at night. Try to cut down on stimulants and consult your GP if you feel you don't sleep well as a side effect of your medication.

- ✔ **Physical causes:** If you have additional medical symptoms, such as getting up frequently because of chronic pain, breathlessness or having to go to the toilet, a physical cause may be the reason for your sleepless nights. See your GP for further assessment when you suspect an underlying medical cause.

- ✔ **Sleep habits:** Sleep problems are common in people who regularly have to sleep at different times, for example shift workers. Whenever possible, try to go to bed at more or less the same time each day and avoid daytime naps if you can.

Feeling that everything is 'spinning around'

Dizziness is a feeling of light-headedness when you get up from sitting, kneeling or lying down. Feeling dizzy can be similar to feeling faint (you can read about causes of feeling faint earlier in this chapter). When you feel that everything is spinning around you, or that you're moving despite standing or lying still, you're likely to be suffering from what's known as *vertigo*. Both conditions make you feel unsteady on your feet and can be very distressing, particularly when you suffer one of them for the first time. Fortunately, in most cases both experiences are due to benign causes and usually settle by themselves.

Vertigo can be due to any of the following conditions (starting with the more common ones):

- ✔ **Labyrinthitis:** Viral infections such as the common cold or flu may spread to the balance organ and cause an infection known as *labyrinthitis*, which can lead to vertigo. This condition can be distressing, particularly if you also suffer from vomiting and feel unsteady on your feet, but it usually resolves by itself. In some cases antibiotics help when the underlying cause is a middle-ear infection, so consult your GP if symptoms are severe, don't settle quickly or if you're unsure.

- ✔ **Benign paroxysmal vertigo:** In this condition small pieces of debris break off inside the fluid-filled balance organ in your inner ear and cause sudden attacks of short, recurrent and intense vertigo that usually don't last for much longer than 10–20 seconds. Simply rolling over in bed or turning your head may be enough to bring on symptoms, but you don't usually have any problems with hearing or ringing in your ears. Symptoms often settle after a few days but can sometimes last for weeks or even months. Visit your GP, who may perform a simple sequence of head movements (called the *Epley Manoeuvre*), which can help relieve symptoms dramatically.

✔ **Vestibular neuritis:** Sometimes an inflammation of a nerve in the inner ear (called *vestibular neuritis*) can cause ear pain and vertigo, which may last anything from a few hours to several days. With this condition, you don't normally have any hearing problems or ringing in the ears.

✔ **Ménière's disease:** Severe vertigo may be due to *Ménière's disease*, which experts think is caused by increased pressure in the inner ear. In addition, you may notice loss of hearing and ringing in your ear (called *tinnitus*). The tinnitus of Ménière's disease often progresses over weeks and months, and hearing loss may sometimes be permanent. If you suspect you have the disease, consult your GP, who's likely to prescribe medication and may consider specialist referral. For further advice and information contact the Ménière's Society on 0845 1202975 or visit the website at `www.menieres.org.uk`.

If you take medication for another condition, remember that some prescribed drugs can cause dizziness or vertigo. Examples include aspirin-type drugs, blood pressure lowering medication, antidepressants or sleeping tablets. See your pharmacist or GP for advice about how to deal with any unwanted side effects.

You can try to deal with your dizziness or vertigo in a number of ways:

✔ Avoid bending forward and squat instead if you need to reach down.

✔ Avoid reaching up high if doing so extends your neck too much.

✔ Get out of bed slowly and sit on the edge for a little while before standing up.

✔ Move your head slowly and carefully.

On rare occasions, vertigo may have a more serious underlying cause within your brain, such as a brain tumour. If you suddenly feel dizzy or suffer from vertigo, this may potentially indicate a more serious underlying condition such as a heart attack or stroke. (You can find more information on how to spot a heart attack or stroke and other reasons for feeling faint in Chapter 5.) Consult your GP if you're not sure what's going on, your symptoms are severe or they don't settle down quickly. Speak to your GP urgently or consider calling '999' in the following circumstances:

✔ You have central chest pain or tightness, which may radiate to your neck, jaw or left arm and can be accompanied by sweating, nausea, shortness of breath, feeling faint or collapsing.

✔ You suddenly notice odd sensations such as numbness, tingling or weakness in any of your limbs.

> ✔ You can't see properly in one or both eyes, for no obvious reason.
>
> ✔ You have difficulty getting your words out or speak in a strange way.
>
> ✔ You develop a sudden severe headache, particularly if this problem occurs after a head injury.

Vertigo is not the same as a fear of heights (which is called *acrophobia*), although some people feel dizzy when they look down from a high place.

Asking: Can This Be Cancer?

Human bodies are made up of tiny *cells*, most of which keep dividing – which is how bodies grow and adapt. If a cell divides more quickly than it's supposed to, the cells become *malignant*, which leads to tissue growing too fast and out of control. This out-of-control growth is called *cancer* (also often called *malignancy*, *tumour* or *growth*), which can stay in the organ where it started growing or spread to other areas in your body – usually through your blood. When the latter happens, experts call a distant new outbreak of cancer *metastasis*.

Because you may have read about cancer, seen a programme about it on television or you know someone who suffers or died from cancer, you can worry that a new symptom you develop may be due to cancer. You're not alone – in fact, many people worry that their symptoms *must* be due to cancer. The opposite is also true, in that many people who show symptoms of cancer are often not aware that these signals can indicate serious illness – or are too embarrassed to mention it to a health professional.

Being able to spot the signs of cancer is important. Although cancer is a serious – and often very frightening – diagnosis, powerful treatments have emerged in recent years that are able to cure cancers – provided that the diagnosis is made early. Generally speaking, the earlier a cancer is diagnosed, the better the chances of a cure. The cure rates also depend on other things, such as how malignant a cancer is (different degrees exist, depending on the type of cell that's growing out of control) and where exactly it's located, but early diagnosis remains vital.

Although you can see or feel certain cancers (for example, you can typically feel breast cancer and cancer of the testicle as a new lump, and skin cancer you can actually see), other cancers such as cancer of the blood or those located deeper inside your body may be suspected only because of the symptoms they cause. Research shows that these more 'hidden' cancers are frequently diagnosed late, partly because of their location and partly because many people aren't aware of the danger symptoms and signs. So, in this section I give you an overview of important symptoms and signs that may sometimes indicate underlying cancer. Don't worry, you don't need to be able to diagnose cancer yourself, but just know what early features suggest that you need to see your doctor, who can do the 'diagnosis bit'.

At the risk of sounding like a broken record, I say again that developing any of the symptoms and signs that I list here doesn't necessarily mean that you have cancer – they only mean that seeking medical advice from your doctor to find out what's causing them is a really good idea.

If you want to find out more about various types of cancer, check out the CancerHelp UK website at `www.cancerhelp.org.uk` and other Internet resources I suggest in Chapter 25.

Spotting general signs of cancer

Certain circumstances may put you at increased risk of developing cancer. They aren't causes – in other words, they don't necessarily mean that you get cancer – but considering whether any of these risk factors may apply to you can help in assessing your symptoms:

- ✔ **Age:** Many cancers become more common with age. Taking seriously any new symptoms that persist or that you can't explain (this warning of course also rings true if you're younger, but is particularly relevant if you belong to an older age group) is therefore important.

- ✔ **Family history:** You may be at increased risk of cancer when cancer runs in your close family. This situation applies to some cancers more than to others, but if you develop symptoms of a particular cancer then mention this family history to your doctor.

- ✔ **Previous cancer:** If you've had cancer in the past, a recurrence is possible. Even if you see your doctor for regular follow-ups or your regular reviews stopped a while ago, take any unusual and persistent symptoms seriously and seek medical advice.

- ✔ **Smoking:** Smoking increases your risk of developing certain cancers – most commonly lung cancer but also cancer of the cervix and bladder. Time to pack in the ciggies!

- ✔ **Toxins:** Some industrial and occupational exposures may increase the risk of cancer. For example, certain chemicals increase the risk of bladder cancer, alcohol can lead you to develop chronic liver inflammation that can eventually lead to liver cancer, and exposure to asbestos dust in the past puts you at higher risk of developing a certain type of lung cancer.

In addition to being aware of any possible risk factors that may apply to you, consider your symptoms. Cancers can cause a host of symptoms, most of which develop gradually over weeks and months, although sometimes the symptoms start acutely, particularly if a tumour is growing relatively fast. Consider the possibility of cancer if you notice any of the following:

- **Fever and night sweats:** These symptoms are particularly common with blood cancer (such as *leukaemia* – flip to the later section 'Blood cancer' for more details), although of course fever is much more commonly due to an acute infection (perhaps in connection with a cough or a sore throat) rather than cancer. (You can read more on fever in Chapter 7).

- **Nausea and vomiting:** Persistently feeling sick and vomiting may occur with cancers of the stomach but also with other malignancies such as a brain tumour. However, non-serious stomach problems are usually much more likely. (Read more on these in Chapter 11).

- **New, unusual and/or persistent symptoms:** You develop a new, unusual, unexpected, persistent or worsening symptom 'out of the blue' for no apparent reason and are unable to explain it.

- **Swollen lymph glands:** Lymph glands (located, for example, on your neck, in your armpits and in your groins) tend to swell up during certain infections, but if one or more of your glands stays swollen for more than two weeks (particularly if they don't hurt), or they gradually get bigger, this can potentially be a sign of a cancer of the lymph glands (known as *lymphoma*) or one that has spread from elsewhere in your body. (Go to Chapter 8 for more about lumps and bumps.)

- **Tiredness:** Persistent tiredness is a common symptom of many cancers (particularly blood cancer types), but can also occur due to anaemia caused by blood loss from cancer of the stomach or the intestine (for more on anaemia, check out the earlier section 'Experiencing constant tiredness'). But remember that tiredness is in most cases due to other and much less serious causes. (You can read more about this earlier in this chapter.)

- **Weight and appetite:** Consider the possibility of cancer if you lose weight for no apparent reason over a period of weeks or months – with or without reduced appetite. Some cancers can make you lose your appetite, whereas in others you feel more hungry. (Refer to more on weight symptoms in Chapter 7.)

None of these symptoms necessarily mean that you have cancer, but they can do – particularly if they don't go away – and so seek medical advice sooner rather than later if you're concerned.

Recognising different kinds of cancer

When you develop symptoms of cancer, you need to be able to spot these symptoms and visit your GP for further assessment and early diagnosis. This prompt response then allows you to get referred early and quickly for specific, specialist investigations and treatment. In this section I sum up the key symptoms and signs of some of the most common and serious cancers.

Lung cancer

Lung cancer is relatively common – and you're much more at risk of developing it if you're a smoker, particularly if you've been smoking for a long time. Lung cancer also gets more common the older you are.

Consider the possibility of lung cancer if you recognise one or more of the following symptoms and consult your GP:

- ✔ **Cough:** Always take a persistent cough (in other words, one that lasts for more than three weeks) seriously, particularly if you're older, you smoke, or your cough gets worse or fails to respond to any treatment by your GP.

- ✔ **Coughing up blood:** Coughing up blood is an important symptom, particularly if you're an ex-smoker or a current smoker over the age of 40. However, coughing up blood is often due to non-cancerous causes such as a chest infection.

- ✔ **Hoarseness:** Take any persistent hoarseness lasting for three weeks or more seriously, because it can sometimes be a symptom of lung cancer when a nerve that helps work your vocal cords is affected, or it may indicate a possible cancer of your vocal cords.

- ✔ **Other chest symptoms:** Sometimes, lung cancer may lead to persistent and otherwise unexplained chest pain or ongoing shortness of breath, as well as shoulder and arm pain. If you have an ongoing chest problem such as chronic obstructive pulmonary disease (COPD) or asthma (read more on these conditions in Chapter 10) and your symptoms change without an obvious explanation, see your GP for further assessment.

If you're under the age of 40 and have never smoked, the chances that you have lung cancer are really quite slim, even if you have a cough that persists for a couple of weeks or longer. Unless you have any other warning symptoms, in most cases waiting to see if your cough settles by itself is reasonable, particularly if it's obviously due to the common cold.

Cancer of the upper gastrointestinal tract

Cancer of the upper gastrointestinal tract (the upper abdomen, which includes your gullet or *oesophagus*, stomach, liver and pancreas) is relatively common.

Consider the possibility of cancer in your upper abdomen, and see your GP, if you recognise any of the following symptoms and signs:

- ✔ **Gastrointestinal tract problems:** If you have persistent and unexplained upper abdominal pain associated with weight loss, indigestion, difficulty swallowing, black stools or ongoing vomiting without any obvious reason, these important symptoms can indicate an upper gastrointestinal tract cancer.

- ✔ **Anaemia:** If you're persistently tired, feel short of breath on exertion and have been looking pale for a few weeks, potentially this problem can be due to *iron deficiency anaemia* caused by an upper – or lower – gastrointestinal cancer.

- ✔ **Jaundice:** If the whites of your eyes or your skin start to look yellow, this symptom can be due to various reasons – and cancer is one of them.

Bowel cancer

You may find symptoms to do with your bowels embarrassing – join the club! Sadly, because of this embarrassment, many people hesitate to see their doctor when they develop symptoms suggestive of bowel cancer, which often leads to a delay in diagnosis. However, bowel cancer is one of the malignancies in which early diagnosis makes a huge difference to your future health and survival, and so make no excuse and see your GP immediately if you notice either of the following symptoms:

- ✔ **Bleeding from the back passage:** Consider the possibility of bowel cancer if you're over the age of 40 and develop persistent rectal bleeding together with a change in bowel habit towards looser stools, and without any symptoms around your anus such as itching or pain. If you're over the age of 60, regard any blood in your stool as suspicious, particularly when this blood is mixed with your stool.

- ✔ **Change in bowel habit:** If for no apparent reason you develop looser stools and/or pass stools more often than you used to, and if these symptoms last for more than six weeks or so, go to see your GP to get checked out, because this symptom can be a sign of bowel cancer (but plenty of other conditions may also cause it, and so don't panic). The chances of an underlying bowel cancer being present are higher if you also develop bleeding from your back passage at the same time.

Most people who see their GP because of blood in their stools don't have cancer. Fresh blood on the toilet paper or dripping into the toilet pan – which can look quite dramatic – is most commonly due to haemorrhoids – see your pharmacist or GP for suitable treatments. (You can read more about haemorrhoids and other tummy and bowel problems in Chapter 11.) Nevertheless, make sure that you get checked out if your symptoms don't settle, particularly if you belong to an older age group.

Breast cancer

You can sometimes feel the presence of breast cancer. If you're a woman, you need to become *breast aware*, which means that you know how your breasts normally feel. In this way, you can tell if something isn't right. You can find more on breast cancer and breast awareness in Chapter 18.

Visit your GP for further assessment if you develop any of the following symptoms:

- ✔ **Breast lump:** You notice a lump in your breast that persists after your next period, appears after you go through the menopause or gets bigger with time.

- ✔ **Breast shape or size:** You notice any change in the size or shape of one of your breasts.

- ✔ **Nipples:** You notice any change in the shape of your nipples, you get any unusual discharge from your nipples (particularly if this contains blood) or you develop any skin changes on or around your nipples (or other breast areas) that don't disappear by themselves and worry you.

Many men believe that they can't develop breast cancer. In fact, they can – although breast cancer in men is about 100 times less common than in women. So if you're a man and develop a new lump or other change in your breast tissue, go to see your GP to get it checked out.

If you're a teenage boy and develop a – sometimes tender – swelling behind your nipple area, you most likely have little to worry about. This swelling is usually due to hormonal changes in puberty and goes over time.

Ovarian cancer

The *ovaries* are small organs deep in a woman's lower abdomen, near the womb or *uterus*, which produce the eggs released during the childbearing years. Around 6,800 women are diagnosed with ovarian cancer each year in the UK, and unfortunately many of these women don't know much about the presenting symptoms of this cancer. Due to a common misconception, many women think that they're being checked for ovarian cancer through the cervical cancer screening programme – but this programme is for cervical cancer only.

You're at higher risk of developing ovarian cancer in these circumstances:

- ✔ You're aged 50 years or over.

- ✔ You have a history of ovarian cancer in your family.

- ✔ You're overweight.

- ✔ You have no children and therefore have not breastfed.

- ✔ You haven't used the contraceptive pill (the *combined oral contraceptive pill* provides some protection against ovarian cancer if you take it for a number of years).

See your GP for further assessment if you notice any of the following symptoms when they persist for a few weeks or more or get worse over time, or if you can't explain them:

✔ You experience persistent pelvic and stomach pain.

✔ You find eating difficult and feel full more quickly than you used to.

✔ You notice that your stomach has been increasing in size or you feel persistently bloated (not just occasional bloating that comes and goes).

✔ You suffer from other new abdominal or urinary symptoms that start for no apparent reason and don't improve over time – such as needing to go for a pee suddenly or much more often – or that your bowel habits have changed without any particular cause.

✔ You feel tired all the time for no apparent reason.

✔ You suddenly develop lower back pain for no obvious reason.

You and your GP may find that keeping a diary of your symptoms for a week or two is useful.

Urological cancer

Cancer of the waterworks is relatively common, but the symptoms may take a while to develop. In addition, fairly harmless conditions such as bladder infections or a non-serious swelling of the prostate gland in men (known as *benign prostatic hyperplasia*, or *BPH*) can lead to very similar symptoms. So in order to be certain and rule out more serious conditions, consult your GP if you notice one or more of the following (ordered going from the most common to the least), particularly if your symptoms don't settle by themselves or after a course of antibiotics (flip to more about these and similar symptoms in Chapter 12):

✔ **Urinary symptoms:** You develop new urinary symptoms such as having difficulty passing urine, or blood in your urine. Experiencing the latter is always a reason for you to see your GP, as it may potentially be due to bladder cancer (although much more commonly blood in the urine is due to infection).

✔ **Testicular swellings:** Testicular cancer is one of the cancers that's more common in younger men and, similar to breast cancer in women, one of the few cancers that you can actually feel. Therefore, if you're a man check your testicles regularly (perhaps once a month or so) for any new lumps.

✔ **Penis:** If you're a man and notice any persistent sores anywhere on your penis you may have penis cancer, which is rare and more common in older age.

Blood cancer

Cancer of the blood (a common form is called *leukaemia*) is one of those cancers that you can't see or feel. However, you can suspect leukaemia if you notice one or more of the following features, particularly if they occur in combination. If you suspect leukaemia, consult your GP:

 ✔ You develop regular night sweats.

 ✔ You bruise more easily than you used to, or you bleed when you're brushing your teeth without having any obvious gum disease.

 ✔ You've been losing weight for no apparent reason.

 ✔ You itch all over without having a skin condition as such.

 ✔ You suffer from recurrent unexplained infections.

 ✔ You have new and persistent pain in your bones that remains even if you rest, and that may get worse when you drink alcohol.

 ✔ You feel very tired most of the time.

Skin cancer

Most people have *moles* – brownish spots that can be located anywhere on your skin. Usually, moles are light brown in colour, have a clear and well-defined border, don't tend to grow fast in size and usually don't itch or bleed.

Different types of skin cancer exist, and one of them may look like a dark mole: *melanoma* is a type of skin cancer that's linked to sun exposure (which means that you're at a higher risk of melanoma if you had frequent sunburns in the past) and is particularly dangerous because it can spread quickly to other areas of your body.

Generally speaking, consider the possibility of skin cancer if you notice a skin lesion larger than 5 millimetres ($\frac{1}{5}$ inch) or so in diameter that doesn't heal and/or gets larger in size. Two relatively common skin cancers are called *squamous cell carcinoma* and *basal cell carcinoma* (refer to images 1 and 3 in the colour section). Melanoma is a bit different in that it often develops on the basis of a mole – a new one or an existing mole that suddenly or gradually changes. Turn to Chapter 8 for more information about skin cancer and other skin problems.

See your GP if you notice any of the following changes in one of your moles:

 ✔ Your mole changes size, shape or colour.

 ✔ Your mole develops irregular borders.

 ✔ Your mole has different colours in it and is quite dark.

 ✔ Your mole suddenly 'feels' different – for example, it starts to itch or hurt.

 ✔ Your mole starts to bleed for no apparent reason.

As you get older, you may develop what are called *seborrhoic warts*. These warts can resemble melanomas but are completely benign and nothing to worry about. You're likely to have more than one of these warts, and they have a typical 'stuck-on' appearance.

Head and neck cancers

Various cancers may affect areas of your head and neck. Here's a quick guide to the main symptoms for you to look out for. If you notice that you have any of these problems, see your GP:

- ✔ **Hoarseness:** If your voice is hoarse for more than three weeks or so for no apparent reason and doesn't get better, in some cases this problem may be due to cancer of the voice box – which is more likely in heavy smokers or drinkers over the age of 50. However, non-serious causes like infections are much more common.

- ✔ **Lumps:** Treat any persistent lump or other swelling that develops in your neck and which you can't explain as suspicious, particularly if it has been growing over a period of three to six weeks. Single and later on multiple swollen *lymph* glands (lymph is a name for the fluid within your body tissue) that don't hurt and grow over time may be due to cancer of your lymph glands (also known as *lymphoma*) or because another cancer has spread to them (check out the earlier section 'Spotting general signs of cancer' for more on lymphoma).

- ✔ **Pain:** See your GP if you develop a pain anywhere on your head that you can't explain and that doesn't get better over three to four weeks.

- ✔ **Sores:** Persistent sores or lumps in your mouth as well as any patches on the inside lining of your mouth that last for more than three weeks need to be treated as suspicious, especially if you also notice any swelling or bleeding in the affected area. Mouth (or *oral*) cancer isn't as common as many of the other cancers, but it can be more difficult to treat, and so the earlier you can spot it, the better. You're at higher risk of mouth cancer if you're over the age of 50 and a smoker or you drink large amounts of alcohol regularly.

Your lymph glands can sometimes swell up due to throat infection and become painful, which simply means that they're doing their job – filtering the fluid from infected areas and helping fight the infection. If a good reason exists why your glands have swelled up and they settle down as soon as your infection clears, you have nothing to worry about.

Brain tumour

If you suffer from headaches, you may have difficulty not thinking that you have an underlying brain tumour. In fact, although a headache is one of the main symptoms of brain tumour, the chances of your pain being due to a brain tumour are quite slim. For more information on headaches, turn to Chapter 9.

Brain tumours often cause other symptoms in addition to headache, which can help you spot that something more serious may be going on. If you have any of the following problems, see your GP:

✔ You vomit regularly for no apparent reason.

✔ You pass out or have one or more fits (or *seizures*).

✔ You (or others) notice that your personality changes, or you suffer any other mental changes.

✔ You notice a weakness of your muscles or strange sensations in one or more areas of your body (including your face): that is, sensations that don't make sense to you.

✔ You become cross-eyed for no apparent reason.

✔ You develop ear symptoms such as persistent ringing or pain in your ear for no apparent reason.

Other women's cancers

Various other cancers affect only women. Here I list the main symptoms to look out for if you're a woman and suspect a cancer somewhere 'down below' (turn to Chapter 18 for more details on these and other women's health symptoms):

✔ **Bleeding after the menopause:** Vaginal bleeding that starts after you've been through the *menopause* (also known as 'the change') is a sign that you may have genital cancer – such as cancer of the lining of your womb (called *endometrial cancer*) or cancer of the neck of your womb (called *cervical cancer*) – unless you're taking hormone replacement therapy, in which case you may continue to have regular light monthly bleeds, which are nothing to worry about.

✔ **Bleeding between periods:** Bleeding between periods is common and in many cases harmless, particularly in younger women. However, if the problem persists or you bleed after sexual intercourse, see your GP for further assessment and to exclude abnormalities of the neck of your womb (called the *cervix*) as well as infections such as *chlamydia* – a sexually transmitted infection.

✔ **Skin changes on your genitals:** See your GP for any persistent or worsening changes on the skin of your outer genitals (your *vulva*). These changes are most likely due to benign causes, but occasionally a non-healing or intermittently bleeding skin lesion needs to alert you to the possibility of *vulval cancer*. Vulval cancer isn't that common – but the risk of developing it increases with age.

✔ **Vaginal discharge:** This discharge is commonly due to thrush (a common fungal infection also called *candidiasis*), benign vaginal infections (called *bacterial vaginosis*) or sexually transmitted infections (STIs). If you suffer from persistent vaginal discharge – particularly if it's blood-stained – see your GP for a full pelvic examination and inspection of your cervix.

Chapter 7

Covering Symptoms that Affect Your Wider Body

A number of medical conditions can affect almost every part of your body. Being over- or underweight, for example, or having a fever doesn't just affect one part of your body but may involve most or even all of your organs and limbs. It's unlikely that they're all going to spontaneously give up or drop off, or that you're going to go into complete bodily meltdown, but all-over conditions can make you feel pretty under the weather and in some cases they can be quite serious.

All-over conditions may also mean that working out what might be going on can be difficult. For example, weight symptoms and pain can have a number of different causes. In most cases, though, being able to judge when you can manage a symptom yourself and when seeking medical advice is best is more important than working out exactly what's causing your symptoms in the first instance.

In this chapter I pull together symptoms and conditions that tend to involve more than one body part and tell you what to look out for, when you can relax and wait to see what happens, and when you may need to seek medical advice.

Deciding Whether Size Matters: Weight

Although everyone is different as regards body weight and shape, nonetheless each person has an individual 'ideal' or 'normal' weight, at which their body works to its best effect. If you're heavier than this weight, your health may suffer in the long run, with potentially serious consequences. Similarly, losing too much weight for no apparent reason can also cause health problems or indicate a potentially serious underlying condition.

In the following sections I give you the low-down on some of the common health problems that you may develop in connection with weight loss and being overweight, and how to spot when things may be a bit more serious.

Being overweight

If you're overweight or obese, you're not alone. In fact, experts think that more than 50 per cent of people living in the UK weigh too much, with about 4 out of 10 adults being overweight and 1 in 5 being *obese* – in case you're wondering, I define exactly what *obese* means a bit later in this chapter, in Table 7-1. Unfortunately, these figures are going up, and experts are talking about an obesity epidemic.

You may wonder what all the fuss is about, and think that a bit of padding around your waist or hips or a tummy that bulges out a bit surely can't do much harm. Well, they can: lots of health problems may develop over time as a result of weighing too much, and some of them – such as heart attacks or strokes – are among the biggest killers.

Putting your weight into figures

When checking whether you're obese or overweight, simply weighing yourself isn't quite enough: you need to take your height into account, too. To help, health experts have developed a formula known as the *body mass index* (or *BMI*) to relate your body weight to your height.

Your practice nurse can check your weight and height and calculate your BMI for you, but you can calculate your own BMI quite easily by dividing your weight (in kilograms) by the square of your height (in metres). To give you an example, imagine that you weigh 60 kilograms (approximately 9½ stones) and are 1.7 metres tall (just over 5½ feet). To work out your BMI, you make this calculation:

$$60 \div (1.7 \times 1.7)$$

or

$$60 \div 2.89$$

which means that you have a BMI of 20.8.

Alternatively, you can calculate your BMI using an excellent online 'healthy weight' calculator on the NHS Choices website, www.nhs.uk. To see whether your weight puts you at risk of health problems, check your BMI in Table 7-1.

Table 7-1	Health Risks at Different BMI Levels	
BMI	*Weight Level*	*Estimated Health Risk*
Less than 18.4	You're underweight.	You're at some health risk.
18.5 to 24.9	Your weight is normal.	Congratulations – you have no weight- related health risk!
25 to 29.9	You're overweight.	Your health risks are moderately increased.
30 to 39.9	You're obese.	Your health risks are high.
40 and over	You're very obese.	You're at a very high health risk.

Examining reasons for being overweight

In a nutshell, you put on weight when you take in more *calories* (the energy contained in food and drink) than you burn off. This situation means that – in essence – the way to lose weight is to eat less (in terms of food high in calories) and to exercise more. Losing weight isn't always as simple as that – what you eat and how you exercise also plays a role – but the reality really does boil down to this fact for most people.

Occasionally an underlying medical condition may be the cause of your weight gain. Compare your circumstances with these conditions:

- ✔ **Hormonal conditions:** Although less common, hormone imbalances due to an underactive thyroid gland (known as *hypothyroidism* – check out Chapter 6), raised blood sugar (due to *diabetes mellitus* – see Chapter 20) or an increase in steroid hormones (this could be due to excessive *steroid* use in asthma – which I discuss in Chapter 10 – or other conditions, or rarely due to a hormone gland disorder) can lead to obesity. Bear in mind, though, that diabetes may cause weight loss rather than weight gain at the time of diagnosis.

- ✔ **Polycystic ovary syndrome (PCOS):** This relatively common hormonal condition affects women in their reproductive years and can lead to weight problems, absent periods and/or increased hair growth on your body (turn to Chapter 18 for more details on PCOS).

- ✔ **Various other causes:** Other causes exist that can also make you obese – for example, genetic conditions – but they are quite rare.

Consult your GP if you suspect that your weight gain may be caused by one of these conditions. Your doctor can arrange a blood test to help with making the diagnosis and help you identify what may be causing your weight problem.

Becoming aware of obesity-related health problems

If you're overweight or obese, you're at higher risk of developing health problems such as those in the following list, which begins with the more common ones (you can read more about medical emergencies in Chapter 5 and on health problems in later life in Chapter 20):

- **Arthritis:** If you're obese, you're putting a lot of stress on your bones, joints and muscles. Being 10 kilograms (22 pounds) overweight (which doesn't seem a lot) means that you carry extra weight equivalent to one full 10-litre bucket of water around with you, all day and every day! If you're 20 kilograms (44 pounds) overweight (which many people are), this amount equates to the weight of the heaviest suitcase you're allowed to take onto most aeroplanes – just think of the strain on your body if you carry this additional weight with you all the time. No surprise then that your bones and joints suffer (see Chapter 13 for more on this).

- **Depression:** As well as having to suffer the consequences of obesity, such as diabetes or heart disease, being overweight increases your chances of becoming depressed (read Chapter 21 to discover more about depression).

- **Diabetes:** If you suffer from diabetes, your blood sugar is too high, which can lead to both short-term as well as longer-term physical problems (read Chapter 20).

- **High blood pressure:** If you're overweight, you increase the risk of developing high blood pressure, which – if it's too high for a long time and not treated – increases your risk of suffering a *heart attack* or a *stroke* (consult Chapters 5 and 20 for more information).

- **Cancer:** A number of cancers are more common in people who weigh too much (such as cancer of the lining of the womb in women or breast cancer). You can find more on cancer in Chapter 6.

- **Gallstones:** You're at higher risk of developing gallstones, which can cause severe intermittent pain in the upper right area of your abdomen (you can find more on this in Chapter 11).

- **Heart problems:** If you weigh too much, you increase the risk of suffering a *heart attack* (check out Chapter 5).

- **Pregnancy:** Carrying around too much weight isn't great when you're pregnant – it can cause additional health problems and can make your pregnancy and giving birth more strenuous than necessary.

- **Stroke:** A stroke is a *brain attack* – which you're much more likely to suffer if you're overweight or obese.

Feeling lighter – feeling better

Being a healthy weight not only reduces your risk of physical problems, but also helps you to feel better in yourself. Many people who manage to lose weight say that they feel much more positive about themselves as a result and that their quality of life has improved. If you weigh too much and manage to shed some pounds, you're also likely to feel much more energetic, less tired and find that doing exercise is easier.

Losing weight can be difficult. Fortunately, help is available – both from the NHS (see Chapter 25 for a list of useful websites and helplines) and the private sector. Your GP and practice nurse can also advise you about ways to lose weight

and direct you to locally available sources of help and support.

Being realistic about the difficulties of losing weight helps you: losing weight isn't always easy and requires commitment on your part – unfortunately no such thing as a magic bullet or a quick fix exists. Also remember not to expect too much, both in terms of speed and amount of weight loss – but every little helps. Some commercial diets can be successful in getting you to lose weight initially, but you're more likely to achieve and maintain a lower weight if you adopt a healthier lifestyle altogether and maintain this lifestyle in the longer term.

Fading away: Weight and appetite loss

Losing a bit of weight during acute illnesses such as a viral infection or gastroenteritis is common – and as long as you put on the weight again when the illness settles, you've nothing to worry about. However, if you lose weight over weeks or months without any apparent reason (in connection with a reduced appetite or even if your appetite stays normal), you may be potentially suffering from an underlying illness that requires further assessment by your GP.

Compare your situation with the following list of potential causes, which works from the more to the less common:

- **Lifestyle:** A change to your diet can easily lead to weight loss, particularly if you reduce your overall calorie intake. Other lifestyle changes such as moving from office to manual work or cycling to work instead of using the car may in themselves lead to weight loss, unless you match them by eating more to compensate.

- **Medication:** If you take medication regularly, any of your drugs can cause you to lose your appetite. Check the drug information sheet and see your pharmacist or GP if you suspect that your loss of appetite may be due to a drug side effect.

✔ **Mouth problems:** Painful mouth conditions or teeth problems can lead you to eat less, and lose weight.

✔ **Mental health problems:** A number of mental health conditions such as anxiety and depression, or excessive stress – perhaps due to acute life events such as divorce or bereavement – can all cause loss of appetite and weight loss (read more about these problems in Chapter 21). Consult your GP if you feel you suffer from any of these conditions.

✔ **Infection:** Acute infections (caused by viruses like influenza, for example) and other more chronic but less common conditions such as HIV or tuberculosis (TB) (see the later sections 'Approaching HIV and AIDS' and 'Tuberculosis') can cause weight loss – but you usually have other symptoms as well, such as fever and feeling generally unwell. Consult your GP if you think that you may be at risk of HIV or TB: the latter isn't all that common in the UK but is a very common condition in other parts of the world.

✔ **Gastrointestinal causes:** Problems with your stomach or bowels, such as not absorbing food well (known as *malabsorption*), can be caused by various conditions and lead to weight loss. If you also have loose stools, you may have a bowel inflammation or infection. See your GP for further assessment if you think that you may suffer from a bowel-related condition. (Check out Chapter 11 for more on bowel-related symptoms.)

✔ **Cancer:** Unexplained and persistent weight loss is one of the common presenting symptoms of cancer. See your GP if you're losing weight without any obvious reason, particularly when you also show other potential symptoms of cancer (also check out Chapter 6 for more information on cancer symptoms).

✔ **Chronic disease:** A number of chronic medical conditions can cause weight loss. For example, high blood sugar (or *diabetes mellitus*) also causes tiredness and excessive thirst (Chapter 20 contains more information on diabetes). Occasionally, an overactive thyroid gland (or *hyperthyroidism*) can lead to weight loss – but you can also expect to have other symptoms such as a fine shaking of your fingers, increased sweating, diarrhoea and not being able to tolerate warmer environments.

Visit your GP for an assessment if you suspect that you may suffer from a chronic medical condition, or if you've already been diagnosed and feel that the underlying problem may be responsible for your weight loss.

✔ **Eating disorders:** Eating disorders such as anorexia nervosa or bulimia may lead to weight loss, which can be severe, quite dramatic and life-threatening in the case of anorexia. (You can read more about eating disorders in Chapter 17.)

If you suffer from weight loss, look out for the following features that may potentially indicate a more serious underlying disease. If any sound familiar, consult your GP:

- ✔ You lose weight unexpectedly, consistently and/or rapidly.
- ✔ You have other symptoms suggestive of cancer (see Chapter 6).
- ✔ You think you suffer from an eating disorder (see Chapter 17).
- ✔ You feel depressed and have a sense of hopelessness (see Chapter 21).
- ✔ You suffer from additional night sweats and fevers.
- ✔ You also have swollen lymph glands anywhere on your body.
- ✔ You've had cancer in the past.

Checking Out Pain and 'Funny' Sensations

Acute and chronic pain are among the most common reasons for people visiting their GP, which is understandable, because pain is usually an unpleasant sensation that can make you worry that something more serious is going on. As well as pain, you can also suffer from other and perhaps more 'unusual' sensations such as tingling or loss of sensation. In this section I give you an insight into how to interpret pain and other sensations in various contexts, which helps you to decide when to seek assistance and advice from a health professional.

Approaching pain

Pain can strike suddenly (called *acute pain*) or last for three months or longer even when you receive treatment (called *chronic pain*). Actual or potential physical damage to your body tissues is a common cause, but experts now recognise how important social, emotional and environmental factors are in the development and persistence of pain. Suffering from pain for too long can cause you to feel low and unable to sleep properly, making you lethargic and lacking in energy. You may also find mental tasks such as memorising or remembering things or concentrating on your work more difficult.

Although effective medicines are available, controlling pain isn't always easy – for you or for health professionals. Occasionally, even doctors can struggle to find an obvious underlying cause for your pain – which can be quite unsatisfactory and frustrating for everyone involved. If appropriate and necessary, your GP may be able to refer you to a specialist *pain clinic*.

Helping your doctor to assess your pain

If you book an appointment to discuss your pain with your GP, being ready to provide answers to the following questions can help your doctor find out what's causing the pain and decide how best to manage it:

- In which circumstances do you get the pain?

- What (if anything) brought on your pain?

- What do you think may be causing your pain?

- Where exactly is your pain? Does it stay there, or does it move around and spread to other areas? Do you have any pain in adjacent or other areas?

- How severe is your pain (perhaps rate it on a scale from 0 to 10, with 0 being no pain at all and 10 being the worst pain imaginable)?

- Is your pain getting better, getting worse or staying the same? (Generally speaking, pain that gets worse rather than better or that's constant without any periods of relief is potentially – but by no means always – more serious.)

- Does anything make your pain better (for example, painkillers, resting, moving around) or worse (for example, coughing or sneezing, or pressure on the affected body part)?

- How does the pain affect your life? Does it keep you awake or wake you during the night? Does the pain interfere with your ability to get on with your day-to-day activities or stop you from working and enjoying your hobbies?

- How does the pain impact on your mental wellbeing?

- Do you have any financial or other worries because of your pain? Does the pain affect your social life?

If you suffer from pain, consult the chapters in this book dealing with the respective part of your anatomy and consider the following potential causes (ordered from the most common to the least):

- **Trauma:** Any injury – obviously – can cause pain, and generally speaking the more extensive or serious your injury, the more severe your pain (although this situation doesn't always apply). Most pain gets better very quickly, but if your pain is severe or doesn't settle (perhaps due to a bone fracture), consult your GP or go to the nearest Accident & Emergency (A&E) department.

- **Infection:** Skin infections, among others, commonly cause pain. Important additional signs of infection are redness, tenderness and increased skin temperature. Infections deeper inside your body may cause fever in addition to pain, and make you feel generally unwell. Consult your GP if you're not sure what's going on or you can't explain the pain yourself.

✔ **Lack of blood:** You may experience pain if your body tissues don't get enough blood. Fairly common examples of this problem are *angina* (where the blood vessels supplying your heart become too narrow to allow sufficient blood to get through, causing chest pain – see Chapter 10), or *intermittent claudication* (where clogged-up blood vessels cause pain in your legs when you walk a certain distance – check out Chapter 13).

✔ **Inflammation:** Inflammation is common and may be due to overuse of a body part such as a joint, or due to chronic conditions such as arthritis. An inflamed joint or tendon may become swollen and tender, but you wouldn't normally have a fever with inflammation alone. If rest and simple anti-inflammatory medications or gels (your pharmacist can offer advice on suitable preparations) don't work, see your GP for further assessment.

✔ **Nerve pain:** Nerve pain (or *neuropathic pain*) may occur in diabetes because of pressure on a nerve (this can, for example, happen due to a prolapsed disc in your back – see Chapter 13) or for other reasons such as alcohol misuse over a long period of time. Various other conditions may also lead to nerve pain, which tends to be burning or tingling in character. Visit your GP for further assessment.

✔ **Cancer:** Direct pressure of a growing cancer on adjacent tissues or nerves can cause pain. Pain due to cancer is often constant, not relieved by rest and doesn't really get better. However, cancers often don't cause any pain until they're fairly advanced, and cancers may present without any pain at all. You may also suffer from other cancer-related symptoms – see Chapter 6 for further details.

Occasionally, ongoing pain may suggest that you're suffering from a potentially serious underlying cause. Consult your GP if in addition to pain you notice any of the following:

✔ You lose weight and suffer from fevers and/or night sweats.

✔ You feel quite unwell in yourself.

✔ You suspect that your pain is due to violent trauma.

✔ You've already been diagnosed with cancer or HIV.

✔ You use illicit drugs.

✔ You've been told by your doctor that your immune system is suppressed, or you take steroid drugs (often prescribed for asthma, arthritis or other inflammatory conditions).

Pinpointing pins and needles and other 'odd' sensations

You've probably experienced numbness or tingling in various areas of your body in certain situations – perhaps when you've been sitting awkwardly for a while or cycling a lot and your hands and bottom feel a bit numb. Strange sensations such as numbness, tingling or pins and needles in any part of your body without apparent reason, though, may at times (though not always!) be due to an underlying medical condition, and getting some professional medical advice is a good idea.

If you suffer from strange sensations in any area of your body, compare your symptoms with the following descriptions (in order of frequency and/or severity):

- ✓ **Carpal tunnel syndrome:** Numbness in one or both of your hands – particularly at night – that improves when you shake your hands may be caused by *carpal tunnel syndrome* – a condition in which swelling of soft tissues in your wrist leads to pressure on a nerve. Carpal tunnel syndrome is common, particularly if you're a pregnant woman, or if you're overweight. Various treatments are available, and so when the symptoms bother you, visit your GP for an assessment and to discuss the treatment options.

- ✓ **Cervical spondylosis:** If in addition to tingling in your hand you also have neck symptoms such as pain and stiffness, you may suffer from a condition called *cervical spondylosis*. You can imagine this problem as being like 'wear and tear' of the bones in your neck, which may sometimes lead to pressure on the nerves or a blood vessel. Cervical spondylosis isn't a serious condition as such, but see your GP for further assessment and to discuss possible treatments.

- ✓ **Diabetes:** You may start to suffer from numbness, reduced sensation or tingling in your feet or hands if you've had diabetes for a while (called *diabetic neuropathy*). If you've been diagnosed with diabetes, your GP or practice nurse usually checks for this problem at your regular reviews. Consult your GP or practice nurse if you develop any new tingling or numbness.

- ✓ **Hyperventilation:** You may get tingling in your hands if you breathe too fast (called *hyperventilation*) – for example, during a panic attack. Breathe through your nose and take tiny sips of water, which helps to slow down your breathing. (You can find more about anxiety and panic in Chapter 21.)

✔ **Pressure on a nerve:** Numbness or tingling after your body's been in a certain position for a while (such as after sleeping or sitting) can be due to pressure on one of your nerves. The feeling in the affected part usually returns to normal soon, but see your GP if the problem doesn't get better.

✔ **Sciatica:** If your leg feels numb after you suddenly develop back pain that radiates to the leg, you may be suffering from what's called *sciatica*. Contact your GP if your symptoms don't settle quickly, your pain is severe or you have any of the warning signs I list in the discussion on sciatica in Chapter 13.

✔ **Alcohol:** If you've been drinking too much alcohol for long periods of time, you may develop what experts call *alcoholic neuropathy*, which affects the nerves of your body and may be due to direct toxic effects of the alcohol as well as vitamin deficiencies – with various potential consequences. Important symptoms include numbness, tingling, weakness and pain. See your GP for an assessment and to discuss the management options.

✔ **Raynaud's syndrome:** In this condition, the blood vessels of your fingers are very sensitive to a change in temperature. Particularly in winter when the temperature is cold and you go outside, your fingers or toes may start to feel numb and take on a white and then bluish colour, which changes back to normal when the feeling in your fingers returns (although your fingers may swell up a bit). You can develop this condition if you have other problems with circulation of your blood or if you take certain medication, such as beta-blockers. If you're born with the condition, then it's called *Raynaud's Disease*. See your GP for an assessment, and in the meantime try to keep your hands and feet warm and avoid smoking.

✔ **Stroke:** Sudden numbness in a limb or on one side of your face and/or your body can potentially be due to a stroke (you can find more on stroke and how to identify this condition in Chapter 5.) Call '999', particularly if you also experience any of the following symptoms:

- You feel confused.

- You have difficulty speaking and getting your words out.

- You suffer from loss of vision or blurred vision.

- You can't move your arm or leg properly on one side.

Many other medical conditions may also lead to numbness or tingling, and so if you can't recognise what's going on from these descriptions, see your GP for a check up.

Getting Hotter: Fever

A *fever*, which is when your body temperature is abnormally high, is one of the most common symptoms – and so if you develop one, you're likely to be in good company! In this section I cover the potential causes of fever and how to recognise them as well as 'red flag' symptoms that prompt you to seek medical advice. A special case is when you develop fever during or after a trip abroad, and so I cover this situation separately.

Developing a fever

You have a fever when your body temperature goes above 38 degrees Celsius (100.4 degrees Fahrenheit): you can feel hot, cold or shivery, and are also likely to feel unwell. The only way to measure your body temperature accurately is by using a thermometer – Chapter 3 tells you how to do so. (Checking for fever in babies and toddlers can be a bit more tricky – check out Chapter 14 for more information.)

You can develop a fever through being out in the heat for too long (read up on heat exhaustion in Chapter 5), but having an acute infection is the most likely cause. If you think that you may be suffering from an infection, see whether you can identify the underlying problem by comparing your symptoms with the following list:

- **Respiratory infection:** If you develop a fever at the same time as a sore throat or cough, you're likely to be suffering from a *respiratory infection*. Check out Chapters 9 and 10 for more information on identifying relevant conditions such as tonsillitis or a chest infection.

- **Urinary symptoms:** If you have a fever and need to pass urine more frequently than usual or develop other urinary symptoms such as burning, pain or cloudy urine, you may be suffering from a urinary infection such as *cystitis*. You can find out more about this condition in Chapter 12.

- **Viral infection:** If you have aching limbs, a headache, a sore throat and a runny nose as well as a fever, you may be suffering from a non-specific viral infection or the flu (which is short for *influenza*). If paracetamol or anti-inflammatory medications (available without prescription from your pharmacist) don't help, you're severely ill, you keep getting worse or you're worried for any other reason, call the NHS (see Chapter 25 for useful websites and helplines) or speak to your GP or practice nurse.

- **Cellulitis:** Skin infections (particularly one called *cellulitis*) may cause a fever and commonly involve the lower legs. You can discover more about cellulitis in Chapter 8.

Wising up about travel-related illnesses

You can obtain further information about travel-related illnesses from these organisations:

✔ National Travel Health Network and Centre: www.nathnac.org.

✔ NHS Direct: www.nhsdirect.nhs.uk.

✔ Fit for Travel: www.fitfortravel.scot.nhs.uk.

✔ Centers for Disease Control and Prevention: www.cdc.gov/travel (US website).

✔ **Meningitis:** If in addition to fever you suffer from drowsiness, pain on bending your head forward, vomiting or a rash, read the section on headache in Chapter 9, where you can find more information on meningitis and how to spot the danger signs, and refer to image 21 in the colour section.

A fever may occasionally persist for more than a couple of weeks. The cause can be due to prolonged and untreated infections – but other conditions may also be responsible, so see your GP when your fever just doesn't go away. However, occasionally even doctors aren't able to pinpoint the exact reason for a fever.

Getting a fever from travelling abroad

Air travel has made the world a smaller place and travelling has become relatively easy. Vast numbers of people from the UK now travel abroad to hot and sometimes remote locations, which exposes them to the possibility of contracting a whole new range of conditions.

Seeing your GP or practice nurse for travel advice and immunisations against certain infectious diseases before you travel to certain other countries is important. A fever that appears during or after a stay in a hot country (particularly when you didn't see your practice nurse or GP beforehand for travel immunisations or haven't taken medication to prevent malaria) may be a sign of a serious infection – especially if you don't show any symptoms that suggest other conditions common in the UK (covered earlier in the section 'Developing a fever'). In this section I look at the most common exotic illnesses that can bring on a fever.

Providing travelling details for your doctor

When you arrange to see your doctor about a fever developed from travelling abroad, being able to provide the following information helps tremendously:

✔ The exact dates you travelled and where (for example, rural areas, cities), including stop-overs.

✔ The current climate or season in the country you visited.

✔ Whether you were bitten by or exposed to any animals such as insects, mammals or reptiles.

✔ Whether you were in contact with any ill people.

✔ Whether you had unprotected sex with any new partners.

✔ Your vaccination history.

✔ Whether you took anti-malaria or other specific medication before, during or after your trip (bring the packet(s) along if possible).

✔ The type of travel that you undertook and your accommodation.

✔ The type of food and liquids that you consumed, and where these were prepared.

✔ Any illnesses or injuries sustained while abroad, and what treatment you received (particularly with regard to any injections or blood transfusions).

Traveller's diarrhoea

Picking up a tummy bug (leading to *traveller's diarrhoea*) abroad from eating and drinking contaminated food or water is easy – particularly in Africa, Asia and Latin America. The more primitive the conditions in which you live, the higher the chance that you may develop diarrhoea.

Traveller's diarrhoea is in most cases mild and gets better by itself: you don't normally need antibiotics. You're likely to pass 4–6 stools per day for a few days, may develop a mild fever initially and probably lose your appetite as well. Diarrhoea doesn't do much harm when it lasts for only a few days – but make sure that you drink enough clear fluids (to which you can add a rehydration solution), or drink sports rehydration drinks to replace the fluid you lose.

If you develop a high fever or notice blood in your stools (that is, your bowel movements) together with abdominal pain, seek medical help urgently.

Malaria

If you've travelled in the past year or so to a malarial area and you develop a fever, consider the possibility of having contracted *malaria* – a widespread infectious disease present in tropical and subtropical areas, which is spread through mosquito bites. You may recognise these additional symptoms of malaria:

- ✔ You suffer from intermittent (every two or three days) or persistent fevers (the fever doesn't always follow a particular pattern).

- ✔ You get chills and feel sweaty.

- ✔ You suffer from headaches and muscle aches.

- ✔ You feel nauseous or vomit.

A severe form of malaria (known as *Plasmodium falciparum* malaria) can cause muscle weakness, headache, dark urine, unusual sensations and other symptoms. You may also feel confused and short of breath, and finally you may pass out and enter into a coma.

To diagnose malaria, you need to get a blood test, so see your GP as soon as possible if you develop any unexplained fever after a trip into a malarial area.

Typhoid fever

Typhoid fever is a relatively common infectious disease in countries with poor sanitation. As the name of this condition says, fever is the main symptom, but you may also develop a dry cough, initial constipation followed by diarrhoea, and a faint spotty rash (called *rose spots*) on your stomach. The infection usually clears by itself, but you may still have the bug within you, and you can pass it on even when you're feeling better – and so you're still infectious to other people. See your GP for further assessment and treatment if you suspect that you have typhoid fever.

Hepatitis A

Hepatitis A is an infection that affects your liver. You contract hepatitis A from infected food or water but the symptoms can take a few weeks to appear.

Look out for the following features of hepatitis A, which may appear quite suddenly:

- ✔ You develop a fever.

- ✔ You feel very tired and nauseous.

- ✔ You then develop *jaundice*: the whites of your eyes and sometimes your skin take on a yellow colour.

Hepatitis A can make you feel quite ill but you usually recover fully – even if this recovery takes several weeks. Consult your GP for confirmation of the diagnosis.

Tuberculosis

Tuberculosis (TB) is an infectious disease that is present all over the world, but the risk of being exposed to this disease varies between locations. The good news is that TB isn't too easy to catch, and even if you do catch it, only around 5 to 15 per cent of people develop what's called *active TB*, which usually happens within two years or so after getting infected.

You're at increased risk of developing active TB in the following circumstances:

- You're in close contact with one or more people who already have TB.
- You suffer from diabetes (which I describe in Chapter 20).
- You have a chronic kidney condition leading to reduced kidney function.
- You have a diagnosis of cancer (particularly one called *lymphoma* that affects your lymph tissues – I discuss lymphoma in more detail in Chapter 6).
- You take drugs such as *steroids* that suppress your immune system, which your doctor may have prescribed for treatment of asthma or severe arthritis, or other conditions.
- You're HIV positive.

Active TB can sometimes be difficult to diagnose, because the symptoms vary from person to person. However, consider the possibility that you may have TB if you notice one or more of the following:

- You have a *low-grade* (that is, not very high) intermittent or persistent raised body temperature – usually somewhere around 37.5–38.5 degrees Celsius (99.5–101.3 degrees Fahrenheit).
- You suffer a persistent and *productive* (in other words, causing phlegm) cough.
- You sweat a lot at night.
- You're losing weight.
- You feel tired and 'not quite right'.

If you suspect that you may be suffering from TB, visit your GP for further assessment and investigation.

Other infections causing fever

Many other conditions can cause fever in travellers: *yellow fever* (particularly if you're travelling in South America or Africa), *dengue fever* (which you can catch throughout the tropics) and *Lassa fever* (if you happen to travel in Sierra Leone, Liberia or Nigeria), to name just three.

Healthy travelling

You can do a lot to prevent travel-related illnesses. Here's a list of tips to remember so that you can stay fit and well while travelling:

- Always wash your hands after you've been to the toilet and before you touch any food.

- Remember that food and water are common sources for infections, and so if you're not sure whether water is safe to drink, sterilise or boil it first, or use drinks from sealed bottles. (Remember that this precaution includes ice cubes in drinks.) Freshly made hot tea and coffee are usually fine.

- Try to stick to thoroughly cooked food. Avoid food that hasn't been cooked (such as salads, fruit sold on the street, raw fish or mayonnaise) if you're not sure under what conditions this food was prepared. Remember the well-known saying: 'boil it, cook it, peel it or forget it'!

- Use condoms when you have sex with a new partner while abroad to avoid returning home with 'blind passengers' in the form of a sexually transmitted infection.

- Use mosquito nets in malarial areas whenever possible.

- Visit your practice nurse well before you travel to make sure that you're up-to-date with your immunisations and to get further travel information about the country you're travelling to – practice nurses usually have access to the latest travel and immunisation news.

If you suffer from a fever that you feel may be travel-related, consult your GP. Your symptoms may turn out to be due to a minor infection such as a cold or non-specific viral illness, but some 'overseas' illnesses can be unusual and dangerous to your health. As travel-related infections are often unfamiliar to people in the UK, getting your symptoms checked out by a health professional is a wise move.

Seek medical advice urgently if you have a fever and notice any of the following signs:

- You suffer from a severe headache.

- You notice that the whites of your eyes become yellow, or that your skin takes on a yellow tinge.

- You develop a rash.

- You suffer from numbness, tingling, weakness or other 'strange' symptoms anywhere on your body.

- You have ongoing problems with passing urine (such as pain, blood in your urine or passing urine more frequently).

Covering the Whole: Symptoms that Affect the Whole Body

With symptoms that affect wider parts of your body or that don't make much sense to you, various harmless and sometimes serious causes may be responsible. Out of a long list of possible reasons for such symptoms I cover only two of them here: medication side effects – because they're so common but aren't often recognised – and HIV, which is one of the most feared conditions.

Spotting problems with your medication

Medicines can improve your health considerably, but can also lead to unexpected problems you never expected to have. A lot of people take medicines regularly without being entirely aware of the benefits – or the unwanted side effects. I list here some of the issues to consider when you take long-term medication and give you some hints about when to see your GP or pharmacist for a review. Go through this checklist to see whether any of these issues may apply to you (and which your GP would like to hear about):

- **Adverse effects:** Drugs can cause unwanted side effects that impact on your day-to-day life. Problems such as difficulties with erections in men, tiredness and constipation are common with a number of drugs – but many people feel embarrassed or ashamed to mention these side effects to their GP. If you suffer these or other problems and they bother you, see your pharmacist or GP earlier rather than later – in most cases alternative preparations are available that may suit you better.

- **Ineffectiveness:** If you feel that the tablets you're taking aren't effective, or think that you may need a higher dose of any of the drugs you're taking, arrange to see your GP.

- **New medical problems:** If you start to suffer from any new medical conditions, this problem may affect your medication. Your GP may feel that you need a change of medication, or a change of dose.

- **Practical problems:** Tell your GP if you have any practical problems with picking up your prescriptions or taking the medicines (for example, you have difficulties with opening the drug container because of arthritis). Your GP and pharmacist are well aware of such issues and are likely to have a solution up their sleeves.

- **Problems with taking medication:** If you have difficulty taking your medication, perhaps because you forget, don't like the taste, don't believe in taking tablets, can't swallow them or you get unwanted side effects, speak to your GP openly about this issue – you've no need to be ashamed. Your GP doesn't mind and certainly prefers you to discuss any issues that you may have with your prescribed medication.

✔ **Reason for taking your medicines:** After the original problem settles down, you may be able to stop taking your drugs – after discussing the issue with your GP.

✔ **Taking herbal or over-the-counter drugs:** Make sure that you tell your GP about any herbal or other medicines that you buy over-the-counter, without prescription, in case they interact with your regular medication. Your pharmacist is likely to have asked you questions along these lines already, but some people take medicines that have been prescribed to or bought by their family or friends, which can potentially be dangerous.

Consult your GP urgently for a review of your medication if you experience one or more of the following symptoms:

✔ You think that you may have developed an allergy to one or more of your tablets (for more on allergic reactions read Chapter 5).

✔ You suffer severe unwanted effects.

✔ You've stopped taking your medication altogether without first checking with your GP or pharmacist as to whether this course of action is safe.

Approaching HIV and AIDS

Human immunodeficiency virus, or *HIV,* is a virus that can – usually a few years after infection – lead to *acquired immunodeficiency syndrome,* or *AIDS* – a medical condition that causes the immune system to weaken, resulting in life-threatening infections caused by viruses, bacteria and other germs. HIV is spread through body fluids like blood, vaginal secretions, semen or breast milk.

You're at a particularly increased risk of infection with HIV in any of the following circumstances:

✔ You had unprotected (vaginal, anal or oral) sexual intercourse with people who are infected with HIV.

✔ You're an intravenous drug user and share needles.

Remember that you can become infected with HIV only when infected semen, blood or vaginal secretions get into your blood or body. You can't pick up HIV from normal day-to-day contact with people who've been diagnosed with HIV – and so ordinary close contact, sharing food, hugging, touching and shaking hands are all absolutely fine.

If you get infected with the HIV virus, after a few weeks you may develop an acute illness with fever, a sore throat and swollen lymph glands – symptoms that may last for a few weeks and then improve. If you notice these symptoms and feel that you may have been at risk of contracting HIV, see your GP urgently: early diagnosis and treatment of HIV infection can prevent a number of problems that can potentially become very serious.

HIV infection may not cause any symptoms for a few years. After this interval, you may start noticing one or more of the following:

- ✔ You have intermittent and persistent fevers.
- ✔ You suffer from chest and bowel infections.
- ✔ You feel tired all the time.
- ✔ You lose weight.
- ✔ You develop swollen glands.
- ✔ You suffer from blotchy skin.
- ✔ You find concentrating or remembering things more difficult, or you feel confused.

Whether you already know that you have HIV or not, if you notice one or more of these signs, see your GP urgently for further assessment.

You can obtain more information on HIV and AIDS from the National Aids Trust (www.nat.org.uk) or the Terrence Higgins Trust (www.tht.org.uk). You can also find an excellent patient information sheet on HIV and AIDS on the Patient UK website at www.patient.co.uk.

Part III
Going From Top to Toe: Looking at Specific Areas of the Body

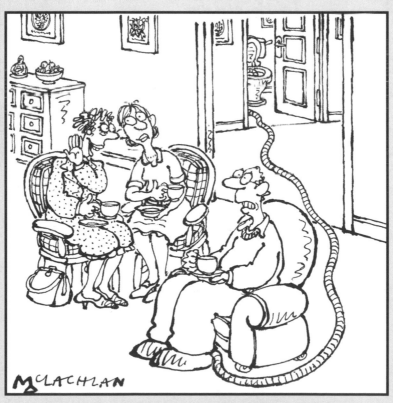

'And has your husband done anything
about his little urinary problem?'

In this part . . .

Many health problems such as earache, skin problems, headaches, tummy symptoms and knee pain affect only certain areas of your body. This part gives you some first-hand tips and advice on how to look at these problems and what you can do about them.

Chapter 8

Sussing Out Skin Problems

· ·

In This Chapter

▶ Looking at various types of rashes

▶ Getting to grips with other common skin problems

· ·

Your skin is the largest organ in your body. Far from being just something that covers you up so that no-one can see your insides, your skin is vitally important for keeping you alive and healthy. For example, your skin plays a major role in keeping your core body temperature and fluid balance constant, and acts as a barrier against infections and injuries.

Many skin conditions exist that can throw a spanner in the works, which is why some doctors, called *dermatologists*, and nurses specialise in diagnosing and managing skin disorders. However, you may be surprised to hear that your regular GP and practice nurse are able to deal with the vast majority of common skin conditions, and people only rarely need a specialist referral.

This chapter helps you to spot symptoms and signs of some major and common skin conditions, and tells you when to consult your doctor or practice nurse. Because skin conditions are so 'visual', be sure to check out the photo section to see what some of them look like.

Checking Out Rampant Rashes

Rashes are a common problem. In particular, infectious diseases in childhood (some of which I cover in more detail in Chapters 14 and 15) often present with a rash. Identifying and working out the cause of a rash can be tricky – even health professionals sometimes struggle – but this section helps you to recognise some of the more common and important ones.

Rashes that itch

The appearance of a rash or skin lesion may not bother or worry you too much, but the itch can drive you mad! This section covers two particularly common itchy rashes – atopic eczema and nettle rash (known as *urticaria*) – that may cause you a lot of concern. Do also check out the 'Skin infections and parasites' section later in this chapter. If you're not sure what to make of a rash, or if you develop itching without a rash, consult your GP.

Atopic eczema

Atopic eczema is an often persistent or recurrent dry skin condition, in which your skin can appear red, swollen, crusty and cracking, commonly leading to itching and even bleeding (see image 4 in the colour section). This condition often starts in childhood and has an allergic component to it, which is why people who suffer from eczema often also suffer from asthma and/or hay fever.

Atopic eczema is very common – about 5 out of every 100 people suffer from this skin disease. In terms of severity, eczema can range from very mild to quite severe, with most people being somewhere in between. Unfortunately, we don't know what causes eczema and, even worse, no known cure exists for this condition, although many effective treatments are available to keep your symptoms at bay. Saying that, many children with eczema 'grow out' of it by the time they reach adolescence.

To find out if you may suffer from eczema check your symptoms against the following list:

- Your skin feels dry most of the time.
- Your skin becomes irritated and red in some areas.
- Your skin creases are mainly affected (such as the front of your elbows and wrists, the backs of your knees and/or your neck).
- Your skin is itchy and the feeling gets worse intermittently; and if you scratch a lot the scratched areas of your skin become thicker.
- Your skin cracks at times, and these cracked areas turn blistery or weepy.
- Your inflamed areas of skin occasionally become infected.
- Your skin condition fluctuates.

Certain factors can make your eczema worse, however, so you can keep it under control by avoiding the following:

✔ **Avoid using soap and bubble bath frequently:** Both can dry out your skin.

✔ **Avoid having long hot baths:** Shower or bathe briefly with lukewarm or even cold (brrr!) water instead. Doing so may be less relaxing and takes a bit of getting used to, but if your eczema is bad this act alone can potentially do wonders for your skin. Some people's eczema improves dramatically just because they change their bathing habits. Give it a try!

✔ **Avoid scratching:** Keep your fingernails short and clean and rub itchy patches of eczema gently with your fingertips rather than scratching them.

✔ **Avoid extremes of temperature:** Too hot and too cold environments can make your eczema worse.

✔ **Avoid wearing certain fabrics that make your eczema worse (such as synthetics):** Try wearing garments made out of cotton instead.

If you find controlling your symptoms difficult, see your GP or practice nurse who can advise you on the best treatment options, which usually include treatment with moisturising creams and ointments (see the later 'Smoothing things over with emollients' sidebar), as well as steroid preparations that you put directly onto your skin. Only rarely is referral to a specialist needed.

For further information, contact the National Eczema Society Helpline on 0800 0891122 or visit the website at www.eczema.org. The Patient UK website (www.patient.co.uk) has a number of patient information leaflets on eczema and its treatment that you may find useful.

Smoothing things over with emollients

Eczema causes your skin to become dry and the dryer your skin becomes, the higher the chances that your eczema symptoms will get worse.

Emollients such as lotions, ointments, creams and shower additives can help because they replace oils that are missing from your skin, keeping it nice and smooth and therefore better protected from irritants. Using emollients regularly, frequently and liberally is the most important part of managing your eczema.

Your pharmacist, practice nurse or GP can advise you about suitable preparations, but you may need to shop around a bit and try different products – different people prefer different emollients, and you can choose from a wide range. Remember that some people are sensitive to the contents (or *bases*) of the emollients – what suits one patient may not suit another. In general, greasier ointments, which contain a high proportion of oils, work better than thinner creams and lotions, which have a higher water content than ointments. Remember, though, that oily bath or shower additives can make your bath tub or shower slippery, and so consider using a rubber mat to avoid slipping and falling.

Urticaria

An itchy rash that develops suddenly, along with raised hives, points to a condition called *urticaria* (also called *nettle rash*). Typically, you develop *weals* – raised, itchy areas on your skin (see image 2 in the colour section). Urticaria often develops because of an allergic reaction to something – you may recognise one or more of the following trigger factors:

- ✔ You have an allergy to a specific food (such as egg, citrus fruits, shellfish or nuts).

- ✔ You react to insect bites and stings.

- ✔ You suffer from a viral infection.

- ✔ You're allergic to drugs such as aspirin, penicillin or others.

- ✔ You react to things that come into contact with your skin, such as creams, lotions, cleaning products or nettle stings.

- ✔ You get urticaria when something firmly rubs your skin.

- ✔ You develop weals when you go out in the cold, or when the temperature is very hot.

Exercise can also bring on this rash, but in many cases you aren't aware of a specific cause. Fortunately, urticaria isn't serious and is likely to go away completely within a day or two, though it can sometimes last for a few weeks. In rare instances, the condition can go on even longer, in which case it's called *chronic* – or persistent – *urticaria*.

Compare your rash with the following descriptions of urticaria:

- ✔ Weals appear on any part of your skin. These areas can take on any shape and are usually up to 2 centimetres (just under an inch) wide, but come in different sizes.

- ✔ Weals look white or red and have a small red area of skin called a *flare* surrounding them. This flare looks a bit like a nettle sting.

- ✔ New weals can appear at any time and may look like they're 'wandering' around your body, even though the rash itself may settle after a day or so.

- ✔ Tissue elsewhere, such as your eyelids or lips, may also swell. This swelling may take a bit longer to settle and can last for up to three days or so.

Urticaria isn't serious and usually gets better without treatment. Some people find relief by taking a cool shower, and you may find taking antihistamines useful. You can buy these without prescription from your pharmacy or get them on prescription from your GP. If the swelling of your tissue is severe, or if you don't get better quickly, see your GP for further assessment because in rare circumstances you may need stronger medication or referral to a specialist.

Rashes that sting or burn

If you suffer from a rash that stings or burns rather than itches, *shingles* (infection with the herpes zoster virus) or an infection with the *herpes simplex virus type 1* may be causing your symptoms. Remember that this virus is transmitted through direct skin-to-skin contact and is different to *herpes simplex virus type 2*, which is the one that causes genital lesions.

Shingles

Shingles is where the *herpes zoster virus* (the same virus that causes chickenpox) infects a nerve (see image 6 in the colour section). The condition is relatively common – about 20 out of 100 people get shingles at some stage in their lives, and usually just the once – but it can happen only if you've had chickenpox at some point in your past.

In most cases, people develop shingles without any obvious underlying cause. However, a compromised immune system – perhaps as a natural result of the ageing process or because you take steroid drugs regularly, you're HIV positive or you're undergoing chemotherapy – makes you more susceptible to developing the infection.

If you recognise the following symptoms, you may have shingles:

- You develop a blistery rash over one area of your body (usually on one side), most commonly appearing on the chest, stomach or the upper part of the face. The blisters eventually dry up after a while and then slowly fade away.

- You develop pain over the area of the rash. This pain has probably preceded the rash by a couple of days, can be of varying severity and may be dull, sharp or stabbing in nature.

- Your skin over the affected area is likely to be tender to touch.

- You may feel unwell and a bit feverish for a few days.

- Your rash usually persists for a couple of weeks, but the pain may go on for longer, particularly if you're over the age of 50.

While you have blisters that haven't dried up, you're contagious. This means that – because shingles and chickenpox are caused by the same virus – your shingles rash can cause chickenpox in people who haven't had chickenpox before. You can minimise the risk of spreading the virus by covering up your rash, but particularly try to avoid close contact with any pregnant woman who's not had chickenpox, as well as people who you know have low immunity. Also avoid contact sports, swimming or sharing towels while you still have the rash.

Complications are rare with shingles, but may include the following:

- ✔ An affected eye (which may appear red), a dislike of the light, a blistery rash on your eyelids or around your eye, and a tender forehead.

- ✔ Infected blisters (you may see some pus – yellowish or greenish thick fluid – and red, tender skin), which indicates skin infection.

- ✔ Persistent pain in the nerve area, which can last for weeks, months or sometimes even longer.

- ✔ The inability to move properly a part of your body that's supplied by the same nerve.

If you develop shingles, make an appointment to see your GP within 72 hours of the onset of the rash for a possible prescription of painkillers and antiviral drugs – the earlier you receive treatment, the better the chance of the medicine working. If you suffer complications, you may also need antibiotics, or referral to a specialist if your eye's affected. Sometimes, you may need additional treatment with other medicines if your pain is severe or you suffer more serious complications, which are fortunately rare. Calamine lotion may help if your rash is itchy.

Although shingles is sometimes called herpes zoster, the condition has nothing to do with genital herpes.

Cold sores

In the UK, 20 in every 100 people suffer from recurring *cold sores* – viral skin infections that commonly start with tingling around your lips or nose, followed by a blistery rash (refer to image 10 in the colour section) that can be irritating and annoying. The *herpes simplex type 1 virus*, which can be passed on through kissing, is responsible for cold sores, and when you've been infected the virus stays with you for the rest of your life. It remains in the background and doesn't cause any symptoms for most of the time, but occasionally – often in particular situations – the typical rash breaks out.

You can recognise cold sores from the following symptoms:

- ✔ Itching, tingling or pain on your lips or nose.

- ✔ Sore blisters develop in the same areas a few hours or up to a day later. They may weep for a few days before scabbing over.

- ✔ The scabs go away over the course of about a week, without leaving any scars behind.

Cold sores may recur in one or more of these circumstances:

- ✔ When you're suffering from an illness such as a cold or flu (which is why they're called *cold sores*).

✔ When you're feeling exhausted, run-down or stressed.

✔ When you've been out in the sun a lot.

✔ When you're a woman of childbearing age, around the time of your period.

If you suffer from cold sores, you can infect other people with the virus, and so avoid kissing anyone or allowing anyone to come into contact with your lips while you have the blisters. In particular, avoid kissing newborn babies or people with low immunity (for example, people who have AIDS, take regular drugs called steroids or are undergoing chemotherapy). Usually, you can't infect anyone else if you haven't got the rash, and you also can't re-infect anyone who already suffers from cold sores.

Although no cure exists for cold sores, you can obtain treatments from your pharmacist or GP to reduce the spread and duration of existing blisters. Simple painkillers such as paracetamol or ibuprofen may also help with relieving your symptoms, particularly when the rash is painful.

Rashes that are simply there

The rashes in this section don't tend to itch, sting or burn as much as the ones I cover earlier in this chapter, but they can nevertheless be irritating and worrying – or both.

Psoriasis

Patches of dry and scaly skin that come and go indicate *psoriasis* – a common skin condition in which the skin cells turn over faster (refer to image 5 in the colour section). The cause isn't known. The most common type is *plaque psoriasis* in which one or more patches (or *plaques*) appear anywhere on your body. Other types of psoriasis exist, which I don't cover here, simply because they're far less common. The severity and frequency of relapses varies between people and ranges from mild to very severe, and about 10 out of 100 people with psoriasis may develop joint problems, which mainly affect the fingers and toes.

Although the lesions of psoriasis can sometimes look quite dramatic, you can't pass this condition on to other people. And you don't need in any way to be concerned that the lesions may develop into skin cancer – they don't.

You may be able to recognise typical psoriasis plaques from these descriptions:

✔ Plaques appear red with flaky silvery scales on top.

✔ Plaques have a well-defined, clearly visible border between their edge and the normal skin.

✔ Plaques usually develop over your elbows and knees as well as your scalp and the lower part of your back. Other parts of your body may also be affected, but your face is always spared.

✔ Plaques may be small or large.

✔ Plaques may only develop in one or two smaller areas, or may be widespread, affecting wider parts of your body.

✔ Plaques may get a bit itchy at times but don't normally cause any symptoms.

If you suffer from psoriasis, you may notice that your condition gets worse in one or more of the following circumstances:

✔ If you're exhausted or stressed.

✔ If you regularly take medicines such as beta-blockers, anti-inflammatory drugs such as ibuprofen or diclofenac, or you drink alcohol regularly.

✔ If you suffer from an acute feverish illness such as a cold or flu.

✔ If you damage your skin because of an injury or because you've been scratching.

✔ If you smoke: sometimes smoking can make psoriasis worse or trigger flare-ups.

✔ If you've been exposed to the sun. Although your psoriasis may in fact improve when you get out into the sun, sunburn and staying out in direct sunlight for too long can make things worse.

✔ If you're a woman, you may notice that your psoriasis gets better when you're pregnant but deteriorates while you're going through the menopause.

Unfortunately, no cure exists for psoriasis. However, a number of treatments are available that can help to treat and keep the skin lesions of psoriasis at bay. If you think you may suffer from psoriasis, consult your GP who can advise you about the various treatment options. For further information and advice, contact the Psoriasis Association on 0845 6760076 or visit the website at www.psoriasis-association.org.uk.

Pityriasis rosea

Pityriasis rosea is a sometimes dramatic-looking rash, caused by a harmless virus, that suddenly develops and commonly affects young adults (see image 7 in the colour section).

You may be able to recognise pityriasis rosea from the following features:

✔ You may first notice a red, oval-shaped patch of about 2–5 centimetres (1–2 inches) in diameter. This mark is known as the *herald patch*, and may appear on your stomach, chest, back, neck or upper arms. A patch, however, isn't always present (or you may not notice it).

✔ You develop, a few days or up to two weeks later and over a period of about ten days, more widespread lesions that are also oval in shape but smaller (about 1–2 centimetres – ½–1 inch – in diameter) and have a pink colour.

✔ You're likely to feel well throughout, although you may feel a bit under the weather or have a mild headache.

No treatment is necessary with pityriasis rosea – the rash gets better by itself, although this may take a few weeks or so. If the rash itches, try using calamine lotion or a mild steroid cream to relieve your symptoms. You can buy both without prescription from your pharmacist.

Identifying Skin Changes: The Good, the Bad and the Ugly

Skin changes – including pigmented moles, ulcers and other lumps and bumps – have different characters: many are benign (and even enhance your appearance), some are a nuisance and the occasional one is outright dangerous. Telling the difference isn't always easy. In this section I tell you about the features of some common and important skin lesions, which helps you to decide whether you need to consult your GP.

Moles

Most people have at least one or more *moles* – areas of pigmented skin in various shapes, forms and sizes. Instead of describing moles in detail, I focus more on describing the 'nasty' type of mole, so that you're able to spot the danger symptoms and signs early on – and be reassured that a mole is unlikely to be serious if none of these features are present.

Benign moles

Harmless, or *benign* moles are often brownish in colour and may be slightly raised, but don't tend to change much in appearance and can make your skin more interesting, which is why some people call them 'beauty spots'.

On the whole, simple moles are entirely benign – that is, harmless – but on rare occasions they can develop into skin cancer. In a nutshell, treat any new, growing or changing mole as suspicious and consult your GP.

Malignant melanoma

Malignant melanoma is a skin cancer that can resemble a benign mole. It's a dangerous type of cancer not because it damages your skin, but because it can spread quickly and cause severe and life-threatening damage to other areas of your body. For this reason, early diagnosis of malignant melanoma is important: spotting the danger signs early enables you to speed up the time to formal diagnosis and treatment. If you get treated early, this type of cancer is entirely curable.

If any of these circumstances apply to you, you're more susceptible to developing malignant melanoma:

- ✔ You had a lot of direct exposure to the sun in the past (for example, you lived in a very sunny country).

- ✔ You suffered severe sunburns in the past, especially in childhood.

- ✔ You have fair or freckled skin.

- ✔ You have red or fair hair.

- ✔ Your skin doesn't tan well or burns before it tans.

- ✔ You have lots of moles (say, more than 100 if you're younger or more than 50 if you belong to an older age group).

- ✔ You (in the past) or someone in your close family have been diagnosed with malignant melanoma.

- ✔ You have low immunity for any reason (for example, you take steroid medication, are HIV positive or you're undergoing chemotherapy).

- ✔ You work outside and your skin gets a lot of sun exposure.

Consult your GP if you notice one or more of the following:

- ✔ A new mole appears.

- ✔ A mole bleeds for no apparent reason, becomes crusty or looks inflamed (in other words, it has some redness around it).

- ✔ A mole changes appearance or increases in size, particularly if it grows to over 7 millimetres (¼ inch) in diameter.

- ✔ A mole has an irregular and/or not well-defined outline.

- ✔ A mole has various types of colour or pigmentation.

- ✔ A mole suddenly causes pain or itching.

These features don't necessarily mean that you've got skin cancer, but you need to seek further medical assessment to get your mole(s) checked when you notice such changes. See your GP urgently if you have any additional symptoms that suggest cancer spread (check out Chapter 6 for more details).

Malignant melanomas can grow anywhere on your body – even in areas that aren't usually exposed to the sun such as your buttocks, the soles of your feet or under your nails. In women, melanomas occur most commonly on the legs, whereas in men they grow often on the back.

Lumps and swellings

Lumps in or under the skin are a common problem and in this section I cover the most common or important causes. However, if you're not sure what's causing a lump on your body never hesitate to see your GP, particularly if the lump is painless, hard and growing fast.

Benign swellings

Most lumps and bumps on your skin are harmless and nothing to worry about unless they cause discomfort, pain or bother you in some other way. The following two varieties are particularly common:

✔ **Lipoma:** *Lipomas* are benign, firm, fatty lumps that develop in the fatty tissues just below your skin for no apparent reason (you know they're under your skin when you can move your skin freely over the lump). They tend to be quite smooth on the surface and when you push them a bit you can move them slightly. Some people have multiple lipomas.

Lipomas don't usually cause any symptoms unless they're quite large or cause pressure on other structures. If they don't change, you don't need to worry, but if for some reason these lumps suddenly grow or become very hard, consult your GP.

Any lumps in your breasts are different – always see your GP about breast lumps.

✔ **Sebaceous cyst:** A *sebaceous cyst* is a lump inside your skin, which means that it moves whenever you try to draw your skin over it. Experts believe that sebaceous cysts are caused by an excessive non-cancerous growth of skin cells within your skin, leading to a foul-smelling build up of cottage cheese-like material.

Sebaceous cysts usually have a tiny hole in the overlying skin, and if a sebaceous cyst becomes infected and appears red and hot – which is quite common – it may eventually burst, leading to pus draining through this hole.

If a sebaceous cyst doesn't cause you any trouble, you don't need to do anything about it, but if it becomes infected or bothers you, see your GP for an assessment.

Swollen lymph nodes

Your *lymph nodes* are part of your *immune system* and have a 'filter' function. You have lymph nodes in various places around your body, such as your neck, your armpits and your groins, and they can swell for many reasons (refer to image 11 in the colour section):

- An infection, such as tonsillitis, glandular fever and others.

- An inflammatory condition, such as some forms of arthritis.

- An underlying cancer, such as a *lymphoma* or a spread from another cancer (you can find more information on cancer in Chapter 6).

If your lymph nodes are painful (commonly below your jaw if you have a sore throat), they're likely to be enlarged and symptomatic of an infection instead of something more serious. See your pharmacist for suitable preparations to ease your symptoms.

Consult your GP in the following circumstances:

- You have one or more swollen lymph nodes that persist for more than two weeks or that get gradually bigger (particularly if they're painless).

- You experience additional symptoms such as night sweats, fever, weight loss, loss of appetite or any other problems that worry you.

Skin ulcers

When your skin breaks down and you can see the underlying tissue, you have a *skin ulcer*. Ulcers can be caused by conditions such as poor circulation, vein problems, injuries and diabetes, and are particularly common on the lower leg or foot, where they can easily be infected. Less commonly, non-healing ulcers may be due to skin cancer.

Foot and leg ulcers

If you suffer from one or more of the following conditions (ordered from the most common to the least), you're at particular risk of developing a foot or leg ulcer:

- **Diabetes:** You have *diabetes mellitus* (read more on this in Chapter 20) and have reduced sensation in your feet and/or poor circulation. You're at greater risk if your diabetes is also poorly controlled. In diabetes, your skin fails to heal as quickly after an injury, compared to people who haven't got the condition. This slow healing makes you more susceptible to developing a foot ulcer even after only a minor injury.

- **Peripheral vascular disease:** You suffer from narrowed arteries (called *peripheral vascular disease*), which I cover in more detail in Chapter 13.

- **Varicose veins:** You have severe *varicose veins*, which are visibly enlarged blood vessels just under your skin.

- **Previous ulcer:** You've had an ulcer in the past.

- **Musculo-skeletal problems:** You tend to be prone to foot problems because of bone, joint or skin problems such as bunions, corns and calluses (flip to Chapter 13 for more information). Or you have problems with your legs that prevent you from walking normally, or you can't reach your feet to look after them. Sometimes, ulcers may also be caused by poorly fitting shoes.

Ulcers are particularly common on the feet and legs (see image 8 in the colour section). Brought on by poor circulation, they tend to hurt, whereas ulcers from vein problems or diabetes are often painless. Regardless, always make an appointment with your practice nurse or GP if you develop an ulcer, particularly in the following circumstances:

- You have any of the factors that put you at higher risk of a foot ulcer.

- Your ulcer shows signs of infection – it may smell, look red or you may notice pus on the surface of the ulcer.

Ulcers tend to get better fairly quickly if they receive prompt treatment. Occasionally they take a long time to heal, particularly if you have diabetes – in which case be sure to attend every scheduled review appointment that your GP surgery normally arranges for you.

To spot ulcers early, check your skin (particularly on your legs and feet) regularly for open spots and see your GP or practice nurse quickly if you notice any signs of an ulcer.

Other serious ulcers

Sores and ulcers anywhere on your body that don't heal, or get worse, can sometimes be due to different kinds of skin cancer, particularly those known as *squamous cell carcinoma* and *basal cell carcinoma*, which are more common in older age (refer to images 1 and 3 in the colour section). Basal cell carcinomas tend to have a 'rolled up' edge and commonly appear on the face. Squamous cell carcinomas often appear as small scaly or crusted skin areas that have a red or pink base. They can develop into wart-like lumps – although can appear in various shapes and sizes, and may even bleed. See your GP urgently for further assessment if you suspect that you may have developed a skin cancer.

Skin infections and parasites

Skin infections and parasites are common reasons why people may visit their GPs. Different types exist – some are minor and get better with no or minimal intervention, whereas others can make you feel quite unwell. In this section, I look at some of the more common complaints.

Boils and abscesses

Boils, or *furuncles* – small collections of pus around a hair follicle – are fairly common and often referred to as *folliculitis*. A larger collection of pus is called an *abscess*. They can appear for no apparent reason but are more common if you have reduced immunity, perhaps due to taking steroid drugs or HIV infection, or if you have diabetes. Boils and abscesses may result from a minor skin infection, but see your practice nurse or GP for further assessment when your boil or abscess doesn't quickly settle after a day or two. You may need a course of antibiotics or, in the case of an abscess, a small incision and drainage of any pus.

Cellulitis

A more widespread skin infection that doesn't lead to collections of pus is known as *cellulitis*. You're most likely to develop cellulitis on your legs, although it can affect any area of your body – a special type of cellulitis called *erysipelas* occurs when you get cellulitis on the face (usually on your cheeks). The severity of cellulitis can vary and ranges from a mild localised skin infection to a serious infection that affects larger areas of your skin and makes you quite unwell.

Cellulitis can develop where bacteria enter your skin and tissues just below your skin through a cut or a graze – which needs only to be tiny – but sometimes it can appear without any obvious underlying cause. The following circumstances make this infection more likely:

- You suffer from *athlete's foot* – a common, mild fungal infection that often causes small and usually itchy cracks in the skin between your toes (see image 12 in the colour section). Check the skin between your toes regularly, particularly if you have swollen legs, you're obese or you have diabetes and the sensation in your feet is reduced.

- You have other broken areas of skin (such as cuts, sores, ulcers, insect bites, scratches or any other injuries) anywhere on your leg. Injecting drugs into your legs also puts you at higher risk of getting a skin infection.

- Your legs are swollen for any reason.

- You have a chronic skin condition such as eczema, which makes your skin dry or more prone to infection.

- You're too heavy for your height (in other words, you're overweight or obese).

- You suffer from diabetes – particularly if your blood sugar levels aren't well controlled (meaning that they're too high for too long).

- You have low immunity, which may be the case if you're undergoing chemotherapy for cancer or you take steroid drugs, which your doctor may prescribe when you suffer from a chronic inflammatory condition.

Being able to recognise the key features of cellulitis is useful, because if you have the condition you need treatment with antibiotics. Compare your symptoms with these features of cellulitis:

- Your skin feels warm or hot and appears red and inflamed – you may also get blisters – and pressing on the affected area probably hurts.

- You notice a sharp border between the red area and your healthy skin, which may spread. (Health professionals often mark out the borders of the inflamed area to be able to assess whether the cellulitis is getting better or not.)

- You feel unwell and have a fever – which may even start a day or so before you notice any of the skin symptoms.

- Your lymph glands in the area nearest to your infection (which are usually your groins if you have cellulitis in your legs) are swollen and tender.

Visiting your GP for further assessment is particularly important in the following circumstances, to prevent the infection from spreading:

- You're suffering from cellulitis around your eye. An infection spreading to your eye can be quite nasty and needs urgent treatment.

- You feel very unwell with a high fever, which can mean that the infection has entered your bloodstream (called *septicaemia*), potentially infecting your heart valves and other organs.

- You notice a collection of pus anywhere close to the infection.

- You get more widespread pain in any muscles or bones close to the infected skin, which suggests that the infection is spreading to deeper tissues – potentially quite serious and needs urgent treatment.

- Your pain is worse than you expect from the appearance of your skin, which looks purple, dusky and/or blistery, and you get worse very quickly, usually within hours or so. The condition commonly known as the 'flesh eating disease' (what experts call *necrotising fasciitis*) may be to blame. This disease is a medical emergency and you need to get to hospital as fast as possible. This condition is quite rare, but if you're in doubt, don't delay seeking medical advice.

Fortunately, getting early treatment for cellulitis increases your chances of a full and quick recovery. Not receiving treatment, however, means that you can suffer any of the above complications as well as long-term problems such as leg swelling and pain. If you don't get appropriate treatment quickly, cellulitis can become persistent, and you may need to take antibiotics for weeks or even months to rid yourself of the infection.

If your cellulitis is severe, extensive or both, you may even need treatment in hospital, where you're likely to receive antibiotics directly into your veins. So the key message is to see your doctor as soon as possible if you think that you're suffering from cellulitis.

To help speed up your recovery, try keeping your affected leg raised higher than your hip when you're sitting down, because this position helps to relieve any swelling. Also, make sure that you treat any athlete's foot promptly – ask your pharmacist for advice on suitable preparations that you can buy over-the-counter or see your GP if you need stronger treatment.

Scabies

Scabies is a contagious skin disease caused by a small mite (see image 9 in the colour section). If you have scabies, you may have picked up the mite through prolonged close skin contact with others, for example by extensive hand-holding or by having sex. (You're unlikely to pick up the mite and develop scabies from hugging or just shaking hands.) Scabies often 'does the rounds' in playgrounds, nurseries, schools and nursing homes, affecting grown-ups as well as children.

You can recognise scabies from the following features:

✔ A lumpy and sometimes blotchy reddish rash appears anywhere on your body, usually most prominently on your stomach, buttocks, genitals, between your legs or in your armpits. Interestingly, this rash isn't caused directly by the mite but is your body's reaction to it, which is why the rash and itch may take a few weeks to develop after you've been infected.

✔ Itching – often quite severe – on your hands or other parts of your body, which tends to get worse after a hot bath or during the night when you're in bed.

✔ Lines on your skin appear, the length of two or three rice grains put in a row. They commonly show between your fingers, over your wrists, or on other parts of your hands, but can appear anywhere else on your body.

✔ Skin damage from scratching, which can lead to skin infection in which your skin becomes red and tender.

Treating scabies is usually straightforward through the application of a special cream or lotion that you can buy from your pharmacist or get on prescription from your GP; but you need to apply it properly for it to work. Make sure that other people in your household or those you've been close to (for example, someone you've had sex with) also get treatment, even if they haven't any symptoms yet, and repeat the treatment a week later. Antihistamines and calamine lotion – both of which you can buy from your pharmacist without prescription – can help to relieve your itch.

Consult your GP if your symptoms don't settle after a course of treatment to make sure that scabies is the correct diagnosis – although the infection may also recur. If someone else or more people in your household develop an itchy rash, however, you can be pretty certain that scabies is the most likely underlying cause.

Don't panic if the itch and/or the rash don't disappear straight away – this process may easily take a couple of weeks or even longer and doesn't mean that the mite hasn't been killed. You may also continue to have some remaining small brownish lumps (particularly on your genitals) that, reassuringly, aren't infectious.

Chapter 9

Trouble at the Top: Head Symptoms and Problems with the Senses

Your head is full of hugely important structures and organs, and therefore symptoms around the head can be worrying. You may be concerned that a headache that refuses to budge must be caused by a brain tumour. And no wonder that you start to panic if something goes wrong with your eyes.

Luckily, problems affecting the head are usually harmless and often go away by themselves. This chapter helps you to recognise the types and causes of problems in this area of the body and to spot the rarer baddies.

Starting at the Top

Headache and facial pain are common head complaints. Immediately sussing out the underlying cause can be quite easy – particularly if your symptoms are due to an injury, a cold or a hangover! In most cases, symptoms soon get better and simple remedies such as painkillers and rest may be all that you need to feel as right as rain again.

High blood pressure: Not guilty

Many people believe that raised blood pressure must be the cause of their headache. In fact, this occurrence is relatively rare, although medicines to treat high blood pressure can lead to headaches. Blood pressure needs to be very high before it causes headache symptoms.

Heading for a headache

Almost everyone suffers from occasional headaches – you're not alone! Fortunately, most headaches – such as migraines and tension headaches – have no serious underlying cause. Headaches can be quite worrying, though, and so here's some reassurance right from the word 'go'. You don't need to be overly concerned if you experience the following:

- ✔ You've always had headaches that come and go and that settle completely between episodes.
- ✔ Your headache is mild and doesn't make you feel unwell.
- ✔ You don't have any other symptoms.

The great news is that the vast majority of headaches are benign and get better themselves. You needn't worry if your headaches come on gradually and settle completely within 24 hours. Rest, relaxation and simple painkillers are often all you need to help relieve your symptoms. Diagnosing the cause of headaches can sometimes be tricky, though, and so don't hesitate to seek medical advice if you're worried or don't know what to make of your headache.

If you're prone to headaches, keep a diary of them to identify your patterns and trigger factors (which could include, for example, stress, alcohol or late nights). For a few weeks, note down the number, duration and frequency of headaches and anything else you think may be relevant. Also record whether exercise, stress or certain foods bring on your headaches. Your findings are sure to come in handy for identifying potential causes or if you want to discuss your symptoms with your GP.

Noticing annoying – but non-serious – causes of headache

Various types of headache can be irritating or even disabling if they're severe, but they don't tend to be dangerous. This section enables you to tell the difference between them.

Tension headache

The usual causes of *tension headache* are stress, lack of sleep or tightening of the neck muscles through bad posture. Tension headache is the most common form of headache, and is more common in women than men. You can identify this type of headache by comparing your symptoms with the following list of typical features:

- ✔ You have a constant ache that affects both sides of your head.
- ✔ You experience a feeling of pressure behind your eyes and tightening of your neck muscles.
- ✔ Your headache lasts for a few hours but sometimes persists for days or even weeks.
- ✔ Your symptoms are usually mild to moderate.
- ✔ Your headache doesn't interfere too much with your day-to-day life.
- ✔ You feel no worse with routine physical activity.
- ✔ You have no more than one additional symptom, such as feeling sick or not tolerating light or sound.
- ✔ You're not vomiting.

A number of effective painkillers such as paracetamol or ibuprofen are available in supermarkets or over-the-counter from your pharmacist, who can also advise you on alternative options. If these drugs don't work, your GP may be able to prescribe stronger medication. Only in rare cases is further investigation or referral to a specialist needed.

Changes in lifestyle, such as reducing stress and your alcohol intake and getting enough sleep, may also help to relieve your symptoms. You can also try applying a hot flannel to your head or neck or pamper yourself by booking in for a massage. Exercising regularly can help ease stress and reduce muscle tension, which may lower the frequency of your headaches.

You may find this fact surprising, but overusing painkillers can itself cause headache! Therefore, always be sure to follow the instructions on the packet and don't take them for longer than a week or two without first seeking advice from your pharmacist or doctor.

Although tension headaches can be distressing, they're never dangerous or life-threatening.

Migraine

Migraine affects about one in ten people in the UK and causes severe and usually recurrent headaches. If you suffer from migraines, the headaches can seriously impact upon daily activities and reduce your quality of life.

Experts think that a temporary widening of the blood vessels surrounding the brain, or a temporary change in certain chemicals in the brain, can cause migraine, but the exact cause isn't known yet. Sometimes, certain trigger factors such as food (for example, cheese or – I know, life's not fair! – chocolate), smoke, noise, menstrual periods or stress may bring on attacks.

Migraines come in different forms, some of which are rare. (Check out the Patient UK website at www.patient.co.uk for more information.) Attacks typically go through five stages, although you don't always experience all five stages during an episode:

1. **Pre-headache:** You may experience a change in your energy levels, mood, appetite and behaviour, and sometimes you notice aches and pains a few hours or even days before the attack.

2. **Aura:** You may have

   - Visual symptoms such as 'blind spots', flashing lights, zigzag lines, not being able to focus properly or a feeling of seeing through a broken mirror.

   - Temporary weakness in an arm or leg, or other nerve symptoms.

   - Stiffness or pins and needles in your shoulders and neck.

   - A feeling of being off-balance or disorientated.

   - Difficulty finding and using words properly.

   - Loss of consciousness, but this is extremely rare.

   Usually, the aura stage starts between 15 and 60 minutes before the headache comes on.

3. **Headache:** The typical migraine headache is throbbing or pulsating and usually affects just one side of your head, though not the same side every time. Feeling and being sick are common, and you may feel very sensitive to bright light, sounds or smells. Lying down in a darkened and quiet room often helps you cope with the symptoms better. This stage tends to last between a few hours and three days.

4. **Resolution:** Most migraines disappear gradually, although sometimes the headache improves quickly after vomiting. Getting some sleep may also help.

5. **Recovery:** You may feel exhausted and weak for a while after a migraine attack.

See your GP for an assessment if you notice any of the following symptoms:

- You have your first migraine when you're over 50 years old.

- You notice a change in your usual migraine symptoms.

✔ Your migraine attacks start to happen more frequently.

✔ Your aura symptoms or migraine headache affect the same side of your body with every attack.

Although no tests are available for migraine, your GP can give you a check over and help with the diagnosis and treatment. And although the tendency for getting migraine attacks is likely to stay with you for life, lots of available treatments may relieve your migraine attacks or prevent them from occurring in the first place. Working out which one of them works best for you may take some time, however.

Your GP or pharmacist can give you advice about treatment options, which include:

✔ Simple over-the-counter painkillers, which work best when you take them at the first sign of an attack.

✔ Anti-sickness medicines, in case you feel sick during a migraine.

✔ So-called special migraine medication (known as *triptans*) or other stronger medicines, for when simple painkillers don't work.

✔ Prevention medicines, if you suffer from severe or frequent migraines.

Some people find that drinking one or two glasses of cold water, or sucking an ice cube, as soon as a migraine attack starts relieves their symptoms.

Very rarely, migraine can lead to blocking of the blood supply in the brain, causing a stroke with sudden and prolonged limb weakness, twisting of one side of the face or other disturbances of movement or sensation. Another risk factor for such a stroke is the contraceptive pill, and so talk to your pharmacist or GP to check whether taking the pill is safe for you in the event that you develop migraines.

You can find more information and advice on The Migraine Trust and Migraine Action websites at www.migrainetrust.org and www.migraine.org.uk.

Cluster headache

The *cluster headache* is one other type of much less common headache. Here are some symptoms to help you spot a cluster headache:

✔ Your symptoms start suddenly, are severe and peak within 10–15 minutes.

✔ You experience a boring and stabbing pain on one side around your eye – you may feel as if your eye is being pushed out.

✔ Your affected eye becomes watery – you may get a runny nose, a sweaty face and feel restless and agitated.

✔ Your scalp and face feel tender, and the pain is so severe that life doesn't feel worth living any more!

With a cluster headache, simple painkillers don't work. Your best option is to see your GP to discuss the treatment options, which include triptan medicines for treatment of an acute attack and various other medicines for preventing recurrences.

Identifying rare, but potentially serious, causes of headache

Although they can be distressing and annoying, harmless headaches are far more common than headaches with a serious cause. On rare occasions, however, an acute underlying condition that requires urgent medical assessment and treatment is to blame.

Meningitis

Meningitis is a potentially dangerous infection of a membrane surrounding the brain. The following symptoms can indicate meningitis:

- ✔ A severe headache of a type that you've not experienced before develops quickly over a few hours, accompanied by fever, vomiting or feeling unusually drowsy. Such a headache can resemble migraine, which I cover later in this chapter, though migraines usually don't come with a fever.

- ✔ A sudden dislike of bright lights.

- ✔ A stiff and painful feeling in your neck and difficulty in putting your chin on your chest.

- ✔ A rash that consists of tiny red or brown pin-prick lesions that don't go away when you press a finger or a glass tumbler against them. The rash may later turn into purple blotches – which may look like bruising or bleeding underneath the skin – or blisters. Such lesions indicate *septicaemia* (blood poisoning) – a life-threatening condition.

A rash may be difficult to spot, particularly on dark skin, and so check the roof of your mouth, the palms of your hands and the soles of your feet for rashes as well.

If meningitis is present, urgent and possibly life-saving treatment is important to prevent long-term damage to your brain. Call your doctor or dial '999' in an emergency. For further information on meningitis, visit the Meningitis Research Foundation or Meningitis Trust websites at www.meningitis.org or www.meningitis-trust.org.

Brain haemorrhage

Very rarely, a headache can indicate a bleeding (known as *haemorrhage*) inside your skull, which is sometimes caused by an injury (leading to a *subdural haemorrhage*) or a malformed blood vessel that bulges and bursts (called *subarachnoid haemorrhage*). In both cases, blood may leak onto the surface of the brain, raising the pressure inside your skull and squashing brain tissue. Unless treated quickly, any damage to your brain may become irreversible.

Bleeding inside your skull can show up in the following ways, and so seek medical advice urgently if you:

- Get a sudden, very severe headache – 'like being hit with a hammer' – of a type you've never had before, particularly if the pain is getting worse.

- Develop a stiff neck, vomiting or speech problems.

- Become increasingly drowsy.

- Feel unsteady on your feet or have problems with your co-ordination.

- Notice a severe discomfort in your eyes when you're exposed to bright light.

Brain haemorrhages can quickly cause serious problems, and so getting medical help immediately is vital.

Spotting other potentially serious causes of headache

Some other rare but potentially serious causes of headache tend to present less acutely than meningitis and brain haemorrhage. Contact your GP urgently for advice if you notice unusual, severe or worsening headache plus any of the following warning signs:

- Your headaches occur more and more frequently.

- You vomit for no apparent reason or have a high fever.

- You continue to have a headache after a blow or other injury to your head. (A mild headache lasting for no longer than a day or two is common after a minor head injury, is usually harmless and should disappear by itself).

- Your headache wakes you or keeps you awake at night.

- Your headache is worse on coughing, straining, bending over, lying down or laughing.

- You experience slurred speech, weakness, numbness or other odd sensations.

- Other people notice and comment on a change in your personality.

If you *suddenly* develop any of these symptoms, they're very severe or they get worse very quickly, contact your GP urgently or call '999' in an emergency.

Fever doesn't necessarily indicate that your headache is serious; quite harmless viral infections are more usual causes of headache and fever.

Temporal arteritis

Temporal arteritis is an inflammation of a blood vessel in your temple area and usually affects only people over 50 years of age. You may experience a new and severe headache that's unusual for you, along with other symptoms such as the following:

✔ Eye symptoms such as sudden blind spots (which can also occur with migraines).

✔ Muscle pains, particularly around the shoulders.

✔ Pain on chewing.

✔ Tender scalp (combing your hair may be painful).

✔ Generally feeling unwell.

Prompt treatment is important to prevent permanent loss of vision – one of the main potential consequences of temporal arteritis – and so contact your GP immediately.

Brain tumour

Consider the very rare possibility of a brain tumour and see your GP urgently for further assessment if you have a persistent headache that gets worse over weeks and months. Also look out for the following:

✔ Changes in personality or other changes in behaviour.

✔ Reduced alertness or unusual drowsiness.

✔ Fits or other symptoms such as tingling, double vision or limb weakness.

✔ Unexplained regular vomiting.

Facing up to facial pain

A new pain in your face can have many causes, and although facial pain can be very distressing it rarely signifies a serious underlying disease. Approaching the problem in a systematic way may give you some clues about the possible underlying diagnosis and whether you need to seek medical advice promptly. Here, I list some typical causes of facial pain:

✔ **Sinusitis:** This problem may show itself with a dull pain and tenderness in the bony bits above or below your cheek bones that gets worse when you bend forward. Sinusitis is an inflammation or infection of the linings of pockets of air in your facial bones, and often occurs after a cold. Simple painkillers can often help relieve your symptoms, but see your pharmacist or GP if they don't work.

✔ **Cluster headache:** Severe pain in the area between your eye and your nose, along with a watery eye and runny nose, can suggest a possible cluster headache (flip to 'Cluster headache' earlier in this chapter), although this condition is rare.

✓ **Shingles:** A blistery rash in the area of the pain may be due to *shingles* – a viral infection of the nerves. Visit your GP if you think that you have shingles, because the infection may affect and damage your eye, and early treatment with antiviral drugs can help.

✓ **Dental problems:** Toothache can spread and cause facial pain. If you have continuous pain, a fever and a tooth that is sensitive to hot or cold fluids, or that just doesn't feel right, you may have a tooth abscess, in which case you need to see your dentist urgently. If you sometimes get throbbing pain in a tooth, which can also be sensitive to touch, dental decay may be the root of the problem. If you get a pain only when you bite or chew, you may have a cracked filling or fractured tooth.

If you're in doubt about the significance of facial pain or if it's severe and doesn't go away, seek medical advice. Consult your GP – or dentist, in the case of a tooth problem – or see Chapter 25 for a list of useful helplines and websites.

Hearing About Ear Troubles

The various parts of the ear are squeezed into a tiny space within the skull, and so any infection with resulting inflammation can lead to considerable discomfort and distress. Almost everyone has had earache at some stage – it really hurts! And if your hearing gets worse, life can become a misery – and other people notice, too.

Tackling ear symptoms

Ear symptoms can range from a mild, dull discomfort, itching or a feeling of the ear being blocked to a severe sharp and throbbing pain. Various conditions can cause earache, and in this section I show how you can tell the more common and important ones apart. Rarely, ear conditions can cause complications, and they may be due to a serious underlying cause such as trauma or a more sinister infection. The following signs should ring alarm bells if you suffer from earache:

✓ A recent injury, burn or blow to your head.

✓ Any lumps or swelling behind or below your ear.

✓ An item stuck in your ear such as an earplug or cotton bud.

✓ An object – such as an insect (yikes!), a twig or sand – in your ear.

✔ A recent exposure to loud noise or music.

✔ A coloured, smelly or blood-stained discharge from your ear.

✔ A hot, red and swollen part of your ear.

If you experience – or have experienced – any of these signs, contact your GP urgently.

Ear canal infection

Earache can be caused by the outer ear canal becoming infected or inflamed. This condition is called *otitis externa*, and is commonly brought on by prolonged immersion of the ear in water – for example, when swimming (hence its other, less scientific, name of *swimmer's ear*). This infection can be extremely painful, and pulling at the earlobe usually makes the pain worse. Symptoms often settle within a few days, but ask your pharmacist or GP for advice if symptoms don't settle or continue to get worse. Antibiotic ear drops may sometimes be necessary.

Try to prevent water getting into your ear and let your ears dry naturally. Use special swimmers' earplugs or a swimming cap to cover your ears.

Infection of the middle ear

Middle ear infections (known as *otitis media*) are common in children but fairly rare in adults. When afflicted, your ear usually feels blocked and the pain can be quite severe. You may also have symptoms of the common cold, such as a runny nose, cough, fever and sore throat.

Take painkillers and consult your doctor for further assessment if your symptoms don't start to improve after two to three days, particularly if you:

✔ Feel unwell.

✔ Notice pus or discharge from your ear.

✔ Have a high fever.

Similarly, visit your GP if you develop any other worrying symptoms such as a tender, boggy swelling behind your ear, neck stiffness or a severe headache, which can mean that the infection has spread beyond your ear.

Ear wax

Excessive ear wax is very common and may partially or totally block your outer ear canal, so that you feel a dull pressure and can't hear properly. Your pharmacist can advise you about using olive oil or ear drops to help soften the ear wax, which then usually works its own way out. If this approach doesn't help, contact your GP surgery to have the ear wax removed.

A word in your ear about 'cleaning'

Your outer ear canal is very sensitive and protected by a thin layer of ear wax that acts as a barrier for infections. 'Cleaning' the ear is usually unnecessary, and doing so may remove the protective wax layer and make your ear more susceptible to infections. Also, cleaning your ear using cotton buds or – even worse – sharper instruments inside the ear canal can be dangerous, and may cause damage to your ear drum. In the worst scenario, you can cause hearing loss. Should your ear feel blocked because of excessive ear wax, refer to 'Ear wax', earlier in this chapter.

You can avoid a build-up of ear wax by keeping your ears dry and not pushing anything into your ear canal.

Pressure-related trauma

You can develop earache during the descent on a plane flight or when you're diving, which is caused by pressures being different on the outside and inside of your ear drum. The pain usually develops suddenly, and you may have a feeling of pressure in your ear (due to a collection of fluid or blood in the middle ear). Visit your GP if the pain doesn't go away after a few days.

If possible, try to avoid flying when you have a cold. If you have to fly, try to yawn, swallow and chew to relieve pressure in your ear. If you're a diver, remember that diving with a cold isn't safe, and you need to wait until the cold clears.

Grappling with sudden hearing loss

Sudden loss of hearing can be distressing but is in many cases due to benign and often short-lived conditions. Here's an overview of the main causes of sudden loss of hearing (for hearing problems that start and progress gradually in later life, flick to Chapter 20):

- ✔ **Ear wax:** A build-up of excessive ear wax is the most common reason for hearing problems and can sometimes suddenly lead to reduced hearing and a feeling of a blockage in your ear. See the 'Ear wax' section earlier in this chapter for ways to deal with this problem.

- ✔ **Common cold:** You may notice temporary mild hearing loss in connection with a cold, because your ear isn't ventilated properly. This loss usually settles down on its own after a few days, and you needn't worry.

> ✔ **Exposure to noise:** Exposure to loud noise – for example, listening to very loud music on headphones or in clubs, or using power tools without ear protection – can affect your hearing in the short term and also cause permanent damage in the long run.

For problems due to other causes of acute hearing loss, see your GP for more investigation.

Checking Out Nose, Mouth and Throat Concerns

Nose, mouth and throat symptoms are very common. The important thing to remember is that most of these problems – such as a runny nose, a sore throat, fever and cough – are simply due to colds, are benign and do go away by themselves.

Developing a nose for trouble

Nose symptoms, such as a blocked nose and nasal discharge, are common and usually clear within a few days. Nosebleeds are also common. This section gives you the low-down on dealing with nose problems.

Nosebleeds

Nosebleeds can be quite worrying. In most cases, they occur because of damage to the lining inside the nose, perhaps caused by dry air, picking your nose or a minor injury. Nosebleeds can also happen during a cold, and occur more frequently during pregnancy.

Raised blood pressure doesn't usually lead to nosebleeds unless the pressure is very high.

If you have a nosebleed, try the following:

✔ Sit up and lean slightly forward. Don't lean back; doing so just leads to the blood trickling back into your throat.

✔ Pinch the fleshy bit of the nose lightly between your finger and thumb, which usually settles the bleeding within a few minutes.

✔ Place a cold, moist flannel on the neck or around the nose and face to help stop the bleeding.

✔ Try not to blow or pick your nose after a nosebleed stops; it may cause the bleeding to recur.

✔ Lie down and on your side if you feel faint and continue to put pressure on your nose.

Nosebleeds aren't dangerous in the vast majority of cases, but seek medical advice urgently or dial '999' if you experience the following symptoms:

✔ Your nosebleed is very severe and you can't get the bleeding to stop within 20–30 minutes.

✔ You feel faint or collapse as a result of a severe or persistent nosebleed.

✔ You can't breathe properly because of the nosebleed.

Blocked nose

A blocked nose is most commonly due to a cold or some form of allergy. Your pharmacist can advise you about over-the-counter treatments that may be effective. If your symptoms persist, see your GP in case of an obstruction – perhaps due to a benign fleshy growth (called a *polyp*) or chronic inflammation of the nose lining – may be responsible.

If your nose feels blocked after you sustain an injury, visit your GP for a check up to assess the situation and see whether you need referral to a specialist.

Runny nose

Discharge from the nose is very common and is usually due to a viral infection, particularly if you also have other cold symptoms such as fever or a sore throat. If the discharge is thick and coloured, and if you also have facial pain, you may have sinusitis (check out the earlier section 'Facing up to facial pain'). If you have itchy, irritated eyes in addition to a runny nose, and you're sneezing a lot, hay fever or another allergy is a likely cause. Antihistamines and anti-inflammatory nasal sprays, some of which you can buy over-the-counter without prescription, can be very effective.

Paying lip service to mouth problems

Minor mouth problems are common, usually harmless and often go away by themselves. Although most mouth conditions tend not to last much longer than a few days, painful areas on the lips, tongue and gums can be very uncomfortable and make your life a misery. Most conditions settle without treatment, but you can buy various preparations over-the-counter to help relieve your symptoms.

If you have any mouth symptoms that last for more than three weeks, visit your dentist or GP. For example, persistent mouth ulcers in later life can potentially be due to oral cancer and need further assessment. Beware of other features, too, such as an increased tendency to infection, weight loss, sweats or fevers, particularly if you smoke or chew tobacco and/or drink alcohol regularly.

Also seek urgent medical advice if you suffer from any of the following:

- ✔ You can't swallow your saliva.

- ✔ You're very short of breath and can't speak in full sentences.

- ✔ You develop a worsening tingling sensation in your mouth with swelling around your lips, mouth, tongue or throat.

- ✔ Bleeding from the lips, mouth, tongue or face.

- ✔ White spots or red patches inside your mouth.

- ✔ A recent injury or burn to your face or mouth that's severe or doesn't heal.

Here are some common mouth problems that are often easy to recognise:

- ✔ **Mouth ulcers:** These look like small craters in the lining of your mouth and can be extremely painful. Mouth ulcers tend to be very sensitive, but are usually harmless and clear up in a week or so. Your pharmacist can recommend self-help medication, such as pain-relieving gels. If they last for longer than two to three weeks, see your GP.

- ✔ **Gum inflammation (*gingivitis*):** This condition is commonly due to poor dental hygiene and may improve by cleaning your teeth more regularly. If not, see your dentist.

- ✔ **Painful tongue:** A sore or painful tongue may be due to an inflammation or fungal infection, which you can recognise because of sore, creamy-yellow patches on the tongue and in other areas of your mouth. Ask your pharmacist for advice on over-the-counter treatments and see your GP if symptoms don't settle.

Becoming sore about your throat

Although a sore throat can be very painful, a minor viral infection or irritation is the usual cause, and the problem fades on its own. However, occasionally other conditions may lead to a sore throat, which then requires you to seek medical advice.

Painful and tender neck swellings below your jaw or on your neck, in connection with a throat infection, aren't due to cancer. They're swollen lymph glands that are just doing their job by filtering tissue fluid from your mouth and thereby clearing the infection. When your throat symptoms have settled, the glands should disappear again.

See your GP if you notice any of the following symptoms:

✔ Your sore throat doesn't start to get better after three to four days or lasts for longer than two weeks.

✔ Your tonsils – the round, red, fleshy blobs at each side of the back of your throat – appear red and inflamed and are covered with white specks or pus, suggesting tonsillitis or glandular fever.

✔ Your mouth develops a very tender swelling inside and you have difficulty opening your jaws; this may suggest that you have developed a collection of pus (an *abscess*) that probably needs antibiotics or draining.

✔ Your throat becomes sore while you're taking medication called *carbimazole* (for an overactive thyroid gland). Here, your sore throat may be a sign that the drug has affected your ability to fight infection.

If you have a fever and pain, freely available drugs such as paracetamol or ibuprofen help to bring your temperature down and ease your symptoms. Be sure to follow the instructions on the pack carefully.

Handling a hoarse voice

The most common reason for losing your voice is a viral infection or inflammation of your voice box, or *larynx,* which connects the back of your throat to your windpipe. This condition is called laryngitis, and may also produce symptoms such as feeling unwell, fever or pain when talking. Laryngitis normally lasts only a few days and usually gets better quickly, although you may be left with a slightly croaky voice for a while until the inflammation has settled completely.

Other causes of hoarseness include:

✔ **Overuse of the vocal cords:** This situation can arise if you use your voice often and continuously, for example if you're a singer or teacher. Shouting at a football match may also be responsible and cause your own voice to score something approaching an own goal! Resting your voice is usually all that's needed, and everything should get back to normal quickly.

✔ **Smoking and drinking:** Smoking tobacco and drinking alcohol may affect your vocal cords and cause inflammation. Go easy on these substances, otherwise the problem can lead to permanent damage if you're unlucky.

✔ **Underactive thyroid:** Occasionally, a gradually developing hoarse voice may be due to an underactive thyroid gland, particularly if you have other symptoms such as dry skin or feeling cold and tired all the time. See your doctor, who can arrange a simple blood test to make a diagnosis.

To relieve the symptoms of a hoarse voice, drink lots of water – even if swallowing is painful. Painkillers such as paracetamol or ibuprofen help with fever and throat pain, and your pharmacist can advise you about suitable throat lozenges and solutions for gargling. Also try to avoid shouting, talking and singing, because resting your voice helps to speed up your recovery.

Occasionally, a hoarse voice can have more serious causes – throat cancer, for example. Visit your GP if the following occurs:

✔ Your hoarseness or loss of voice persists for more than two to three weeks or gradually gets worse.

✔ You have swollen neck glands without symptoms of an infection such as fever, sore throat or feeling unwell.

You're at an increased risk of cancer of the voice box if you smoke, are over the age of 40 or a heavy drinker. Seek medical advice without delay if you have ongoing or worsening problems. But don't panic – benign lumps in your voice box can also be to blame.

Having difficulty swallowing

Difficulty swallowing (called *dysphagia*) may be the result of problems affecting your mouth, throat or gullet (*oesophagus*). Nervousness, nerve-related issues, obstructions in your gullet, reflux of gastric contents, infections and problems with the muscles pushing your food down can all be to blame, too.

In later life, the muscles used for swallowing can become weaker. Don't, however, simply accept problems with swallowing as being a normal part of growing older, because lots of treatments and advice are available to you to help with age-related dysphagia. You may need further investigations such as swallowing tests or direct inspection with a flexible telescope to discover the underlying cause.

Particularly if you're older than 40, ruling out the possibility of cancer is important. Make an appointment to see your GP if you suffer from any of these symptoms:

- ✔ You have persistent pain on swallowing.
- ✔ You can't swallow properly, and the problem is slowly getting worse.
- ✔ You regularly bring food back up.
- ✔ You choke, gag or cough when you eat or swallow.
- ✔ You have a persistent sensation of food being stuck in your throat or chest.
- ✔ You've lost weight for no apparent reason.
- ✔ You suffer from recurrent and frequent chest infections.

Looking at Acute Eye Problems

Eye symptoms, such as discomfort in your eye or problems with your vision, are common. Many non-serious eye infections or inflammation often settle down of their own accord or with over-the-counter treatments that you can apply directly to the eye. However, a number of other conditions can cause more serious eye problems, and so unless things are clear-cut, allow your optician or GP to make the correct diagnosis.

This section deals with acute and sudden eye problems only. For chronic and gradually developing eye problems in later life, take a look at Chapter 20. In addition, I cover eye injuries in more detail in Chapter 5.

Discovering an acute red or painful eye

A number of conditions can cause an acute red or painful eye. Most of these aren't dangerous, but sometimes a red eye may indicate a more serious underlying condition. If in doubt, see your GP for further assessment.

Seek medical advice immediately in the following circumstances:

- ✔ You notice a sudden pain in one of your eyes together with partial or total loss of vision (this can in rare cases be due to *acute glaucoma* – a condition in which the pressure inside your eye is raised).

✔ You suffer a blunt or penetrating eye injury, or get chemicals in your eyes (turn to Chapter 5 for more on the management of eye injuries).

✔ You have a red and painful – rather than just uncomfortable – eye.

✔ Your eyes suddenly become uncomfortable in bright light.

✔ Your *pupil* (the black, round central part) in your affected eye has a different size or shape from that of the unaffected eye.

Here's an overview of common and important eye conditions:

✔ **Blepharitis:** This problem is an inflammation of your eyelids in which both lids are usually sore and red, and may stick together (refer to image 14 in the colour section). Your eyelashes become crusty, you feel a gritty, burning sensation in your eyes and sometimes you may have a small boil (called a *stye* – refer to image 16 in the colour section) at the base of an eyelash. Clean your eyelids every day, use cloths or cotton wool soaked in warm water to loosen up crusting over your eyelids and avoid using make-up. Symptoms often disappear after about a week or so, but may come and go for a while. See your pharmacist or GP to discuss alternative treatment options if things don't improve. Blepharitis is not infectious, in contrast to conjunctivitis.

✔ **Conjunctivitis:** Conjunctivitis is an inflammation of a membrane covering the white of your eye and the inside of your eyelids and may be due to infection, allergies or irritants. Symptoms include a red and watery eye with a sticky coating of the eyelashes. Soreness is common, and your eyelids can be slightly swollen. Wipe your eyes regularly with clean, moist cotton wool and don't share your towels with other members of your household, to prevent the infection from spreading. See your pharmacist or GP if your symptoms don't improve after about five to seven days or if they are severe. (Refer to image 15 in the colour section.)

✔ **Bloodshot eye:** A burst blood vessel in the white of your eye commonly causes a red eye, which may look dramatic but is usually harmless. A bloodshot eye doesn't tend to cause any discomfort or problems with your vision. You don't need any treatment because it gets better by itself.

Experiencing sudden loss of vision

Suddenly losing your vision can be extremely worrying and may be down to any one of a long list of possible causes. You may suffer from a condition relating to the eye itself, or on rare occasions you can have a potentially serious problem such as meningitis, a blockage of a blood vessel supplying your brain or eye, or an inflammation of a blood vessel on your skull. Visual symptoms are also common in migraines, in which case they're usually not serious.

Here are some other important symptoms that should prompt you to seek medical advice immediately, particularly if you notice sudden total or partial loss of vision:

- ✔ Flashes along with a sensation that small objects are floating in front of your eyes.
- ✔ Sudden weakness in a limb or your face on one side of your body.
- ✔ Sudden double vision.
- ✔ Tenderness over one of your temples with pain on combing your hair or when chewing, especially if you're over the age of 50.
- ✔ Headache (with or without a high fever) along with neck stiffness or a rash.
- ✔ Loss of central vision only – which feels like looking through a tunnel.
- ✔ A missing area of vision, such as a 'blind spot'.
- ✔ A feeling that a curtain has appeared in front of your eyes.

A sudden loss of vision is rare, and so seeing your doctor or going to an Accident & Emergency (A&E) department straight away is essential. Early treatment can, in many cases, prevent permanent loss of vision.

Aim to see an optician every two years to make sure that your eyes are healthy. If you wear glasses or contact lenses or have another eye problem, ensure that you follow your optician's recommendations and have regular follow-up appointments.

The Eyecare Trust website (www.eyecaretrust.org.uk) provides lots of useful advice on looking after your eyes and about eye-related disorders.

For long-term problems with vision in later life, check out Chapter 20.

Chapter 10

Exploring Chest Problems

In This Chapter

▶ Recognising when chest complaints may be serious

▶ Reassuring yourself when they're not

▶ Checking breathing problems and coughing

Chest symptoms such as sudden shortness of breath or chest pain often appear in medical television dramas, mainly because they're always good for a bit of excitement in a storyline! Perhaps because of this exposure, a niggling pain in the chest can make you worry that you're having a heart attack, and a persistent cough can lead you to fear lung cancer. If you get scared by chest problems in this way, you're not alone.

Be reassured by the fact that chest symptoms in real life are more likely to be benign. Pulled muscles and vague chest discomfort due to viral infections are incredibly common and usually harmless. Taking chest symptoms seriously is important, however, because they may indicate a problem with your heart or lungs, and the fact that you need to seek medical help quickly. The trick is knowing how to tell the difference between something benign and something serious, and being able to decide whether to just have a hot bath and relax or to call '999'. Making an initial assessment of chest symptoms may feel daunting. To help, this chapter looks at how to troubleshoot chest symptoms such as palpitations, chest pain, breathing problems and coughing, and enables you to decide what to do next if you experience any of them.

Checking Out Chest Concerns

This section is about the symptoms that may make you fear that something's wrong with your heart. If you suffer from *heartache* though, you're looking in the wrong place – try Chapter 21 on anxiety and depression instead!

Heart-rending matters: Chest pain and tightness

Chest pain is a common symptom and comes in different forms, ranging from a mild discomfort to a severe crushing tightness that makes you feel extremely uncomfortable. Reassuringly though, most chest symptoms are harmless and get better by themselves. In this section, I cover common and usually non-serious types of chest pain first, before moving on to chest symptoms that should make you seek medical help quickly.

Considering chest pains unrelated to the heart

Don't jump straight to conclusions when you experience chest pain; the heart is rarely to blame. Here is a list of other underlying causes that may be at the root of the problem, starting with the most common:

- **Chest wall pain:** Injury or a persistent cough can lead to inflammation or a sprain of your chest muscles or ribs, and a cracked rib may be the cause if you feel very tender to the touch over your chest. Although you may be in pain, however, rib sprains and cracked ribs usually aren't dangerous, and heal by themselves. The pain may take several weeks to subside, though.

  See your GP or go to your local Accident & Emergency (A&E) department when you have a severe chest injury, when your pain doesn't improve or gets worse, or when you suffer from additional symptoms such as shortness of breath.

- **Stomach problems:** Heartburn, indigestion and reflux of stomach contents may lead to chest pain. Look at the section, 'What goes up must come down: Heartburn and reflux', later in this chapter for more info.

- **Chest infection:** A *productive cough* – one in which you bring up yellow or green secretions – together with a fever can indicate that you have an infection of your lung (called *pneumonia*) or airways in the chest (known as *bronchitis*), which may sometimes be accompanied by chest pain. Chest infections can be dangerous when you're older or suffer from poor health. See your GP for further assessment and treatment.

- **Shingles:** A blistery rash appearing on one side of your chest a few days after the onset of chest pain may indicate that you're suffering from a viral infection of the nerves, called *shingles*, or *herpes zoster* (refer to image 6 in the colour section and Chapter 8 for more info). Your GP may prescribe painkillers or antiviral preparations to speed up your recovery.

A heart-to-heart about chest pain

Blood vessels can become narrow because of fatty deposits inside their walls. These deposits build up slowly over the years, and eventually they block up the blood vessels completely. The effect is a bit like a blocked sink – you don't notice the sludge building up, but then the sink may drain increasingly slowly over time, until one day suddenly nothing can get through and you end up in a right old mess.

In a similar way, chest pain can indicate that your heart muscle isn't getting enough oxygen because of problems with the blood supply. In the case of a complete blockage (a *heart attack*), the quicker the blood supply is restored with clot-busting drugs or other interventions, the better. Just like leaving a plant without water for too long, the heart can survive for some time but not indefinitely. For this reason, heart doctors sometimes say 'time is muscle' – which means that the faster you get treatment, the better!

✔ **Panic attacks:** Suddenly feeling anxious, uneasy or frightened can be enough to bring on chest pain. When for no apparent reason your heart begins to race, you feel faint or you can't catch your breath, your symptoms may be due to a panic attack. Speak to your GP, who can exclude other potential causes and talk about what you can do during such attacks to help minimise the pain, as well as how you may be able to prevent them in the first instance. Flip to Chapters 5 (on 'emergencies') and 21 (covering 'anxiety and stress') to find out more about panic attacks – and what to do if you get them.

✔ **Collapsed lung (*pneumothorax*):** A lung may partly or fully collapse for no apparent reason or sometimes because of a serious chest injury. This condition is rare but tends to be more common in young and tall men, but you're also at increased risk if you suffer from chronic lung disease. A sudden breathlessness and chest pain that tends to be worse on breathing can indicate a collapsed lung. See your GP for further assessment.

Suspecting angina or a heart attack

Angina and heart attacks are more serious causes of chest pains. *Angina* is occasional or regular pain or tightness in the chest caused by *coronary heart disease* – that is, reduced blood flow in one or more blood vessels that supply your heart with oxygen. Angina pain commonly feels like a 'tightness' – as if someone is sitting on your chest. A *heart attack* is a complete blockage of that blood supply – and an emergency situation (refer to Chapter 5 for more information on how you can spot a heart attack). The likelihood of experiencing these conditions increases in later life; both are very rare in otherwise healthy people under the age of 40.

Dealing with the bad guys creeping up on your heart

You can do a lot to try and prevent coronary heart disease:

✔ **High blood pressure:** Get your blood pressure checked by your pharmacist or practice nurse. If it's too high, you may benefit from treatment.

✔ **High cholesterol:** Try to keep your cholesterol down by eating at least five portions of fruit and veg per day, and fewer meat and dairy products. Particularly avoid or reduce your consumption of foods with a high fat or sugar content.

✔ **Lack of exercise:** To prevent heart disease, exercise regularly and briskly for at least 20 minutes a day. Swimming, jogging, cycling and gardening are particularly good for you.

✔ **Obesity:** Try to shed some pounds if you're overweight.

✔ **Smoking:** Smoking accelerates the build-up of fatty sludge in your coronary arteries and at least doubles your risk of having a heart attack.

The British Heart Foundation website (www.bhf.org.uk) has more information about heart disease.

Depending on which area and how much of your heart is affected, symptoms can range from a mild discomfort behind your breast bone to severe crushing chest pain. Less commonly, you may experience angina just by feeling sick or short of breath, without any chest pain at all. Heart attacks, though, sometimes occur completely out of the blue and are cripplingly painful and life-threatening (see Chapter 5).

Angina

Compare your symptoms with the following ones, which suggest angina:

✔ You get intermittent chest pain in the centre of your chest that comes on when you exert yourself – for example, when walking up a hill.

✔ Your pain usually gets better with rest and lasts for no more than ten minutes.

✔ You may notice that the pain spreads to your jaw, neck, arms or stomach.

✔ You can bring on your symptoms by eating a large meal, experiencing stress or going out into the cold.

If you think that you may have angina, make an appointment to see your GP. If she confirms the diagnosis, she can talk you through the many treatments available that can improve your symptoms and reduce your risk of heart attack. If these treatments fail, your doctor may refer you to a heart specialist for possible further tests and treatment.

Heart attack

Dial '999' immediately if you suffer from central chest pain that feels like a band around your chest or an elephant sitting on you and your pain doesn't get better after resting for a few minutes, particularly if:

- ✔ Your pain spreads to your neck, jaw, shoulder or arm.

- ✔ You're experiencing such symptoms for the first time.

- ✔ You notice that your heart is beating very fast or irregularly.

- ✔ You vomit or feel short of breath and sweaty, or you faint.

Exploring blood clots on the lung

A blood clot may form inside a blood vessel in your leg – a condition called *deep venous thrombosis* (I explain the reasons for this further down in this section, but flip to Chapter 13 for further details on thrombosis and leg pain). The clot (known as *pulmonary embolus*) can dislodge and then travel through your heart into your lung where it gets stuck – a condition known as *pulmonary embolism*.

Symptoms of pulmonary embolism include:

- ✔ Feeling suddenly short of breath together with a sharp pain in your chest that gets worse when you breathe in.

- ✔ Also coughing up blood, feeling faint and your heart seems to be racing.

Pulmonary embolism is rare and in most cases isn't the cause of chest symptoms. However, you're at higher risk of suffering from a blood clot on your lung in these circumstances:

- ✔ You notice pain and swelling in one of your legs.

- ✔ You've had a recent surgical operation.

- ✔ You've been in bed for more than a day or two.

- ✔ You're pregnant or have just had a baby.

- ✔ You're obese or overweight.

- ✔ You take the oral contraceptive pill or hormone replacement therapy (HRT). (The risk from these medications is very small, however, and the vast majority of women don't get any complications as a result of taking them.)

- ✔ You've been diagnosed with cancer.

- ✔ You've had problems with blood clots in the past.

Pulmonary embolism may cause mild symptoms where it affects only a small blood vessel, but you're likely to be severely ill if a major blood vessel is involved. In most cases, symptoms appear suddenly over a few minutes, although small clots can lead to more longstanding and less dramatic symptoms that come and go over weeks or months.

Contact your GP urgently or dial '999' in an emergency if you feel unusually unwell with any symptoms suggesting pulmonary embolism, particularly if you're at increased risk because of the circumstances mentioned in the preceding bulleted list.

Looking into leaking blood vessels

Rarely, the large blood vessel, or *aorta*, in your chest and abdomen can swell up like a balloon (called an *aortic aneurysm*), and then develop a tear and leak. This rare medical emergency, which is more common in later life, requires immediate admission to hospital. Consider this possibility if you experience both the following symptoms and dial '999' in an emergency:

- ✔ A sudden severe pain in your chest or stomach that also goes down your legs, to your back or from your back towards your abdomen.

- ✔ A pulsating sensation in your abdomen that may be accompanied by a tearing- or ripping-like pain between your shoulder blades or along your back bone.

Beat it! Palpitations and the racing heart

Palpitations – the sensation that you get when you're aware of an unusually fast, strong or irregular heartbeat – can be very worrying, particularly when you experience them for the first time. The good news is that usually you don't need to panic, because most palpitations are benign and not due to any problems with your heart.

Anxiety and nervousness are common culprits, as are caffeine-containing drinks and smoking (due to nicotine). In these instances, the palpitations usually clear up on their own when you avoid or remove the cause. Your palpitations may also be caused by medication, such as antidepressants.

Less commonly, another medical condition such as an overactive thyroid gland or an underlying heart disorder may be the cause. In these circumstances you're likely to show additional symptoms. See your GP if, in addition to your palpitations, you notice the following symptoms, which may suggest an overactive thyroid (known as *hyperthyroidism*):

- ✔ You've been losing weight for no reason, despite an increased appetite.
- ✔ You feel restless.
- ✔ You sweat more than you used to.
- ✔ Your eyes start to look bigger and may appear to 'bulge' in the later stages of hyperthyroidism.
- ✔ Your pulse is irregular.
- ✔ You feel more breathless than you expect.
- ✔ You feel tired or weak, with no obvious explanation.
- ✔ Your stools, or bowel movements, have become looser.

Without wanting to get your heart rate going, you need to seek medical advice urgently or, in an emergency, dial '999' if you experience a sudden onset of palpitations and feel unwell, particularly if you also have the following symptoms:

- ✔ You feel dizzy or faint.
- ✔ You collapse and don't feel better after resting for a few minutes.
- ✔ You become short of breath.
- ✔ You experience chest pain.

Also seek medical advice when you're just not sure what's going on, particularly if your palpitations are frequent or they go on for a long time. Occasional 'missed' or 'extra' beats (medics call them *ectopics*) are common and usually harmless. See your GP if you're worried about them, particularly if you have symptoms such as those mentioned earlier.

What goes up must come down: Heartburn and reflux

Reflux of digestive stomach juices (also called *gastro-oesophageal reflux disease*, or *GORD*) into the part of your throat called the gullet is probably the most common cause of discomfort in the lower chest and upper abdomen. Your gullet's lining isn't as tough as the lining of your stomach, and so when the acidic fluids that usually stay in your stomach reflux into your gullet, they can cause inflammation and a burning pain known as heartburn, or *dyspepsia*. However, as unpleasant as most heartburn is, it tends not to last long.

With heartburn, in addition to feeling a burning pain or discomfort behind the breastbone or in the upper abdomen, you may notice the following:

- You get a burning feeling or acidic taste in the back of your throat or mouth.
- You belch frequently and get a lot of wind from your stomach.

Various causes can bring on heartburn or make it worse. Here are some of the more common ones:

- Eating certain foods, such as fried or fatty meals.
- Eating large meals late at night (causes night-time symptoms).
- Drinking bubbly soft drinks, coffee or alcohol.
- Bending forward.
- Smoking.
- Being overweight.
- Being pregnant.
- Taking certain medicines, such as aspirin-type drugs or antidepressants.

Tackling these more usual causes of heartburn should reduce the frequency and severity of attacks.

Here are some top tips for trying to relieve your symptoms:

- **Eating habits:** Eating smaller portions more frequently instead of large meals and not having your last meal late at night both help to prevent heartburn and reflux. Also look out for and avoid anything that brings on your symptoms – coffee, spicy or fatty foods, alcohol and chocolate are common offenders. Why do the tasty foods always get the blame?!
- **Sleeping position:** If you suffer from night-time symptoms, you can try putting some blocks under the head of your bed to raise it – but make sure that your bed stands safely. Using extra pillows doesn't always work: in fact, this attempt can sometimes make things worse by increasing the pressure on your stomach.
- **Medication:** If your symptoms persist, ask your pharmacist about over-the-counter medication that you can take to relieve your symptoms. Your GP can also prescribe other preparations if you still have problems.

Reflux is incredibly common, but don't accept it as part of your life – many effective treatments are available. Because pain in your lower chest and heartburn may sometimes be symptomatic of a more serious underlying cause, such as an ulcer or, in rare cases, a stomach cancer, check for the following symptoms and seek medical advice if you suffer from heartburn and in addition notice any of the following:

- ✔ You find swallowing difficult.
- ✔ You suffer from unexplained fevers, weight loss or sweating.
- ✔ You feel very tired and your skin and nailbeds look pale – may indicate ongoing blood loss (known as *anaemia*) from your stomach.
- ✔ You've been passing black tar-like stools, which may indicate a stomach bleed (but remember that taking iron tablets can also make your stools appear black – in which case this is harmless).
- ✔ You develop persistent reflux and heartburn when you're aged 50 or over.
- ✔ You had a stomach ulcer in the past.

Heartburn and reflux are rarely serious, but seek medical advice from your GP or call '999' in an emergency if you notice the following symptoms:

- ✔ You experience severe, persistent, worsening and unexplained upper abdominal pain, particularly if this pain occurs together with chest pain, shortness of breath or sweating (also check out the section 'Heart-rending matters: Chest pain and tightness' earlier in this chapter). Various causes may be responsible.
- ✔ You vomit persistently, bring up blood, pass black stools while you feel faint or have collapsed. All may indicate bleeding in your stomach.

You can experience heartburn for various reasons, and most of the time the cause is entirely benign. Visit your GP for further assessment when problems with heartburn and reflux go on for a prolonged period of time or interfere with your life. If your reflux or heartburn doesn't get better with treatment, your GP may arrange tests and in some cases refer you for further investigations, which may include looking down your gullet with a flexible telescope (called *gastroscopy*).

Taking Your Breath Away: Breathing Problems

Most of the time, people aren't aware of their breathing – it just happens – so breathing symptoms can be very frightening. You can feel short of breath for a variety of reasons, but regular breathing problems may indicate a more serious underlying heart or lung condition. On rare occasions, breathing symptoms may even suggest a life-threatening illness. The intensity of breathing problems varies from feeling a bit puffed out to – in the worst case – having a sensation of choking to death. You may also experience coughing, wheezing or shortness of breath alone or in combination.

Contemplating coughing

Coughing is a natural defence to anything that enters or irritates your throat or lungs and is a way of getting rid of the stuff. Being able to cough is therefore very important in maintaining your health. Common causes are colds, smoking, asthma and dust. Coughs can be dry, or they may produce phlegm.

Harmless cough

However they come, coughs can be very annoying but are, in most cases, harmless and nothing to worry about. If you have the sniffles and a sore throat as well as an acute cough, the most likely cause is a simple *cold* – a viral infection of your upper airways, which include your mouth, throat, windpipe and lungs. You may also have a fever for a few days and headache as well as general aches and pains.

The symptoms of an acute cough often start to improve after a few days. However, because your throat and windpipe have become inflamed, the cough itself may last for up to three or four weeks even though the infection has already cleared. This dry cough can be hugely annoying, but usually isn't dangerous and doesn't have any lasting effects.

When suffering from a cough due to the common cold, taking paracetamol or ibuprofen usually helps to make you feel better. Your pharmacist can suggest alternative preparations that may work for you, although little evidence exists to suggest that over-the-counter cough medicines do much good. Visit your GP if your cough lasts for longer than two weeks or if it steadily gets worse.

Most infections clear without treatment, and letting your body get on with fighting the infection is often your best option, making sure that you drink plenty of clear fluids. You probably don't need antibiotics – they may even make you worse by causing sickness, diarrhoea, a rash or a more severe allergic reaction such as *anaphylaxis* (see Chapter 5 for further information).

Other causes of cough

Sometimes, however, coughing may be due to a more serious underlying cause in the throat or lungs, so check for the following symptoms:

- ✔ You have a persistent or very high fever (flip to Chapter 7 for information on how to spot and assess a fever) for more than a few days, which can suggest a *chest infection*.

- ✔ You cough up blood (this can also occur with harmless viral infections such as colds).

- ✔ Your cough lasts for more than three weeks without seeming to improve.

- ✔ You have other unexplained symptoms such as weight loss, loss of appetite, feeling tired all the time, night sweats, fevers and feeling unwell for no apparent reason.

When you're coughing up blood

Coughing up streaks of blood when you have a cold usually means that a tiny blood vessel in your lung has ruptured, which isn't much to worry about. Do see your GP, though, if you cough up blood regularly or if it comes out in larger amounts. Chest infection, fluid on the lungs, tuberculosis (TB), a blood clot on your lung or a lung cancer are some of the causes that your doctor may want to exclude.

The following causes can be responsible for these symptoms:

- ✔ **Chest infection:** An infection of the deeper airways is known as a *chest infection*, sometimes also called *lower respiratory infection, pneumonia* or *bronchitis*. Compared to the common cold, symptoms of a chest infection include a persistent high fever, feeling more unwell than you'd expect, becoming confused (particularly if you belong to an older age group) and breathing much faster than usual.

If you've been coughing for more than three weeks, or if you suffer from other additional symptoms, you may want to look at the following list for potential causes (starting with the common ones):

- ✔ **Smoking:** Smoking is one of the most common reasons for a persistent cough, which often is worse in the mornings. Smoking leads to a chronic inflammation of the airways but may also cause chronic airway infection or even lung cancer.

- ✔ **Medication:** If you take blood pressure-lowering medication, check whether it belongs to a group called the angiotensin-converting enzyme (ACE) inhibitors. These drugs can bring on a dry cough – a relatively common and often annoying side effect. See your doctor for a medication review if you're suspicious.

- ✔ **Asthma:** Asthma (flip to the later section, 'Wheezing and noisy breathing: Asthma' for more details) is a common cause of chronic cough – remember that you may not always notice a wheeze.

- ✔ **Lung cancer:** Persistent cough can sometimes be a sign of lung cancer, particularly if you smoke. See your doctor if you also notice unexplained sweating, weight loss, loss of appetite, tiredness, neck swellings or hoarseness, particularly if in addition you've been coughing up blood. Lung cancer is rare under the age of 40, but smoking increases the risk dramatically, being responsible for over 90 per cent of lung cancers.

- ✔ **Other causes:** Less commonly, allergies, reflux of stomach contents into the gullet or tuberculosis (TB) may cause a persistent cough.

Not going up in smoke

The problem with tobacco smoke is that it contains a number of toxic substances, including nicotine, tar and carbon monoxide. Smoking increases the risk of your arteries clogging up and of you suffering a heart attack or stroke in the future. You're also about 15 times more likely to die from lung cancer than non-smokers. Giving up smoking is therefore one of the best things you can do to maintain your health, and can reduce this risk after a few years to that of a non-smoker. You may also save several hundred pounds a month if you're currently a heavy smoker.

Visit `http://smokefree.nhs.uk`, on the National Health Service website, or contact your local surgery to find out more about all the other benefits of a smoke-free life and ways to help you stop smoking – loads of support is available to you.

The bottom line is that most coughs aren't dangerous and settle by themselves, even though you may need two or three weeks to clear them completely. Be aware of the danger signs, however, and see your GP if you're unsure or concerned about possible underlying problems.

Feeling short of breath

You probably don't worry when you feel a bit puffed out after running for a bus or pushing yourself in the gym. But if you start to feel uncomfortable when, in theory, you should be breathing normally, you may begin to wonder what's going on. Common and benign reasons for breathlessness are feeling anxious or nervous, being overweight or lacking fitness. However, shortness of breath may in some cases indicate a problem with your heart or lungs, or lack of blood (called *anaemia*), among other things.

Acute, sudden shortness of breath

If you're suddenly and acutely short of breath, and any of the following conditions apply to you, see your GP:

- ✔ **You have a fever:** A temperature of over 38 degrees Celsius (100.4 degrees Fahrenheit) suggests some form of chest infection, such as bronchitis or pneumonia (which I cover in the preceding section, 'Contemplating cough'). Coughing up green or yellow phlegm is also highly likely if you have a chest infection.

  If you're in poor health or belong to an older age group, you're at higher risk of suffering complications from a chest infection, and so see your GP for further assessment and treatment such as antibiotics. If your infection is severe, your GP may in rare cases need to admit you to hospital. The good news is that – if you're normally healthy – you're likely to get better quickly.

✔ **You're pregnant:** Although you may find that getting around is harder and you become more puffed out in the weeks prior to giving birth, you shouldn't really feel breathless in the earlier stages of pregnancy. See your GP or midwife if you're pregnant and find yourself becoming short of breath.

✔ **You're under a lot of stress or feel anxious:** Your shortness of breath may be due to a panic attack. If you've never experienced this symptom before, contact your GP for advice. If your breathing problems go away quickly but you continue to suffer from symptoms of anxiety, depression or stress (turn to Chapter 21 for more), book a routine appointment to see your GP – lots of treatment options are available.

If you suddenly feel breathless, unwell and notice any of the following symptoms, seek urgent advice from your GP or call '999' in an emergency:

✔ You think you may be experiencing an allergic reaction, for example to antibiotics or nuts, which can cause sudden noisy breathing (or wheezing).

✔ You also have chest pain (take a look at the 'Checking Out Chest Concerns' section, earlier in this chapter).

✔ You feel faint or have collapsed.

✔ You cough up blood.

✔ You've been short of breath for a while but suddenly get worse.

✔ You're coughing up frothy phlegm (or *sputum*) and feel better only when you sit up, which may indicate problems with your heart.

✔ You have an unexplained swelling in your leg and suddenly become breathless (see 'Exploring blood clots on the lung' earlier in the chapter).

If you feel breathless, keep calm, remove any tight clothing and sit the wrong way round on a chair with your arms supported by the back rest instead of lying down flat. Turn to Chapters 5 and 24 for advice on how to deal with emergencies.

Persistent shortness of breath

Symptoms of breathlessness may progress slowly, or you may not even notice that your breathing is getting worse until people close to you mention it. See your GP for further assessment to discover the underlying cause. The first step is usually to check whether your symptoms are due to problems with the heart, the lung or both, or if something else may be causing trouble.

Persistent (or *chronic*) breathing problems become more common in later life, with heart and lung conditions being the main underlying causes. Here are some of the causes, starting with the commoner ones:

✔ **Obesity:** Being overweight is a common cause for persistent breathlessness. Someone who's 20 kilograms (44 pounds) over a healthy weight carries around the equivalent of two buckets full of water – or the heaviest suitcase you can check in with most airlines – all day and every day.

✔ **Medication:** Occasionally, certain drugs – such as beta-blockers, medications like aspirin, ibuprofen or diclofenac and others – can cause breathlessness, particularly if you suffer from asthma. Check the drug information leaflet or speak to your pharmacist or GP if you feel your medication may be the cause.

✔ **Chronic obstructive pulmonary disease:** Smoking puts you at higher risk of developing *chronic bronchitis* or *emphysema* (also collectively known as *chronic obstructive pulmonary disease*, or *COPD*). In this condition your airways become tighter, making it more difficult for the air to pass through. In addition, more and more of the tiny bubbles that make up your lung tissues burst, so that the overall surface area of your lung – which helps to shift oxygen from inhaled air into your blood – reduces in size. The severity of this condition ranges from very mild symptoms of cough, shortness of breath and wheeze (if the damage to your lung is small) to severe shortness of breath (in advanced disease) – in which case you may even need treatment with oxygen.

If you're diagnosed with COPD, the best thing you can do to help yourself is to try and stop smoking. Many other treatments are available to help relieve your symptoms and prevent things from getting worse, so see your GP for further assessment and management.

✔ **Heart problems:** If you regularly wake up at night because you can't breathe and have to use more than one pillow to be comfortable, your breathing problem may be due to underlying heart disease. In some cases, the heart not pumping properly may be the problem, leading to fluid building up within your lung, which shows itself through shortness of breath. Many people are surprised that heart problems can cause shortness of breath. To get to the bottom of this symptom, see your GP for further assessment.

✔ **Thyroid disease:** Rarely, an overactive thyroid gland may cause you to feel short of breath. In this case, you may also feel edgy or nervous, get palpitations, feel sweaty or lose weight for no reason. See your GP for further assessment and a simple blood test to confirm the diagnosis.

✔ **Possible lung cancer:** See your GP if – in addition to a persistent shortness of breath – you cough and feel tired all the time, are off your food, have lost weight, cough up blood or suffer from unexplained sweats, particularly at night. These symptoms may sometimes be due to underlying lung cancer, which is much more common in smokers and in older age groups. Remember that these symptoms may also occur in other more benign conditions, and so ask your GP to assess you, as you're likely to need an X-ray of your chest.

Information about the severity of your breathing problems is important when your GP makes her assessment. Making a note of which activities – such as talking, climbing stairs, hobbies, dressing, washing, cleaning or anything else that you can think of – are affected by your breathlessness can help.

Wheezing and noisy breathing: Asthma

Wheezing is a gasping sound that indicates that you're breathing with difficulty. If you suffer from wheezing or noisy breathing that comes and goes and makes you feel short of breath, you possibly suffer from *asthma* or another lung condition such as *chronic bronchitis*. You may know quite a few people with asthma, who all seem perfectly well. So, do you need to be concerned?

Asthma is a condition in which the smaller airways of your lung sometimes become inflamed and narrow – hence the wheezing. The squeezed airways cause difficulty in getting air out of your lungs, which is why the wheeze mainly occurs on breathing out. The condition often starts in childhood but may develop at any age. The degree and duration of the narrowing can vary, and your symptoms may only be mild.

Signs that you suffer from asthma can include intermittent:

- ✔ Coughing.
- ✔ Shortness of breath.
- ✔ Tightness in your chest.
- ✔ Wheezing.

When you first notice these symptoms, see your GP for an assessment and to confirm the diagnosis.

Viral respiratory infections, exercise, going out into the cold, allergic reactions or hay fever can bring on the symptoms of asthma, but you're unlikely to have any problem for most of the time. With asthma, breathing is typically worse at night and early in the morning, and the coughing and wheezing may wake you from your sleep. The extent and duration of these symptoms varies from one episode to another, and your breathing problems can last anything from an hour or so to days or even weeks.

Aspirin-type medicines, contact with certain animals and a group of drugs called beta-blockers (which come in tablet form as well as eye drops used for the treatment of glaucoma) are common triggers that can cause wheezing and bring on asthma attacks – try to avoid these. If you don't know what triggers your asthma, see your GP who may possibly arrange further testing. The effect of triggers varies from person to person, and what sets off an attack in one person may not in another.

No cure exists for asthma, but effective treatments are available to treat and prevent your symptoms. You get a lot of benefit from using inhalers as prescribed by your GP or asthma nurse, but sometimes you need to take other medicines as well. Asthma UK, which aims to improve the health and wellbeing of people with asthma, offers further information and help on its website at www.asthma.org.uk.

Asthma can make you so unwell that it becomes a medical emergency and you need assessment and treatment in hospital. In rare cases, asthma can kill, so taking the illness seriously is important. Fortunately, a number of pointers suggest when your asthma is getting worse and you need to seek medical advice. These symptoms may develop quickly, without much notice:

- You use your inhalers more and more often.
- You wake at night feeling short of breath, coughing, wheezing or having a tight chest.
- You take time off work or school due to your asthma symptoms.
- Your asthma symptoms increasingly affect your day-to-day life.

Sometimes, asthma can strike suddenly and severely. Turn to Chapter 5 to find out more about these attacks and how to deal with them.

Chapter 11

Untangling Tummy and Bowel Problems

In This Chapter

▶ Sussing out nausea and vomiting

▶ Dealing with diarrhoea and constipation

▶ Assessing abdominal pain and other related symptoms

*M*ost people experience nausea, stomach ache, vomiting or diarrhoea at some stage in their lives. Such symptoms can really make you feel sick and be, quite literally, a pain in the bum! As well as being annoying, abdominal problems can be quite worrying, particularly when they last longer than you expect, or if they make you feel very unwell or uncomfortable. Reassuringly though, most tummy problems are benign and go away by themselves.

Stomach and bowel infections are among the most common causes, but abdominal symptoms can also mean that a problem is brewing elsewhere in your body. (For example, you may be surprised to hear that a problem with your ear can cause vomiting!) Sometimes, abdominal symptoms can be due to a more serious underlying cause, such as appendicitis, inflammation of your gall bladder or one of many other conditions.

This chapter identifies the clues to look out for when tummy trouble strikes so that you're in a position to decide whether you're safe to wait and see, or whether you need to seek medical help sooner rather than later.

Going Out and Staying In: Problems With the Digestive Tract

Now for a brief anatomy lesson: when you swallow, anything that passes your throat initially enters your gullet, before reaching your stomach and finally your small and large bowels (also called your *intestines*). All these tube-like organs help to digest the food you eat. Leftovers, and other substances that your body wants to get rid of, come out the back passage as stools, or *faeces*. Life can become rather uncomfortable when things go wrong in this department.

Taking the lid off nausea and vomiting

Nausea is a sick feeling in your tummy that often precedes vomiting. When you vomit, your stomach muscles contract suddenly and bring up what's inside the stomach – sometimes for good reasons, for example when you eat food past its sell-by date or you have a tummy bug.

Becoming utterly sick of it!

Lots of things can make you feel sick or vomit, many of which are obvious and benign. You probably aren't too concerned when you feel sick or vomit after drinking too much alcohol or overeating a particularly heavy meal, especially if you feel better after vomiting. But in less clear-cut situations, when the underlying reason isn't so obvious, check whether your symptoms fit with any of the following conditions:

- ✔ **Gastritis:** This problem is an inflammation of the stomach lining that, among other things, can be caused by irritation from alcohol or food poisoning. You may know immediately what's been causing your symptoms, which tend to go away by themselves after a day or two. See your pharmacist for advice on over-the-counter medications if you need symptom relief.

- ✔ **Gastroenteritis:** This condition is an infection of the stomach and bowel, which in many cases is caused by a virus. Typically, you may have been in contact with someone who has similar symptoms, although that may not always be the case. Vomiting and diarrhoea are the main symptoms, and you may also have a mild fever. To combat gastroenteritis, drink plenty of fluids (in small sips if you have difficulty keeping things down) and eat only small amounts of light food at a time. You should start to get better after a couple of days, but symptoms can last for seven to ten days. Seek medical advice if you don't start to improve within 24 hours or you can't keep fluids down, and wash your hands frequently to avoid spreading the infection. (The later section 'Enduring acute gastroenteritis' has more on gastroenteritis.)

- ✔ **Inner ear problems:** Conditions affecting the balance organ in the inner ear may cause a feeling – called *vertigo* – of the world spinning around, which is often accompanied by acute vomiting (Chapter 6 has loads more on dizziness). Motion sickness when travelling is also common. Visit your GP for a check-up and to discuss the treatment options; a number of drugs are available to help relieve your symptoms.

✔ **Medication:** Various drugs – and, occasionally, drug allergies – can cause nausea and vomiting, particularly aspirin-type medicines (including ibuprofen and diclofenac). If you feel that your medication may be responsible, discuss your concerns with your GP.

The main risk of severe vomiting and diarrhoea is losing too much body fluid, or *dehydration*, and so drinking plenty of fluids is important.

Feeling sick all the time

If you've been vomiting intermittently or persistently for a while, consider other causes. The possibilities are almost endless, and so the following list contains only a selection of important causes, starting with the more common ones:

✔ **Pregnancy:** If you're a woman of child-bearing age, always consider the possibility of being pregnant, particularly if your period is late and you show other symptoms of pregnancy such as tender breasts or feeling tired. You can buy a testing kit from your pharmacy to check whether you're pregnant or not. Alternatively, contact your GP surgery for further advice.

✔ **Regular alcohol misuse:** If you drink alcohol regularly and over the recommended limits (check out Chapter 23 for further information on alcohol-related problems and safe limits), ongoing stomach inflammation due to the toxic effects of alcohol is possible. Try to reduce your alcohol intake and ask your pharmacist for over-the-counter remedies. See your GP in case your symptoms persist and/or you struggle to kick the booze.

✔ **Reflux:** Reflux of stomach contents into your gullet or an ulcer in your stomach can cause vomiting and nausea: turn to Chapter 10 for more on reflux. Consult your pharmacist for suitable over-the-counter remedies and see your GP if your symptoms don't settle.

✔ **Gallstones:** Gallstones often cause intermittent pain that's worse on the right side just below your ribcage and often occurs after a meal. See your GP to confirm the diagnosis as you may need an operation (called a *cholecystectomy*) to remove your gall bladder.

✔ **Appendicitis:** Pain in the area of your navel that moves into the right lower tummy, or abdomen, suggests possible appendicitis (see the 'Exploring abdominal pain' section later in this chapter), particularly if you also have a mild fever and feel unwell. Seek medical advice immediately.

✔ **Liver problems:** Rare liver infections and other conditions can cause vomiting: look out for the whites of your eyes turning yellow (which is known as *jaundice*). Visit your doctor for further assessment if you suspect these conditions.

Spotting dehydration

Vomiting a lot can make your body become too dry (which is called *dehydration*), so be on the lookout for these early signs of dehydration:

- ✔ Dry tongue and lips.
- ✔ Headache and thirst.
- ✔ Urine that gets darker.

If you spot these signs in yourself, drink a lot of fluid as soon as you can to replace those you've lost through vomiting. Drinking water is usually fine, but if you vomit a lot – particularly if the weather is hot and you feel sweaty too – get some special sports drinks (available from most supermarkets) or rehydration solution from your pharmacist to help replenish your body salts.

If you don't pass urine for 8–12 hours and your eyes start to look sunken, you may be suffering from more severe dehydration. Don't delay seeking medical help when you feel that you're dehydrated and can't keep anything in, particularly if you become unusually drowsy. This situation can develop into a medical emergency.

Identifying symptoms of more serious underlying disease

Occasionally, more serious underlying problems can cause persistent vomiting. Here some scenarios that should prompt you to seek medical advice immediately – phone your doctor or see Chapter 25 for details of useful helplines and websites:

- ✔ You vomit following a head injury.
- ✔ You experience general symptoms such as weight loss, loss of appetite, sweating, fever and feeling unwell over weeks or months – particularly if these symptoms are getting worse.
- ✔ You notice red or black blood in your vomit.
- ✔ You suffer from prolonged and severe vomiting with no obvious underlying cause.
- ✔ You become severely dehydrated.
- ✔ You notice a persistent and worsening headache, particularly if you experience additional symptoms such as weakness in a limb, reduced sensation, fits, speech problems, or loss of balance.
- ✔ You have severe pain in one eye (on rare occasions, this symptom can be due to glaucoma – see Chapter 9 for more on this).

Occasionally, nausea and/or vomiting can be due to acute and potentially dangerous underlying conditions. Seek medical advice urgently or call '999' in an emergency if you experience the following in addition to vomiting:

✔ You suffer from chest pain or tightness (check out Chapter 10 for more on chest problems).

✔ You have a high fever over 38 degrees Celsius (100.4 degrees Fahrenheit) and a rash (suggesting *meningitis* – see Chapter 9).

✔ You develop neck stiffness and can't tolerate bright light (which also suggests meningitis).

✔ You have severe abdominal pain that isn't relieved by vomiting.

✔ Your tummy becomes swollen and tender.

✔ You feel extremely and unusually drowsy or confused.

✔ You have a severe headache that starts before the vomiting (unless you regularly suffer from migraine and vomiting is one of your usual symptoms).

Diarrhoea in a nutshell

Your stools should ideally be just right – neither too hard nor too soft – but a huge variation exists in what's normal for people, in terms of how frequently their bowel movements occur and how hard or soft the stools are. Some people 'go' only once every few days, whereas other people have up to four or five bowel movements a day. Your own bowel habits can also vary from time to time and be affected by stress, a change in diet, travelling and not drinking enough fluid.

Diarrhoea means that your stools are unusually loose and frequent, though it may sometimes occur in cases of severe constipation, when loose bowel contents bypass the hard stool in the blocked-up back passage. Diarrhoea can be due to a number of causes, ranging from anxiety to bowel cancer, but when it hits suddenly, the most likely cause is a viral infection. In this case, the symptoms often start to improve within 48 hours, you don't normally need any treatment and most of the time the problem goes away on its own. If your symptoms haven't settled after about a week, or if you continue to be unwell, contact your GP for advice. Replacing the lost fluid is very important.

Enduring acute gastroenteritis

An infection called *gastroenteritis* is the most common reason for the onset of diarrhoea. People suffering from gastroenteritis may have picked up the infection from contact with someone else who has similar symptoms, but this scenario isn't always the case.

The main symptoms of gastroenteritis are usually relatively mild. Beginning with the more common, these symptoms include:

- Needing to rush to the toilet.
- Cramp-like abdominal pains which improve after opening your bowels.
- Feeling sick or vomiting.
- Loss of appetite.
- A short-lived fever, usually lasting not much longer than a day or so.
- A mild headache without neck stiffness or intolerance of light.

You often get better after seven to ten days without receiving any specific treatment, but a few weeks may pass before your stools return completely to normal.

Diarrhoea due to tummy bugs can make you feel rotten but usually isn't dangerous – as long as you make sure that you drink enough fluids to replace those you lose. If you have acute short-term diarrhoea, you don't normally need any treatment or tests. However, if your symptoms persist for a week or more, your GP may arrange for you to have stool or other tests.

Seek medical advice if your diarrhoea is severe and you notice the following additional symptoms:

- You become dehydrated (see the 'Spotting dehydration' section, earlier in this chapter).
- You feel thirsty and have a headache, a fast pulse or feel unusually drowsy.
- You have a persistent high fever (above 38 degrees Celsius, which is 100.4 degrees Fahrenheit).
- You notice blood in your stools.
- You have to get up during the night to open your bowels.

Also visit your GP if you develop diarrhoea after travelling abroad, particularly if your symptoms don't settle by themselves after a few days or you have blood-stained diarrhoea together with fever and abdominal pain. In very rare and severe cases – usually when you're dehydrated – you may need hospital treatment so fluids can be administered to you through a drip.

Anti-diarrhoea medicines such as loperamide (available from your pharmacist) may sometimes help by slowing down the movement of bowel contents, but they also have the potential to prolong your illness, because diarrhoea is your body's way of getting rid of the bugs. Taking such medicines can mean that the bugs remain in your body for longer.

Step away from the kitchen!

Don't handle food intended for other people if you have diarrhoea due to an infection. Therefore, if you have a job in the catering industry, you may need to take time off until your infection clears. If you have gastroenteritis, always wash your hands thoroughly, clean the toilet seat with disinfectant and don't share towels so you keep the risk of spreading the infection to other people to a minimum.

Although experts used to advise not eating anything for a day or two while you have diarrhoea, research shows that no harm exists in eating foods high in carbohydrates (bread, potatoes, rice or pasta) or fruit as soon as you feel like it. Salty soups, too, are fine and can help you by replacing the salt lost through the loose stools. However, if you don't feel like eating anything, don't worry. Not eating for a couple of days does no harm, and your appetite is likely to return soon.

If you're a woman, severe diarrhoea that lasts for more than 24 hours can make the combined oral contraceptive pill less effective, and so you're at an increased risk of becoming pregnant. If this situation applies, you need to use additional contraceptive precautions during and for seven days after recovery.

Continually having 'the runs'

Ongoing diarrhoea can be annoying and embarrassing. Consider this list of important and common causes if you suffer from persistently loose and frequent stools:

- ✔ **Alcohol misuse:** Too much alcohol drunk over a prolonged period of time can cause persistent diarrhoea. Reduce the amount and frequency of your drinking.

- ✔ **Antibiotics:** Antibiotics that are used to treat infection may also lead to diarrhoea. Discuss the options for managing your symptoms or changing treatment with your GP.

- ✔ **Laxative misuse:** Taking too many stool softeners (known as *laxatives*) can cause loose and frequent stools. Reduce the number you take, or discuss alternatives with your GP.

If diarrhoea is affecting your life to the extent that you're always running to the toilet or don't like socialising anymore because of the problem, get your GP to check you over. See your GP to rule out more serious underlying causes such as infection, immune conditions or bowel cancer if, in addition to diarrhoea, you experience any of the following symptoms:

✔ You experience unintentional weight loss over a few weeks or months, prolonged fever, persistent loss of appetite and fatigue, a feeling of being unwell and sweats that last for more than seven to ten days.

✔ You notice a persistent change in your bowel habit to looser stools, particularly along with blood-stained stools, weight loss or abdominal pain. These symptoms may suggest bowel cancer, which gets more common in people over the age of 40.

These symptoms don't necessarily mean that something serious is going on, but they should prompt you to visit your GP. Don't panic, because numerous other causes from food intolerance to diabetes, bacterial bowel overgrowth and problems with food absorption can be responsible. In general, if you have uncertainty over what's causing your symptoms, see your GP.

Pulling the plug on constipation

Constipation is when your stools become hard and you find it difficult or even painful to pass them when going to the toilet. Being constipated once in a while is common and usually completely harmless. Often, a good reason exists for getting 'bunged up'. Check if any of the following possible causes of constipation apply to you (ordered from the most common to the least):

✔ **Lack of fibre in your diet:** To combat what's probably the most common reason for constipation, make sure that you take plenty of fibre in your diet. Foods high in fibre include cereals, bran, wholemeal bread, fruit and vegetables.

✔ **Postponing going to the toilet:** Resisting the call of nature when you have a busy lifestyle is easy, but try to avoid doing so. Ignoring the urge to poo, or *defecate,* means that your stool stays longer in your bowel, where it becomes drier and harder.

✔ **Drugs:** Some painkillers, particularly the stronger ones that contain codeine or similar substances, can reduce your bowel activity and cause constipation. Other drugs that may be responsible include antidepressants, iron tablets, calcium supplements, water tablets (also known as *diuretics*), medicines for treating epilepsy and acid-reducing medication. See your pharmacist or GP for advice if you think any of these items may be responsible for you living with 'slow motion'.

✔ **Lack of exercise:** Not moving about much (for example, through illness) can bring on constipation. Exercising can be very effective in improving bowel function, but if you can't be active make sure that you drink plenty of water and have lots of fibre in your diet.

✔ **Overuse of laxatives:** Regularly using laxatives can lead to your bowel becoming lazy. See your pharmacist for advice on safe levels of laxative use and alternatives you can try. Some slimming diets can also cause constipation.

✔ **Conditions affecting the anus:** Anal disorders, such as a tear in the lining of the back passage (called *anal fissure* – see the section 'Turning your back on anal problems' later in this chapter for more information) or haemorrhoids, may make opening your bowels difficult or uncomfortable. Don't delay going to the toilet because of this discomfort: doing so may only make things worse. See your pharmacist or GP for advice on how to deal with this problem.

✔ **Irritable bowel syndrome:** Changes in your bowel habits may indicate a common condition called *irritable bowel syndrome*, particularly if you also pass mucus and suffer from abdominal bloating and discomfort. See your GP for advice.

✔ **Pregnancy:** Constipation is common in pregnancy and usually improves after giving birth.

✔ **Drinking too much alcohol or caffeine-containing drinks:** These drinks can cause dehydration, and so ensure that you don't overdo it and drink plenty of water as well.

✔ **Other causes:** On rare occasions, other conditions can cause constipation. See your GP for further assessment if none of the preceding causes seem to apply to you, so she can rule out these more unusual possibilities.

In most cases, constipation is short-lived and settles by itself. Increasing the amount of exercise you do and eating plenty of fruit and vegetables – at least five portions a day – often helps to keep things moving. See your pharmacist or GP if your symptoms persist for more than two weeks or you're worried for other reasons.

High-fibre diet – what's in it for me?

Most plant foods such as cereals and vegetables contain some indigestible material called *fibre*, or *roughage*. Having enough fibre in your diet is important, because it ensures that your stools are bulky enough to pass through your bowels and stay nice and soft. A high-fibre diet also reduces the risk of bowel cancer and other bowel conditions. And by eating plenty of fibre you may also find losing weight easier – because you feel full without the extra calories.

Fruit, vegetables, beans and pulses, as well as unrefined cereals and bran, contain a high proportion of fibre. Don't overdo it with these foods though, because too much fibre can sometimes lead to unpleasant bloating and tummy-rumbling.

Do visit your GP, however, if your constipation doesn't improve after 10–14 days or if you notice any of the following symptoms – particularly if you're over the age of 50, have never suffered from constipation before or if these symptoms persist for six weeks or more:

- ✔ You experience blood in your stools and don't have any anal symptoms such as bleeding or pain.

- ✔ You lose weight for no apparent reason.

- ✔ You feel tired all the time.

- ✔ You feel sweaty, feverish or just not 'right'.

- ✔ You have a feeling of incomplete emptying of your bowels.

Getting a Feel for Stomach Ache and Other Problems

Abdominal pain anywhere between your lower ribcage and your groin is common and can be due to a variety of possible causes. Such pain may occur together with nausea and vomiting or just by itself, and the causes of these symptoms can overlap. Rest assured that most of the time abdominal pain is due to benign causes such as a mild stomach upset or overeating.

Sometimes, though, abdominal pain indicates a more serious underlying cause. This section enables you to assess abdominal pain, and to spot some of the danger symptoms and features of the more common underlying conditions. (For abdominal pain in children, take a look at Chapter 16.)

Exploring abdominal pain

When you're ill, the main thing for you to determine is how serious your condition is – whether you can safely 'wait and see', or whether you need to seek medical help. Quite often, the exact cause of abdominal pain may be hard to fathom, and so taking a systematic approach when making an assessment is helpful.

To start your assessment of the problem, ask yourself these two questions:

- ✔ **When did the pain start?** The acute onset of a pain that you've never had before – as opposed to a pain you've had for a long time and that doesn't bother you too much – is more likely to need assessment by a medical professional.

✔ **Where is the pain?** Identifying the area of the pain can often – though not always – help you with identifying the possible underlying causes. Table 11-1 gives an overview of which conditions or organs are related to individual areas of the abdomen.

Abdominal pain isn't always related directly to the underlying organs, but can originate in other areas, such as the chest or the testicles (also known as *referred pain*). Pain from inside the abdomen can also spread to other parts of the body. For example, you may feel pain caused by gallstones or inflammation of your pancreas in your back as well as your front.

Table 11-1 Areas of Abdominal Pain and Some Possible Causes

Location of Pain Within the Abdomen	*Possible Underlying Conditions*
Right upper corner	Gallstones; inflammation of the pancreas
Upper middle part	Stomach problems such as indigestion, an ulcer or reflux of stomach contents into the gullet; heart problems; inflammation of the pancreas
Central area	Appendicitis (initially; pain then typically moves from there down to the right lower area); ruptured blood vessel (called *abdominal aortic aneurysm*, or *AAA*; rare, and usually in older people)
Both lower corners	Bowel, kidney and female organ problems
Lower middle part	Bladder problems such as urine infection or female organ conditions such as period pains

Getting to the bottom of your abdominal pain can be tricky, and many more causes than those listed in Table 11-1 may be responsible. To list all the potential causes here is impossible, but you may be able to recognise some important conditions from your symptoms:

✔ **Drugs:** Some drugs such as aspirin and ibuprofen can cause abdominal pain. If you take medicines regularly and get abdominal symptoms, check the drug information leaflet and speak to your pharmacist or GP if you're concerned. Be aware that drugs called *steroids*, sometimes prescribed for treatment of arthritis or other chronic conditions, can mask abdominal symptoms – which means that you may experience less pain than you would if you weren't taking the medicines. Therefore, seek medical advice sooner rather than later.

✔ **Gallstones:** If gallstones get stuck in the tube that connects the gall bladder to your bowels, you may suffer from intermittent pain that waxes and wanes (called *colicky* pain). You're also likely to feel sick or vomit when you get the pain. Consult your GP.

✔ **Gastroenteritis:** Abdominal pain is a common symptom when you have a tummy bug (also known as *gastroenteritis*). Typically, the illness starts quickly and you may feel quite unwell with nausea, vomiting and loose stools. You may also have a fever. Gastroenteritis pain tends to get better after opening your bowels and is usually cramp-like. You can find more on this condition in the earlier section 'Enduring acute gastroenteritis'.

✔ **Hernia:** A swelling in your groin area is due to a break in the muscular wall of your abdomen, leading to bowel contents being pushed through (called an *inguinal hernia*), which can get worse on coughing or straining when the hernia gets trapped. In most cases, you can push the swelling back – although it usually recurs quickly. Flip to Chapter 12 for more about hernias, and see your GP for more assessment.

✔ **Indigestion:** Pain or abdominal discomfort after eating is known as *indigestion*. Speak to your pharmacist about over-the-counter preparations to relieve your symptoms. However, if your symptoms don't settle or are severe, do consult your GP.

✔ **Irritable bowel syndrome:** Intermittent abdominal pain may be due to what's called *irritable bowel syndrome*, particularly if you also have other bowel symptoms such as diarrhoea, constipation or wind. See your GP for further assessment.

✔ **Pregnancy:** If you're a woman of childbearing age, consider pregnancy as a possible cause for your abdominal pain, particularly if your period is late and you have other pregnancy-related symptoms such as tender breasts, passing urine more frequently or feeling very tired. You can get a home pregnancy test from your local pharmacy to find out if you're pregnant. Contact your GP immediately if the test confirms that you're pregnant or if you could possibly be pregnant but haven't done a test. Although most abdominal pain in pregnancy is harmless, some of the potential underlying causes are serious and need urgent assessment and treatment. For further information, check out the relevant sections in Chapter 18.

✔ **Urine infection:** Urine infections (most commonly due to bladder infection, or *cystitis*) can cause pain in the middle of your lower abdomen – the area where your bladder is. Other symptoms of urine infection are burning or stinging when urinating and passing urine frequently. Your urine may look cloudy or even blood-stained. Contact your GP because you may need antibiotics, particularly if the pain spreads towards your *loins* (the areas below your bottom ribs on your back and your sides), which can indicate an infection of your kidney (known as *pyelonephritis*) – particularly if you also have a fever and feel lousy. Turn to Chapter 12 for more on urinary problems and bladder infections.

If your abdominal pain isn't too severe, drinking fluid in small amounts regularly, and taking simple painkillers such as paracetamol, may help to relieve mild pain. Perhaps also keep a bowl ready in case you need to be sick. If your symptoms resemble the conditions in Table 11-1, however, or in the preceding bulleted list, seek medical help, especially if you also notice any of the following:

- ✔ You lose weight for no reason and experience night sweats, fevers, constant pain, excessive tiredness and/or bleeding from the back passage.

- ✔ Your pain is getting worse all the time.

- ✔ Your pain is constant, without any periods of relief.

- ✔ You develop back pain in addition to abdominal pain.

- ✔ You also suffer from severe diarrhoea or constipation.

- ✔ You have a fever. (With abdominal pains, however, young children and people who are very old or severely ill may not always develop a fever, even if they have a severe underlying infection.)

- ✔ You notice a lump or other swelling in your abdomen.

Occasionally, your abdominal pain may be due to a more serious underlying cause. Speak urgently to your GP or consider calling '999' in the event of a true emergency when you get worse very quickly if you experience severe tummy pain plus any of the following symptoms:

- ✔ You have a very painful and rigid tummy that's tender on pressure.

- ✔ You suddenly feel faint or drowsy.

- ✔ You're pregnant and you develop a sudden onset of abdominal pain. Take action particularly if this pain is in the lower abdomen in early pregnancy, if you feel faint or have collapsed and if you notice dark vaginal discharge.

- ✔ You also experience chest tightness, shortness of breath, nausea or vomiting.

- ✔ You also have a rapid pulse and cold, clammy or sweaty skin.

- ✔ You vomit blood, have bleeding from the back passage, notice blood in your urine or, if you're a woman, suffer from any non-menstrual vaginal bleeding.

Tummy pain can be tricky to suss out, and so if you're unsure about the cause or you have any additional symptoms not covered in this section, speak to your doctor.

Attacking abdominal swelling

Have you ever noticed that your tummy swells up for no apparent reason, and then goes down again as if nothing has happened? If so, don't worry – you're not the only one. Many women and – less commonly – men suffer from intermittent swelling of the abdomen, an unpleasant symptom that may make you feel embarrassed. Fortunately, usually no serious underlying cause is to blame.

Common causes of abdominal swelling

Persistent or increasing swelling of the abdomen, however, is one of those symptoms that you do need to take seriously. If your swelling comes on gradually or occurs regularly, consider the following causes:

- **Constipation:** If your stools are hard and dry, abdominal swelling may be due to constipation (check out the 'Pulling the plug on constipation' section earlier in this chapter).

- **Excessive wind:** Acute swelling of the abdomen may simply be due to excess wind in your bowels – you often notice rumbling noises. Getting rid of the wind through your mouth or back passage usually relieves the swelling and discomfort.

  Excessive wind is hardly ever anything to worry about, and is usually brought on by eating certain foods such as cabbage or beans, or due to swallowing air. Speak to your pharmacist about over-the-counter medications that can relieve your symptoms and consult your GP if you fail to improve.

- **Fluid retention:** Rarely, a build-up of fluid (also called *fluid retention*) due to heart, liver or kidney problems can cause swelling of the abdomen. Where this problem is the cause, your ankles may also be puffy – check whether you can produce indentations when you press into the swelling for a few seconds with your fingertip. If you think that you may be accumulating fluid, ask your GP to check you over.

- **Hormonal changes:** If you're a woman and the swelling comes on at the same time as your period or at some other regular time in your cycle, it may be due to hormonal changes. Such changes aren't dangerous, but do see your GP if you're concerned.

- **Obesity:** Simply being overweight is one of the most common causes of a swollen abdomen (check out Chapter 7).

- **Pregnancy:** If a chance exists that you may be pregnant, do a home pregnancy test (you can buy these kits at your local pharmacy) and contact your GP surgery for pregnancy-related advice if the test is positive.

✔ **Urine retention:** A sudden painful swelling in the lower abdomen may be due to retention of urine in the bladder. Enlargement of the prostate gland in men is a common cause of this problem. Contact your GP immediately. Chapter 12 has more on prostate problems.

Contact your GP or call '999' in an emergency if you suffer from an acutely swollen abdomen and any of the following symptoms:

✔ Sudden onset of persistent severe pain, where passing wind doesn't relieve your pain. This pain may, in rare cases, be due to an obstructed bowel.

✔ You vomit and feel very unwell and unusually drowsy, or have passed out.

Ovarian cancer

The *ovaries* are small grape-size organs close to the womb that produce eggs in women of childbearing age; in rare instances, abdominal swelling may be due to ovarian cancer. Although cancer of the ovaries can develop at any age, it appears more commonly in older women and where another family member has developed ovarian cancer.

This condition has in the past been known as 'the silent killer', but new research shows that many women with ovarian cancer start showing early symptoms for about a year prior to getting a formal diagnosis. So, by knowing and being able to spot the signs of ovarian cancer early on, you stand a better chance of dealing with it successfully.

Symptoms of ovarian cancer are often vague, but are present almost all the time – not just on occasional days – and may include:

✔ Constant, persistent bloating (not bloating that comes and goes).

✔ Difficulty eating, and feeling full quickly.

✔ Increased abdominal size.

✔ Persistent pelvic and abdominal pain over weeks and months.

Occasionally, ovarian cancer can lead to other additional symptoms such as:

✔ A change in your bowel habit.

✔ A feeling of being tired all the time for no apparent reason.

✔ New and unexplained back pain.

✔ Urinary symptoms, such as going for a wee more frequently than usual or having to go suddenly.

Remember that if you experience any of these symptoms, ovarian cancer is unlikely to be the cause; lots of other, benign conditions can bring them on. But if symptoms persist, get worse, are very frequent or appear out of the blue without an obvious cause, do consult your GP to rule out ovarian cancer. For further information and advice, check out the Ovarian Cancer Action website at www.ovarian.org.uk.

Battling with the Back Passage

Unlike Paul Simon's song, in which you have '50 ways to leave your lover', stools can leave you in only one way! Although problems with the back passage and the *anus* – the short bit of your intestine that connects the end of the bowel to the outside – are common, most people would really rather ignore them, if it wasn't for the discomfort or pain they can cause.

Not surprisingly, speaking to a pharmacist or GP about any issues involving this part of your body can take a lot of courage. But you're not alone, and don't worry – doctors have heard and seen it all before, and they all prefer that you come and speak to them about your problem instead of sitting at home suffering in silence. Don't hesitate to ask for advice or further assessment from your GP if you can't make out your underlying problem from this section.

Turning your back on anal problems

A ring of muscles called the *sphincter* closes the anus, and as long as it's intact the sphincter prevents bowel contents from spilling out. This area of the body is very sensitive, and so even minor conditions here can cause considerable discomfort and reduce your quality of life considerably. The good news is that most conditions affecting the anal region are fairly straightforward to identify. (Because you can't see your back passage, you can place a hand-mirror on the floor and have a look that way.) Here are some of the common conditions:

- **Anal fissure:** If passing stools is painful, you may be suffering from an *anal fissure* – a small tear in the anus, or from haemorrhoids. Anal fissures may develop after passing a very hard or large stool. Medicines (available from your pharmacist or GP) for making the faeces softer can assist, but helping your anus to heal and preventing recurrences by eating a diet high in fibre is the best way forward (you can find more information about this subject in the earlier sidebar 'High-fibre diet – what's in it for me?').

✔ **Anal warts:** Warts around your anus (also called *genital warts*) are caused by a viral infection of your skin, and can be transmitted sexually. You may only have one or two, or more of them. See your GP to discuss the various treatment options.

✔ **Haemorrhoids:** Swollen veins around the anus are called *haemorrhoids*, or *piles*, and are extremely common. They frequently cause itching, irritation and intermittent bleeding from the back passage and, if present, you may see fresh blood on the toilet paper or even notice it dripping into the toilet pan.

Pharmacists can help you find available treatments – many over-the-counter preparations are available without prescription. In severe or persistent cases, however, see your GP to discuss the treatment options and to rule out other causes of anal symptoms. Also, check out the later section 'Bleeding from the back passage'.

✔ **Skin infection:** A sore area just above your anus is most likely due to an infected skin pouch (called *pilonidal sinus*), which is sometimes caused by an in-growing hair or a collection of pus known as an *anal abscess*. These conditions may heal by themselves or with antibiotics, but often need an operation to clear the infected area, and so getting your GP to check you out is always a good move.

✔ **Skin inflammation:** Sometimes, the anus may be very itchy and sore without any apparent reason (a condition called *pruritus ani*). Although resisting may be difficult, try not to scratch if possible. Your pharmacist or GP can advise you with regard to soothing ointments.

Avoid using soapy water to wash your anus and instead just let cool or warm (not hot) water run over your back passage. Some people find that wearing cotton underwear helps to reduce the itching.

✔ **Threadworms:** Itching around the anus and small white threads in your faeces indicate that you've acquired threadworms, either through touching contaminated surfaces, such as toilet seats which haven't been disinfected in a household where someone has threadworms, or from contaminated food. This common infection is harmless and easily treatable with over-the-counter medicine from your pharmacist, or on prescription from your GP. Usually your whole household need to be treated.

Make sure that you wash your hands carefully after going to the toilet and before you prepare food and clean potentially infected areas (such as toilet seats, door handles and basin taps) with disinfectant.

Bleeding from the back passage

Bleeding from the back passage (or *rectal bleeding*) is a common symptom. Particularly if you belong to a younger age group (that is, under the age of 50), rectal bleeding is rarely serious though it can be. The chance of a more worrying underlying cause (such as bowel cancer) increases with age, so it's best to consult your GP to get checked.

In this section I give you the low-down on possible reasons as to why you may bleed from your back passage, and what you should do about it.

Benign causes of rectal bleeding

If you bleed from your back passage at the same time as or just after painful or uncomfortable emptying of your bowels, the chances are that you have a benign underlying cause such as an *anal fissure* or *haemorrhoids* – particularly if the blood looks bright red or drips into the toilet pan. Check out the previous section 'Turning your back on anal problems' for more information on anal fissures and haemorrhoids.

Other non-cancerous causes of rectal bleeding

A number of other conditions can cause rectal bleeding, some benign and some more serious. Here's an overview of some causes of rectal bleeding, starting with the least serious one:

- **Diverticular disease:** Constipation – when you persistently have to strain to defecate – can cause small pouches, or *diverticula*, the size of a pea or a grape to form inside the wall of your bowel. These pouches can become inflamed or infected – a condition called *diverticulitis*. This problem can cause pain over the lower left side of your abdomen that opening your bowels or passing wind often relieves. Intermittent diarrhoea or constipation are common signs of diverticular disease, and you may also pass blood from your back passage. Distinguishing diverticular disease from other conditions without further tests can be impossible, and so make sure that you ask your GP to check you over.

- **Inflammatory bowel disease:** Ongoing rectal bleeding together with loose stools may be due to an inflammation of the bowel. The two main conditions are called *ulcerative colitis* and *Crohn's disease*, and diagnosis is usually made by a specialist after referral by your GP. Diagnosing these conditions usually involves looking at the inside of your bowel with a flexible fibre-optic telescope and taking some tiny tissue samples.

Bowel cancer

Cancer of the large bowel (which can be *colon* or *rectal* cancer) is one of the most common cancers in the UK and is the second leading cause of death from cancer. Rectal bleeding may be the only symptom of bowel cancer (particularly as you get older from the age of 40 onward), and the chances of you having bowel cancer increase if you have additional symptoms.

Consulting your GP to rule out bowel cancer because of rectal bleeding is especially important if the following circumstances apply to you:

- ✔ You're over the age of 40.
- ✔ You notice a change in bowel habit to looser stools and/or increased frequency of opening your bowels.
- ✔ You notice blood mixed in with your stool.
- ✔ You have rectal bleeding with no anal symptoms.
- ✔ You suffer from persistent abdominal pain.
- ✔ You experience general symptoms such as weight loss, loss of appetite, tiredness, sweats, feeling unwell and sweats.
- ✔ You leak faeces in the absence of an acute bowel infection.

Remember that haemorrhoids and cancer may sometimes co-exist – particularly as you get older.

Most people feel worried and embarrassed when visiting their GP with problems of the back passage, perhaps because they worry it may be cancer or because they dread the thought of being examined or investigated in such an intimate area. The quicker your GP checks your symptoms, however, the better – if caught in its early stages, bowel cancer can be cured completely!

Chapter 12

Getting Lower: Urinary and Other Disturbances 'Down There'

....

....

*M*edical stories are always popular – they're often shared between friends and family, and regularly come up during dinner conversations. But the talking quickly dries up when the subject turns to urinary problems. Why? Urinary problems are incredibly common, and yet many people feel too embarrassed to talk about them. Discussing back pain or flu with other people is easy – anyone can do it – but leaking urine or rushing to the toilet all the time is a different matter. Research shows that people can take many years before they talk to a health professional about their urinary problems – which is a shame, because so much can be done about them.

This chapter gives you the basic low-down on urinary problems and I hope encourages you to seek medical help early if you're affected.

Going With the (Urinary) Flow

Urinary symptoms are often due to problems with your *bladder* (a thin-walled hollow organ like a balloon) or your *pelvic floor* (a thin layer of muscles deep in your pelvis that supports your internal organs like a hammock and helps prevent your bladder from leaking). Sometimes, other more 'mysterious' causes may be responsible. For example, passing urine frequently can occasionally be an early sign of diabetes or indicate a problem with the heart. This section gives you the low-down on troubles with the waterworks and what you can do about them.

TECHNICAL STUFF

Producing and getting rid of urine

You produce urine in your kidneys, which filter your blood to produce it. The urine then flows from your kidneys through small tubes (known as *ureters*) into your bladder for storage. At certain intervals your bladder becomes full, and the increasing tension in the lining of the bladder signals through nerves to your brain that you need to find a toilet. You then pass urine through another tube (called the *urethra*) that empties the bladder. Simple as that!

Experiencing urinary symptoms

Problems with the organs that produce and store your urine – particularly the bladder – can cause a number of symptoms that can make your life a misery. Fortunately, many effective treatments are available.

Cystitis and urethritis

Pain and discomfort while passing urine are very common and in the vast majority of cases are due to an infection of the bladder, called *cystitis*. Cystitis is much more common in women than in men because the urethra in women is much shorter, meaning that infections can more easily enter the bladder. You may also be at an increased risk of developing bladder infections if any of the following situations apply to you:

- ✔ You're a woman going through the menopause.

- ✔ You have an abnormality of the urinary tract organs involved in producing or storing urine.

- ✔ You're prone to getting infections; for example, if you suffer from diabetes, are in the later stages of life or take drugs – such as steroid medication – that suppress your immune system.

Some common telltale signs of cystitis are as follows:

- ✔ You experience an increased urge to pass urine, giving you less time to get to the toilet.

- ✔ You have a pain in the lower abdomen over the bladder area.

- ✔ You notice a burning sensation when you pass urine.

- ✔ You pass urine little and often.

- ✔ Your urine looks cloudy or blood-stained.

- ✔ In addition, you don't feel well in yourself and you may have a fever.

If your symptoms are mild, see your pharmacist for advice and consider trying over-the-counter medicines first. If your problems are severe, or they start to affect your quality of life, contact your GP or practice nurse. You may need to have your urine tested and take a short course of antibiotics. Seeing your GP is also important for reducing the risk of getting recurrent bladder infections.

The following, more serious, symptoms indicate that you need to see your GP:

- ✔ You pass blood in your urine – particularly if this problem persists (blood in the urine, however, is common in cystitis and can be acceptable in this circumstance).

- ✔ You get severe or recurrent pain in your lower abdomen, in the softer parts of your back and sides just below your ribcage (called the *loins*), or in your lower back.

- ✔ You feel very unwell.

- ✔ You notice an unusual discharge from your genital area.

- ✔ You have a fever together with your urinary symptoms.

Urinary symptoms can have more likely causes depending on whether you're male or female. If you're a woman and have pain on passing urine, your problem can be due to a number of reasons. Here are some common ones:

- ✔ **Itchy and dry genitals:** Inflammation and itching of the genital area (or *pruritus vulvae*) is common, and often has no obvious underlying cause. Due to falling hormone levels you're more likely to develop a dry vagina when you're past the menopause (or 'the change'). Using perfumed soap or experiencing sexual anxiety may also be responsible. When this happens, you are more likely to develop urinary infections or 'irritation' down below, causing burning and stinging when you pass urine.

- ✔ **Thrush:** Vaginal thrush (also called *candidiasis*) is a common fungal infection and usually shows up with a profuse thick white vaginal discharge. You may also notice soreness around the outside of your genitals (known as the *vulva*). Taking antibiotics or certain types of oral contraceptive pill, or suffering from diabetes, makes you more likely to develop thrush. You can treat thrush yourself, and over-the-counter preparations are readily available from your pharmacist, but if your symptoms persist or are unusual, do visit your GP or practice nurse.

- ✔ **Urethral syndrome:** This inflammation of the *urethra* – the tube that empties your bladder – may occur after sexual intercourse and is due to mild bruising. You may experience an uncomfortable burning sensation when you pass urine, or find yourself going to the toilet more frequently. If your symptoms don't settle by themselves, see your GP to get your urine tested. You may be prescribed a course of antibiotics in case you have an underlying urine infection.

Keeping cystitis at bay – for women

If you're a woman and suffer from cystitis, taking the following steps may help to relieve your symptoms or prevent them from recurring:

- ✔ Take paracetamol or ibuprofen for pain relief; placing a hot water bottle over your lower abdomen may also make you more comfortable.

- ✔ Drink plenty of non-sugary drinks and avoid drinks that contain caffeine, particularly in hot weather.

- ✔ Empty your bladder before and after intercourse and consider using an additional lubricant.

- ✔ Empty your bladder frequently, wherever possible.

- ✔ Keep your genital area clean but avoid vaginal douches, heavily scented soaps and deodorants.

- ✔ Avoid wearing nylon tights or underwear: cotton is usually better.

- ✔ Wipe from front to back after using the toilet.

Remember to see your GP if your symptoms don't go away or are very severe.

Urinary symptoms in women

If possible try not to scratch for any reason when you have itching or soreness 'down below'. Doing so often makes things worse. Use lukewarm water only for a gentle daily wash. Soothing creams from the pharmacy may help, but try to avoid perfumed bath salts, deodorants and talcum powder. You may also want to avoid wearing synthetic underwear – cotton is usually better. Also consider using lubricating jelly if your vagina is dry during intercourse. If the symptoms persist, see your GP for further assessment.

Urinary symptoms in men

Urinary problems in men become more common in later life, when enlargement of a chestnut-sized organ called the *prostate gland* is often responsible. The prostate gland sits deep inside your lower abdomen and surrounds your urethra where it leaves the bladder. As men get older and past 50 years old the prostate gland may enlarge and press on the urethra. Although a normal part of ageing, the symptoms can become troublesome.

If you have an enlarged prostate gland, you may have some of these symptoms:

- ✔ Your urine doesn't flow as fast as it used to.

- ✔ You pass small amounts of urine frequently.

- ✔ Your urine takes a while to come out.

- ✔ You dribble at the end of urination and lack full control when you try to stop.

> ✔ You urinate in stops and starts.

> ✔ You have a sensation of not completely emptying your bladder.

> ✔ You have to get up more often at night to pass urine.

Usually, difficulties with passing urine are due to a benign swelling of the prostate, called *benign prostatic hyperplasia.* Much less commonly, but importantly, the same symptoms may be due to *prostate cancer,* so do see your GP for an assessment and further tests. Your GP probably needs to arrange a simple blood test (called *Prostate Specific Antigen,* or *PSA,* test) that can help with diagnosing prostate cancer, and check your prostate gland with a gloved finger via your back passage. This procedure called *rectal examination* is best done afterwards as it can raise the PSA and, in case you're worried, it may be a bit uncomfortable but usually doesn't hurt.

The following additional symptoms may sometimes suggest prostate cancer:

> ✔ Blood in your urine or semen.

> ✔ Constant, worsening pain in your back, hips, pelvis or other bony areas.

> ✔ Pain on passing urine.

> ✔ Problems with achieving or maintaining erections.

The CancerHelp UK website (at www.cancerhelp.org.uk) provides more information on prostate cancer.

If you're suddenly unable to pass urine despite feeling a strong urge, you may have gone into what experts call *urinary retention,* which means that you can't pass urine, usually due to an obstruction. Taking a warm bath can sometimes ease your symptoms, but seek medical advice immediately if this approach doesn't help straight away.

Problems due to kidney stones

Sometimes, certain waste chemicals in the urine can crystallise and form small *kidney stones* in the bladder, urethra or the *ureters* (the small tubes that carry urine from your kidney to your bladder). Kidney stones are common and vary in size. Often they aren't problematic, but when they get stuck in one of these structures they can cause considerable pain (also known as *renal colic*).

If you have renal colic, you may suddenly experience one or more of these symptoms:

> ✔ Agitation and restlessness.

> ✔ Blood in your urine.

> ✔ Frequent, painful urination.

> ✔ Nausea and vomiting.
>
> ✔ Pain that comes and goes (but can be constant) and radiates to your groins or genital area.
>
> ✔ Sudden onset of severe loin pain that comes and goes.

If you suffer from renal colic, you're more likely to be pacing around the room rather than lying still, which is one of the main differences compared with other causes of abdominal pain.

If you suspect renal colic, visit your GP, who usually checks your urine and may arrange more tests such as an X-ray or scan. Symptoms often settle quickly if the stone is passed, but sometimes specialist referral is needed for further treatment.

To help prevent problems with kidney stones, drink regular glasses of water to help your body dissolve and flush out any stones.

Kidney infection

Rarely, a urine infection may spread towards your kidneys. In addition to your urinary symptoms, you may feel unwell and have pain in your back or sides, and a raised temperature. Treatment with antibiotics is necessary to prevent any damage, so see your GP who can assess you and start treatment as appropriate. Further tests, which may include taking scans of your kidneys, are sometimes necessary for checking out your urinary system.

Sexually transmitted infections

Pain while passing urine can sometimes be due to a sexually transmitted infection. If confirmed, you're likely to need antibiotics, and any sexual partners also need treatment. Chapters 18 and 19 have details of how to spot the symptoms and signs of sexually transmitted infections.

Leaking urine

Leaking urine (also called *urinary incontinence*) and poor bladder control can be very distressing. Because of feelings of shame, embarrassment, fear or the loss of independence, many people with this problem avoid talking about it.

Incontinence becomes more common in older age and can range from leaking a few drops and dribbles to a continuous flow of urine. As you get older, incontinence can often lead to other problems such as falls, social isolation and depression, which can be severe enough for some people to say that 'Incontinence doesn't kill, but it takes your life away'. Urinary incontinence does also occur in younger women, however, and is frequently caused by weakened pelvic floor muscles after childbirth.

Urinary incontinence is very common and contrary to common belief can be cured in about 70 per cent of cases. Even where a complete cure isn't possible, many treatments are available to improve things considerably.

If you're a woman and you find that holding your urine is difficult, here are some possible causes to consider:

- ✔ You may have suffered damage to your bladder neck muscles in pregnancy or during labour.

- ✔ Your urethra and pelvic floor muscles may have become weaker in the menopause.

- ✔ You may have developed a prolapsed womb, which you can notice by feeling a discomfort or 'heaviness' between your legs.

The following causes can affect both men and women equally:

- ✔ Your bladder may be more irritable because of recurrent bladder infections, anxiety or other nervous problems.

- ✔ You may suffer lack of bladder control if you have diabetes or a problem affecting your spine.

- ✔ You've suffered a stroke or have dementia.

Various types of incontinence exist, which all require different forms of treatment. In men, problems with the prostate gland are common – refer to the 'Urinary symptoms in men' section earlier in this chapter.

Stress incontinence

Think of your bladder as a balloon that's filled with water. If the knot doesn't seal properly and you squeeze it a bit, water starts to leak out. In a similar way, your bladder is sealed by muscles. If these muscles weaken or get distorted – in women this is particularly common during pregnancy or after childbirth – any increased pressure can then lead to urine leaking out, which is called *stress incontinence*. You may experience the following:

- ✔ You leak urine when you laugh, cough, sneeze or exercise.

- ✔ You can't hold urine for very long.

- ✔ You have a feeling of your bladder not emptying properly.

In stress incontinence, urine leaks tend to be fairly small at a time, and you don't normally have to rush to the toilet or get up at night to pass urine.

Several treatments can help when you suffer from stress incontinence:

✔ **Pelvic floor exercises:** These exercises aim to make the muscles that seal your bladder stronger. Your GP may be able to refer to you to a special continence physiotherapist who can provide more information and show you how to do pelvic floor exercises correctly. You can also download a good information leaflet on how to do pelvic floor exercises from the Patient UK website at www.patient.co.uk.

✔ **Vaginal or other surgery:** Your GP can refer you for surgery to repair or correct any distortion of the muscles, or other anatomy, down below.

Talk to your GP, who assesses and refers you for investigation and treatment if appropriate. In the meantime, or if your symptoms are only mild, speak to your pharmacist for advice. If you're overweight, losing weight may also help, and special sanitary devices including tampons are available for women.

Urge incontinence

Leaking urine caused by involuntary contractions of the bladder muscles is called *overactive bladder*, which can lead to *urge incontinence*. The following signs can indicate urge incontinence:

✔ You find that you can't hold urine in as long as you used to.

✔ You have 'accidents' when you don't get to the toilet in time, because you have such an urge to pass urine.

✔ You're always on the lookout for toilets, wherever you go.

✔ You may get up twice or more at night to pass urine.

✔ You often have to rush to the toilet and don't get much warning.

✔ You may accidentally leak larger amounts of urine and not be able to stop the flow.

Any of these situations may indicate an overactive bladder, particularly if you have no other symptoms that suggest a bladder infection or other problem.

If you suffer from urge incontinence, try to avoid the following:

✔ **Alcohol:** Alcoholic drinks can make you run to the toilet more often.

✔ **Being constipated:** Eat plenty of fruit and fibre, make sure that you drink enough water and see your pharmacist for advice on laxatives in case you need them.

✔ **Caffeine-containing drinks:** Drinking lots of water is good, but tea, coffee and some fizzy soft drinks contain caffeine, which tends to increase urine production and make your bladder more sensitive.

✔ **Going to the toilet just in case:** Only go when your bladder is full, and empty your bladder completely every time. Bending forward at the waist when sitting on the toilet may help.

If your problems are mild, bladder training – trying to hold on to your urine for longer and increasing the time between visits to the toilet – can be effective and may give you back some control. Pelvic floor exercises and medication can also help. See your GP for more advice on treatment options.

To help your GP with making a diagnosis, consider keeping a 'bladder diary' for a few days in which you record your fluid intake and output. For each day, write down the time and amount of any fluid you drink and the amount of urine you pass. To measure the latter, use an old measuring jug or go out and buy a cheap one. Also note down any times that you leak urine together with some description of the circumstances in which it happened.

Speak to your GP urgently if you suddenly lose control of your bladder, particularly if you also have back pain or leg symptoms such as weakness or other odd sensations, which may indicate pressure on the nerves in your spine.

Suffering from frequent urination

Lots of different causes can be behind a need to go to the toilet more frequently than you're used to, many of them quite normal. Being cold, anxious or excited are common benign causes for going to the toilet often, and drinking more alcohol, tea or coffee can also be responsible.

Here's how you can spot the features of some other underlying conditions, starting with the more common ones:

✔ **Urinary tract infection:** Passing urine frequently is a common symptom of a bladder or urethra infection, usually along with other symptoms, too.

✔ **Pregnancy:** Frequently passing urine is a common early sign of pregnancy and isn't usually due to infection unless you also suffer pain or discomfort. Symptoms usually improve after you're more than four months pregnant.

✔ **Narrowing of the urethra:** This condition is more common in women and can be a result of childbirth or frequent bladder infections. Passing urine frequently in small amounts and (usually) a slow urinary stream with no pain or discomfort are signs that a narrowing of the urethra may be the cause. See your GP because you may need to be referred to hospital for tests. A simple surgical procedure is sometimes all you need to sort things out.

If you pass larger amounts of urine frequently, a possibility exists that you may have developed *diabetes*, a condition caused by your body not producing enough of a hormone called *insulin*. Contact your GP immediately if, in addition to the above urinary symptoms, you also notice the following:

- ✔ You feel tired all the time for no apparent reason.
- ✔ You always feel more thirsty than you think is normal.
- ✔ You're losing weight without any change in your eating habits.

Your GP or practice nurse can check for diabetes with a simple blood test, and getting treatment for this condition as soon as possible is important. You can find out more about diabetes in Chapter 20.

Finding blood in your urine

Blood-stained urine is a common symptom and in many cases is due to common causes such as cystitis. Cystitis is particularly likely where you also notice burning or stinging when you pass urine or if you're going to the toilet more frequently. In most cases, infection isn't too much to worry about and settles when the infection is treated. However, do see your GP for a confirmation of the diagnosis and treatment.

Your GP can exclude other potentially serious causes, such as infection or cancer of the bladder, prostate or kidney, injury to your genital area, kidney stones or cysts and taking certain drugs (some antibiotics and aspirin-type medications can cause blood in the urine). Taking medicines such as warfarin, which thins the blood, can cause problems with reduced blood clotting and blood in the urine, although the drug alone is rarely to blame.

Assessing Groin Problems

The *groin* is an area where blood vessels, nerves, bones and other structures such as bowel – and in men, tubes running to and from the testicles – lie close together. Groin symptoms may therefore not always immediately point to the underlying cause.

Experiencing groin pain

Here's a list of common groin problems and how they may show up:

- **Genital problems:** Infection, inflammation or other problems with the testicles in men can cause pain that mainly affects the groin. See your GP.

- **Groin strain:** Pain in your groin can come on when you engage in certain forms of exercise, such as high-impact sports like running, tennis, football or squash. Rest and pain relief are usually all that you need (speak to your pharmacist for suitable over-the-counter preparations) but see your GP if the problem doesn't settle or your symptoms are severe.

- **Hernia:** This condition is a bulging of abdominal contents, such as fat, or bowel through an area of weakness in your abdominal wall. Groin pain may sometimes be the only symptom. The 'Addressing groin swelling' section later in this chapter has more details. See your GP.

- **Kidney stones:** Pain from kidney stones usually comes on suddenly, waxes and wanes, and is often accompanied by urinary symptoms such as pain on passing water or blood in the urine. Visit your GP. (For more info, flip to the earlier section 'Problems due to kidney stones'.)

- **Osteoarthritis of the hip:** Gradual onset of pain in the groin as you get older may indicate *osteoarthritis* – 'wear and tear' – of the hip. Contrary to common belief, hip joint problems usually make their presence felt in the groin and may radiate to the leg and knee; they're not usually felt over the hip joint itself. See your GP if your symptoms don't settle and don't respond to painkillers available over–the-counter. (You can read more about osteoarthritis in Chapter 13.)

Consult your GP if you notice any of the following:

- A sudden or gradual onset of severe pain in the groin, which can sometimes be due to a strangulated hernia.

- A severe pain in your testicle.

- Unexplained general symptoms such as fever, weight loss, not 'feeling right', tiredness or sweats, in addition to the groin pain.

If you're a man, seek medical advice immediately if you develop sudden, severe pain in a testicle and groin pain, which may indicate that your testicle has twisted, affecting its blood supply (called *testicular torsion*). This condition is more common in boys and young men, and an urgent operation is necessary to prevent permanent damage to the testicle. Common additional symptoms include nausea or being sick, lower abdominal pain and feeling faint. The testicle is usually very tender to touch and may be slightly swollen.

Addressing groin swelling

The most common cause of a swelling in the groin is a *hernia,* which means a bulge of abdominal contents through a weak spot in the muscles. Hernias may occur in different places; in the groin, a hernia is called an *inguinal hernia.*

Hernias usually develop where the weaker muscle areas can't withstand an increased pressure in your abdomen. Imagine yourself holding a balloon the size of a tennis ball in your hands. When you close your fist, the pressure in the balloon increases, and when you press hard enough and leave small gaps between your fingers, parts of the balloon squeeze through these gaps. A hernia develops on the same principle. Persistent coughing, lifting heavy objects or straining when opening your bowels increases the pressure within your abdomen and leads to the weaker points of muscles in the groin being stretched. Fatty tissue or part of the bowel can then push through like a balloon between your fingers.

Hernia symptoms may occur suddenly or develop gradually over a period of days, weeks or months. Typical features are:

- A lump in your groin that may go away when you lie down and comes back on straining or coughing. You may or may not be able to push this lump back yourself.
- An aching or dragging sensation (a feeling of 'heaviness') in your groin.

If you develop a hernia, your usual options are to wait and see or to have it repaired with a surgical procedure. You can discuss your options with your GP; what you ultimately do depends on the severity of your symptoms, the size of the hernia, the presence of other symptoms and your general health.

Rarely, you may develop what's called a *strangulated hernia.* Seek medical help immediately if you develop a sudden severe pain in a previous swelling and if you vomit in connection with groin pain and swelling.

Many other causes may be responsible for a swelling in your groin, so visit your GP for further assessment when you're concerned.

Chapter 13

Groaning Bones and Moaning Muscles

....

In This Chapter

▶ Assessing bone, muscle and joint symptoms

▶ Checking out problems with your spine

▶ Looking at shoulder, arm, elbow and hand trouble

▶ Answering questions about hip, leg, knee, ankle and toe complaints

....

*Y*our body has to be able to put up with sometimes considerable strain as you move about, play, exercise and work. Therefore, injuries and problems caused by 'wear and tear' or the overuse of joints, ligaments and muscles are common.

This chapter explains some important causes of problems with these body structures and helps you to manage them. (For further information on injuries, also check out Chapter 5.)

Having a Word About Bone, Muscle and Joint Problems

No doubt you know that you can keep your muscles and joints in shape by exercising them regularly, assuming that you're able to do so. Not moving enough, or putting too much strain on those joints and muscles, can mean that you end up with aches and pains, and sometimes joint swelling and inflammation. Muscular, bone or joint symptoms can affect any part of your body – not just your 'head, shoulders, knees and toes' as the old song goes – and so these problems can severely impair your quality of life.

This section tells you how to spot some important clues when looking for the causes of joint and muscle symptoms.

Hot tips for checking out a swollen joint

If you suddenly develop a hot and swollen joint, the chances are that this problem is due to some form of injury or inflammation. Joint infection is also a possibility, though this is very rare. When one of your joints becomes hot and swollen, consider the following causes:

- **Bursitis:** A number of fluid-filled cushions surround certain joints to prevent overlying muscles and ligaments from rubbing. When these cushions become inflamed due to overuse or direct pressure, you may develop a soft swelling around or close to the joint, called *bursitis* (see image 18 in the colour section). Common locations include your elbow or knees. Rest, as well as prescribed or over-the-counter (such as ibuprofen) anti-inflammatory medication, can help to bring the swelling down. Antibiotics may sometimes be needed to treat or prevent infection.

- **Gout:** *Gout* is where uric acid (a chemical substance that your body produces as part of its normal metabolism) is raised in your bloodstream and crystallises in a joint, leading to inflammation and tenderness (see image 17 in the colour section). Big toes are often affected in gout, and your pain may be so severe that you can't even tolerate a blanket over your foot at night. If you suspect that you have gout, consult your GP, who may give you a prescription for drugs such as anti-inflammatory painkillers or medicines that lower your uric acid blood levels to prevent gout attacks from recurring. If you suffer recurrent attacks, also try to avoid potential triggers such as alcohol or rich foods.

- **Injury:** Injury is one of the most common reasons for a swollen and painful joint – particularly with knees and ankles. If you suffer a mild injury (commonly referred to as *sprain* or *strain*) to a joint, rest the affected body part and cool it down, for example with a packet of frozen peas wrapped in a thin towel. Painkillers and anti-inflammatory gels to help relieve your symptoms are available over-the-counter from your pharmacy. If you suspect a more serious injury, seek medical advice – refer to Chapter 25 for a list of useful helplines and websites or contact your GP surgery.

- **Osteoarthritis:** *Osteoarthritis* is a common cause of joint pain and swelling in later life, and is a condition often said to be due to 'wear and tear' of a joint (see image 20 in the colour section). You don't, however, necessarily develop osteoarthritis just through using your joints a lot; in fact, exercise that doesn't excessively impact upon your joints is beneficial. Other factors may also contribute, such as increased pressure on a joint due to being overweight. Your GP can help to exclude other causes and advise you on suitable painkillers. Physiotherapy and certain exercises can help to relieve the pain, but if things are really bad joint replacement may be the only means of getting rid of your pain and enabling you to go onto the dance-floor again.

✔ **Reactive arthritis:** Bacterial or viral infections in another part of the body (such as the gut or lungs) can sometimes lead to inflammation of one or more joints in your body, which is called *reactive arthritis* (also known as *Reiter's Syndrome*). Knees, ankles and toes are most commonly affected, and your joints are likely to feel stiff before you develop any pain and joint swelling. Other seemingly unrelated symptoms may include inflammation of your eyes and difficulty passing urine. In such cases, antibiotics (if an infection is still present) and anti-inflammatory medication may help. If you suspect reactive arthritis, consult your GP for confirmation of the diagnosis and appropriate treatment.

✔ **Rheumatoid arthritis:** *Rheumatoid arthritis* is a long-term condition that can affect many parts of your body and not only your joints. The joints of the wrists, hands and fingers are commonly involved, but hip, knee and ankle joints may also become stiff and painful (see image 19 in the colour section). Your GP is likely to arrange some blood tests and possibly X-rays if he suspects that this condition may be responsible for your symptoms. If the diagnosis is confirmed, various drugs and other therapies may help to keep the inflammation at bay.

Doctors always keep an eye out for the possibility of joint infection for good reason, because infections can potentially cause permanent damage to a joint if they're missed and not treated properly. Consider the possibility of a more serious joint infection (called *septic arthritis*) if you develop an acute joint problem, particularly under the following circumstances:

✔ You develop a single hot and swollen joint.

✔ You're very reluctant to move the affected joint.

✔ You're unable to bear weight or perform basic essential tasks.

✔ You also have a fever and feel unwell.

✔ You suffer from diabetes.

✔ You have a suppressed immune system (for example, you take steroid medication, undergo chemotherapy, are HIV positive or you suffer from another significant illness).

✔ You've had a recent joint or bone operation, such as a hip or knee replacement.

A number of other causes may be responsible for a hot and swollen joint, and so visit your GP for help with the diagnosis and to get the right treatment if your symptoms are more severe or don't settle by themselves. As a general rule, if your pain is severe and gets worse, or you can't move the affected limb, seek medical advice earlier rather than later.

Aching muscles

For your muscles to ache after playing sports, or when you engage in any other unusual activities such as DIY projects, is normal. Ongoing muscle pains, however, can be frustrating for you and your GP because sussing out the exact underlying cause can be difficult. They can also be very unpleasant and affect your quality of life considerably.

Here are some conditions that may cause muscular aches, starting with the more common ones:

- ✔ **Viral infections:** Viral infections such as influenza-type illnesses (often referred to as *the flu*) commonly cause muscle aches and tend to occur at the same time as other symptoms like sore throat, cough and fever. Taking paracetamol usually helps to relieve these symptoms.

- ✔ **Medication:** Muscle pains can sometimes be a medication side effect, for example, of cholesterol-lowering medication or other drugs. See your pharmacist or GP for a medication review if you think that your muscle aches may be related to the tablets you take.

- ✔ **Underactive thyroid gland:** Chronic muscle aches can be a symptom of an underactive thyroid gland (known as *hypothyroidism*). Usually, you have additional symptoms such as tiredness, always feeling cold, putting on weight, problems with passing stools, low mood and heavy periods in women. See your GP for further assessment and a blood test which will help with making the diagnosis.

- ✔ **Chronic fatigue syndrome:** You may be suffering from *chronic fatigue syndrome* when you feel tired all the time or at intervals without any obvious cause, particularly if you get very tired from exercise after a delay of about 24 hours. Additional symptoms include sleeping problems, headache, painful lymph glands that aren't swollen, feeling unwell and problems with memory or finding words. If your symptoms persist, consult your GP.

- ✔ **Fibromyalgia:** In a condition known as *fibromyalgia*, you may experience widespread tenderness and have an increased sensitivity to pain. Other symptoms include feeling low, a sensation that your joints are swollen although they don't appear so, difficulties with memory or finding words, headaches and sleeping problems. Consult your GP.

- ✔ **Polymyalgia rheumatica:** In people over the age of 50, this condition may sometimes be responsible for muscle pain around the shoulders, hips or neck. In addition, you may feel tired all the time, suffer from morning stiffness (well, more than you expect normally), weight loss, low mood and a mild fever. See your GP for confirmation of the diagnosis. Symptoms usually respond well to a course of steroid tablets.

✔ **Temporal arteritis:** *Temporal arteritis* is an inflammation of a blood vessel over your temple area, which may cause muscle pains in connection with headaches, intermittent or permanent loss of vision, or pain in your jaw when you chew. See your GP for urgent assessment and treatment – which is usually with steroid tablets if the diagnosis is confirmed.

If your muscle pains are severe, last for more than a few days or you notice any of the following symptoms at the same time, you need to seek medical help. In particular, look out for:

✔ Muscle aches combined with swollen joints.

✔ Chest symptoms, such as breathing problems or chest pain.

✔ Unexplained weight loss, tiredness, sweats or swollen glands.

✔ Muscle weakness, particularly if this situation has been getting worse over time.

✔ Other unusual symptoms, such as numbness or tingling.

Muscle aches and pains aren't a normal part of later life. See your GP for further assessment and help with the diagnosis if you're not sure about the cause and when simple over the counter remedies aren't working for you. Various other treatments are available.

Problems With Your Spine: Stripped to the Bone

Your spine is made up of bones called *vertebrae*, between which lie cartilage-like cushions called *discs* that make your spine mobile and act as shock absorbers. Muscles and ligaments hold everything together.

Most of the time, these components work perfectly in harmony with each other, and the good news is that in the majority of cases spine problems aren't due to any serious underlying conditions.

Struggling with back pain

Back pain is very common and a frequent reason for people having to take time off work. Common causes of back pain are as follows:

- **Mechanical back pain:** This type of pain is usually due to muscular tension or abnormal stress or strain on the muscles and ligaments in the lower back.

- **Sciatica:** A pain caused by pressure on a nerve that goes from your back into your leg (the *sciatic nerve*), *sciatica* often occurs because one of the discs between the bones in your spine pushes out temporarily, or sometimes permanently.

Although back pain can be quite severe and disabling, in the vast majority of cases it's not due to any serious underlying problem and usually gets better by itself within a matter of days or a couple of weeks. Rarer causes of back pain, however, include injury to your spine or inflammation of the joints in your back, among other problems.

Seek medical advice as soon as possible if you have back pain, particularly in any of the following circumstances:

- Back pain that travels higher up into your chest area.

- A history of cancer or a depressed immune system due to taking steroid drugs, chemotherapy or HIV infection.

- Loss of sexual function.

- Major trauma, such as a road traffic accident or a fall from a height, or a minor trauma if you suffer from weak bones (known as *osteoporosis*).

- New back pain when you're older than 50 years or younger than 20.

- Night-time pain that prevents you from getting to sleep or that keeps you awake.

- Numbness or loss of sensation around your bottom ('saddle area'), anus or genitals.

- Problems with walking.

- Sudden muscle weakness.

- Trouble passing urine or opening your bowels.

- Unexplained night sweats, fever, weight loss or tiredness.

Even if no clear diagnosis can be made for your back pain, you don't necessarily need further testing and you certainly don't always need a scan or X-rays. No such thing exists as a standard cure for back pain, and you may have to try different approaches before you find something that works for you. Doctors don't advise bed rest anymore, because it can slow your recovery. Gently getting moving again is much better. Only a very small minority of people with back pain need surgery and, in many instances, you don't necessarily even have to stay off work if you suffer from back pain.

Adequate pain relief is very important in helping to speed up your recovery from back pain. Your GP and your pharmacist can advise you about suitable preparations. If your symptoms don't improve by themselves or get worse, though, consider seeing a chiropractor or osteopath, or speak to your GP about other forms of treatment such as physiotherapy, as well as different types of medication.

Check out the Arthritis Research Campaign's website at www.arc.org.uk for further information on back pain and how to prevent it.

Dealing with a pain in the neck

Neck pain is incredibly common. One reason is that your neck muscles become tense when you're stressed which, if it goes on for too long or your neck doesn't get much of a chance to relax, can lead to short-term or longer-lasting neck pain. Other important causes of neck pain include muscular strains from exercising (some sports such as rugby or gymnastics increase the risk of a neck injury), wear and tear of the upper spine and a *whiplash injury*. Whiplash can result from a car accident, when your head is suddenly pushed backward or forward. Only very rarely is a more serious cause such as meningitis or bleeding inside your skull responsible for neck pain.

In the event of minor causes of neck pain, speak to your pharmacist about available over-the-counter preparations like anti-inflammatory drugs or gels, which can help with relieving your symptoms. If your pain is muscular in nature, then a massage can help, too.

Neck pain due to whiplash injury as a result of a car accident is almost never due to injury to the spine itself, but instead is caused by muscle strain and stiffness. X-rays therefore are rarely helpful or necessary.

If you suffer from neck pain, consult your GP in the following circumstances:

- Your pain is very severe.
- Your pain starts as a result of a high-speed or high-impact injury.
- Your pain keeps you awake at night.
- You're tender over one or more of the bones in your neck.
- You're suffering from additional general symptoms such as unexplained fever, night sweats or weight loss.
- You're also experiencing swollen lymph glands in your neck.

> ✔ You're also suffering from weakness or numbness in your arms or legs.
>
> ✔ You've fallen as a result of your neck symptoms.
>
> ✔ You develop tingling or numbness in your shoulders or arms.
>
> ✔ You've been diagnosed with rheumatoid arthritis, cancer, infection or tuberculosis (TB).
>
> ✔ Your immune system is suppressed, for example if you've been diagnosed with HIV, you're undergoing chemotherapy or you're taking steroid medication.

Also visit your GP for further assessment when you can see no obvious explanation for your neck pain, simple over-the-counter remedies don't help, the pain just doesn't get better or you have any other symptoms that you can't explain.

Checking Out Arms, Shoulders and Hands

If you have problems with simple day-to-day activities such as getting dressed, preparing a meal or doing household chores because your arms or shoulders are painful, stiff or just don't work properly, this section ensures that you're not out on a limb for too much longer.

Wrestling with shoulder and arm pain

If you suffer from pain and stiffness in your shoulders or arms, your problem may originate from the shoulder joint or its adjacent muscles, ligaments or tendons, which can easily become inflamed from injury or overuse. Shoulder pain may also occasionally be due to *referred pain* (in other words, pain that originates elsewhere but you feel in your shoulder) from the neck, heart or other structures inside your chest or abdomen. Your shoulders and arms may also ache because of conditions such as frozen shoulder, tendon inflammation or arthritis.

When suffering from shoulder and arm pain and deciding what to do about it, one of the main questions to ask yourself is 'how much does the problem affect my day-to-day life?'. If your symptoms are mild and perhaps due to overuse from sport or work, rest and pain relief with soothing gels or painkillers from your pharmacy may be all that you need. However, if you suffer severe pain and don't know what's going on, and the pain really affects your ability to function as normal at home or at work, your best course of action is to visit a physiotherapist or your GP.

Shoulder problems are most likely to develop in these situations:

✔ Where your job involves repetitive movements and/or vibration (for example, using vibrating tools), or other manual work.

✔ Where you habitually do a lot of sports and exercise involving the shoulders (for example, throwing, swimming or rugby).

✔ Where your shoulder went out of joint at some point in the past (called *shoulder dislocation*).

✔ Where you suffer from arthritis in other joints.

Compare your symptoms with the following list. If any of these scenarios sound close to what you're experiencing, seek medical advice from your GP:

✔ You also suffer from general symptoms such as unexplained fever, weight loss, feeling unwell, night sweats or excessive tiredness.

✔ You also have pain in your chest or abdomen (which can sometimes indicate problems with your heart or gall bladder).

✔ You've had a cancer in the past.

✔ Your skin overlying your shoulder is red and inflamed.

✔ You're unable to use your shoulder or arm.

✔ You experience other unexplained and potentially worrying symptoms such as numbness, tingling or weakness in your arms.

✔ You've suffered significant trauma to your shoulder with the sudden onset of pain.

If you suffer a significant shoulder injury or you suspect that your shoulder may have gone out of joint, go straight to your local Accident & Emergency (A&E) department to get it checked.

On rare occasions, shoulder or arm pain may be the main symptom of a heart attack, particularly if you're at higher risk because you belong to an older age group, smoke, have high blood pressure, are diabetic, have raised cholesterol, or have had heart problems in the past.

Call '999' if you develop sudden shoulder or arm pain at the same time as:

✔ Central chest pain or tightness.

✔ Feeling faint or having collapsed.

✔ Nausea or vomiting.

✔ Shortness of breath.

Tackling elbow problems

Among the most common elbow problems are overuse injuries that cause the inflammation of tendons and other structures around your elbow. You may have heard of *tennis elbow* and *golfer's elbow*, conditions that are in fact more commonly caused by doing DIY work or other activities around the house as opposed to playing tennis or golf. Elbow pain may also be due to referred pain from the neck or shoulder.

Elbow problems can be very disabling and specialise in making life difficult. One of the main factors to help you decide whether you need to see your GP or not is the degree to which you can't use your elbow. You can treat minor elbow problems with over-the-counter preparations from your pharmacy, but when your symptoms are severe, don't improve or significantly affect your daily life, seeking medical advice is usually the way to go.

Compare your symptoms with those I describe for the following conditions:

- ✔ **Elbow injury:** If, after taking a fall or having another injury from sport or work, you have severe elbow pain or can't move your arm well, visit your GP or local A&E for further assessment, because even minor fractures can cause longer-term problems.

- ✔ **Golfer's elbow:** Golfer's elbow is very similar to tennis elbow (check out the last item on this list) but affects the inner side of your elbow.

- ✔ **Olecranon bursitis:** At the back of your elbow joint is a small fluid-filled cushion that prevents tendons from rubbing on the bone. If overused or injured, this cushion may become inflamed and swell up, sometimes to the size of a tennis ball (see image 18 in the colour section). Typically, you don't notice any significant reduction of movement in your elbow joint. Usually, the swelling disappears with rest and over-the-counter anti-inflammatory medication from your pharmacist. But if the problem doesn't improve or you notice signs of infection such as fever, swelling or redness and you feel unwell, consult your GP.

- ✔ **Tennis elbow:** This condition is an inflammation of the outer aspect of your elbow. You probably notice a tender area close to the bony outer bit of your elbow, and the pain tends to get worse with rotational movements such as using a screwdriver or opening a jar. DIY weekend projects are often responsible, particularly if you're not very used to manual work. Rest your arm, try to avoid activities that make the pain worse and see your pharmacist for anti-inflammatory preparations. Your GP can help if your symptoms don't improve after a few days.

Wising up to hand and wrist pain

Many activities can become tricky when your hands don't work properly. Lose the function of one finger or your thumb, and even mundane activities such as unscrewing a bottle or brushing your teeth become difficult. Needless to say that your ability to work may also be greatly affected.

Hand problems are commonly due to overuse, sporting or other injuries, many of which tend to be short-lived and get better by themselves.

Here, I list some common causes and signs of hand and wrist problems, and ways to deal with them:

- **Arthritis:** *Osteoarthritis* – a form of wear and tear of your joints – is more common in older age, but *rheumatoid arthritis* (due to an auto-immune process) may start when you're younger (see image 19 in the colour section). Typical features include joint pain and swelling, which vary from day to day (see image 20 in the colour section). In rheumatoid arthritis, you may experience additional symptoms, such as feeling tired and unwell. Paracetamol and anti-inflammatory medication often help, but do see your GP for more assessment because rheumatoid arthritis often needs more intensive treatment.

- **Carpal tunnel syndrome:** Tingling in the tips of your thumb, index, middle and one half of your ring finger as well as over the thumb-side of your palm and back of your hand suggests *carpal tunnel syndrome*, which is due to pressure on a nerve running through your wrist. Carpal tunnel syndrome is more common if you're overweight or pregnant, or if you do a lot of manual work, but in most cases the cause is unknown. Symptoms are often worse at night and get better when you shake your hands. You may have become clumsier with fine hand movements, and in severe cases you may have lost your full grip strength. Certain hand movements and positions can also make your symptoms worse. Consult your GP if you suspect carpal tunnel syndrome; treatment options include splints, steroid injections or an operation.

- **Dupuytren's contracture:** Painless lumps in the palm of your hand and problems with straightening one or more fingers – which looks like 'clawing' – may be due to this condition. *Dupuytren's contracture* is a fairly common problem that affects the hands, and experts think that the condition is linked to excessive alcohol intake, diabetes and the use of vibrating machinery, but the condition can also occur for no particular reason. If you can't use your hands properly as a result, see your GP for further assessment. In severe cases, an operation may be necessary to straighten your fingers.

- **Tendonitis:** Tendon inflammation (called *tendonitis*) is usually due to overuse through activities such as DIY projects, typing or housework. Resting the affected wrist or hand and using anti-inflammatory gels or medication – speak to your pharmacist for advice on over-the-counter preparations – can help to deal with your symptoms. Sometimes, a wrist splint may relieve the pain. If at all possible, try to avoid activities that make your pain worse until your symptoms settle.

Wrist fractures are common, particularly as you get older. Go to A&E for further assessment if you have a fall or other injury causing pain in your wrist that doesn't get better or is severe, particularly if your wrist looks out of shape. If you feel tender in your wrist near the base of your thumb, this may be due to a fracture of the bones of your forearm or of the *scaphoid bone*, which – if missed and not treated properly – can lead to long-term problems with your wrist.

I cover only the main causes of wrist and hand symptoms in this section – many more possible causes exist. If your problems are severe or persist, you suffer significant loss of function or you're just not sure what's going on, do get your GP to take a look.

Running Through Lower Limb Problems

Your legs are, in many ways, similar to other parts of your body, but they don't always make spotting the underlying cause of a problem all that easy. One of the reasons is that the list of potential causes of leg symptoms is long . . . very long! Sometimes the diagnosis is obvious, but occasionally even experienced health professionals find that getting to the bottom of a leg problem is challenging. In this section, I take a closer look at some of the most important problem areas.

Getting hip to hip conditions

Many conditions can be responsible for hip pain, something that becomes more likely as you get older. Here, I list a selection of some of the more important causes. Bear in mind that hip problems often show up with pain in the groin or knee rather than in the hip itself:

- ✔ **Arthritis:** 'Wear and tear' to joints (known as *osteoarthritis*) is common in later life, whereas *rheumatoid arthritis* often affects people at a younger age. Pain that's often worse when getting up after resting is the main sign of osteoarthritis, and walking may become difficult. See your GP if your pain doesn't get better with over-the-counter painkillers such as paracetamol and ibuprofen, or if walking becomes difficult.

- ✔ **Overuse of the joints:** When you play more sport or walk more than you're used to, overuse of your hips can be the cause of your pain. Overuse pain is common and often gets better by itself with rest and painkillers. Consult your GP if your symptoms don't improve.

- ✔ **Spine problems:** Hip symptoms may be due to problems with the lower spine, particularly if you also have back pain. See your GP for further assessment.

✔ **Trochanteric bursitis:** The inflammation of a fluid-filled cushion over the hip bone (known as *trochanteric bursitis*) can cause hip pain, which may settle by itself with rest. In trochanteric bursitis, the sides of your hips become painful and tender to touch, but usually there's not much else to see. Anti-inflammatory gels or tablets available from your pharmacist may also help. See your GP if your symptoms don't start to improve after a few days.

See your GP for more assessment if you notice the following signs:

✔ Your hip pain is severe and affects your life and mobility considerably.

✔ You develop pain in your hip after an injury or other trauma.

✔ You belong to a younger (under 20 years) or older (over 70 years) age group when you develop hip pain.

✔ Your hip problems seem to get worse over time rather than better.

✔ You've had cancer in the past.

✔ You also experience general symptoms such as unexplained fever, feeling unwell, excessive tiredness or weight loss.

The following symptoms may indicate a hip fracture, particularly if you belong to an older age group, so either speak to your GP or call '999' for an ambulance if you can't walk:

✔ You develop sudden and constant hip pain after a fall.

✔ You can't weight-bear on your affected side.

✔ Your painful leg seems shorter and is rotated inwards.

Some people with ongoing hip problems wrongly believe that nothing can be done about hip pain, that they need to avoid exercise or that surgery is always successful. In fact, a lot can be done about your hip pain, so consult your GP to discuss appropriate treatment options, which often initially involve adequate pain relief and physiotherapy.

Suffering with painful and/or swollen legs

Having your leg pulled often hurts on the inside, but plenty of physical things can go wrong with your legs, too: problems with your skin, blood vessels, nerves, muscles, joints and bones can all cause leg trouble. Sussing out leg symptoms can be tricky, and even health professionals often have problems deciding what may be wrong, because leg pain and swelling can occur alone or in combination with other problems.

Causes of leg pain accompanied by leg swelling

A leg that's both painful and swollen may be caused by any of the following conditions:

- **Cellulitis:** Skin infections (called *cellulitis*) on the leg are common. They may develop without reason but are more likely if you already suffer from *athlete's foot* (an itchy fungal infection that commonly occurs between your toes) or if you have diabetes or poor circulation. Having a tender leg is a sign that you may have cellulitis. You also have a red patch on the skin that may spread, and you may have a fever and feel generally unwell. See your GP, because you'll probably need a course of antibiotics if the diagnosis is confirmed.

- **Thrombosis:** A *deep vein thrombosis* (or DVT) is a blood clot in one of your veins, usually in your leg. This clot can be dangerous, because if it dislodges and travels within the bloodstream to your lung (called *pulmonary embolism*), it can cause severe breathing problems – a medical emergency.

  You're at an increased risk of developing a DVT in these circumstances:

  - You've had major surgery within the last four weeks.

  - You've recently travelled a long distance without moving about much.

  - You're overweight or obese.

  - You're a pregnant woman.

  - You've had a thrombosis in the past.

  - You're a woman taking the combined oral contraceptive pill or hormone replacement therapy (HRT).

  - You've been confined to bed for more than a day or two.

  - You have your leg in plaster because of a leg injury.

  - You have a diagnosis of active cancer.

  Call '999' if you have a swollen and/or painful leg and notice the following signs, which may indicate a lung problem due to a dislodged blood clot from your leg:

  - You suffer from unexplained chest pain or shortness of breath.

  - You feel faint or have passed out.

  - You notice that your heart's beating very fast.

- **Varicose veins:** Veins that lie just beneath your skin and are enlarged because of impaired blood flow are called *varicose veins* and may lead to aching legs, particularly after standing for prolonged periods. Varicose

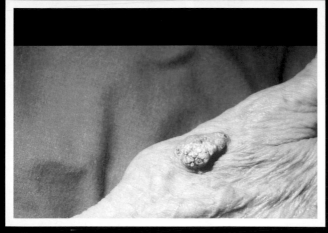

1. Squamous cell carcinoma (Ch 8): Detected and treated early, this skin cancer is usually curable.

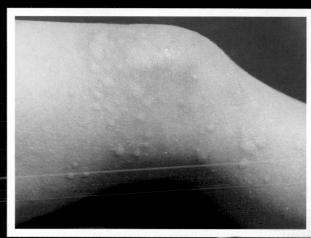

2. Nettle rash (urticaria) (Ch 8): Antihistamines are used to treat this raised and itchy rash.

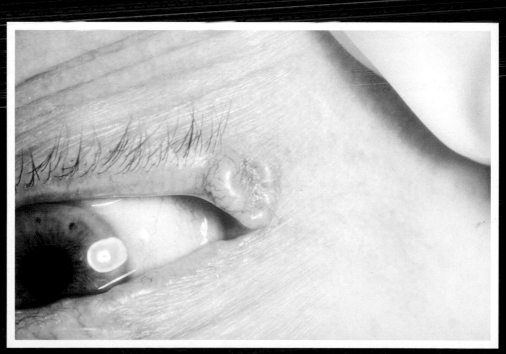

3. Basal cell carcinoma (Ch 8): Characteristic for this localised skin cancer is the 'rolled' edge.

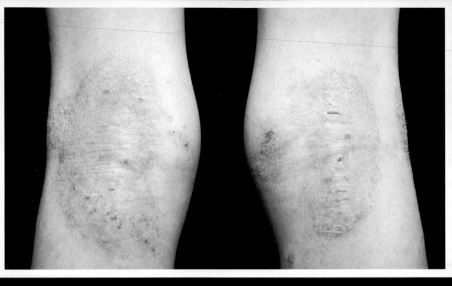

4. Atopic eczema (Ch 8): This common chronic skin inflammation usually starts in childhood.

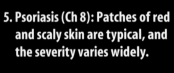

5. Psoriasis (Ch 8): Patches of red and scaly skin are typical, and the severity varies widely.

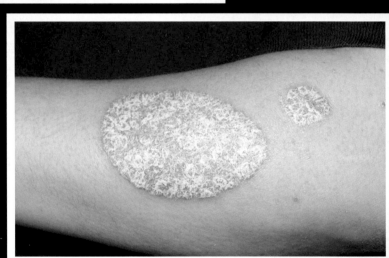

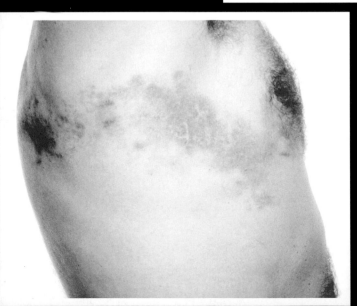

6. Shingles (Ch 8): This painful blistery rash is caused by a viral nerve infection.

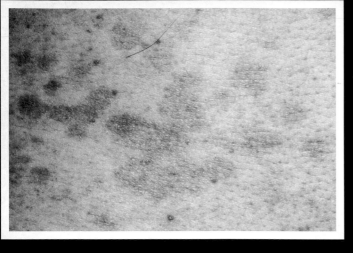

7. Pityriasis rosea (Ch 8): Although the rash can look dramatic, the illness is harmless.

8. Diabetic foot ulcers (Ch 8): These sores can be due to nerve damage and poor circulation.

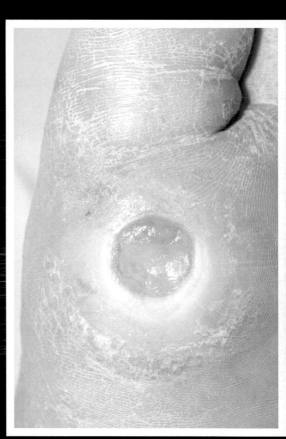

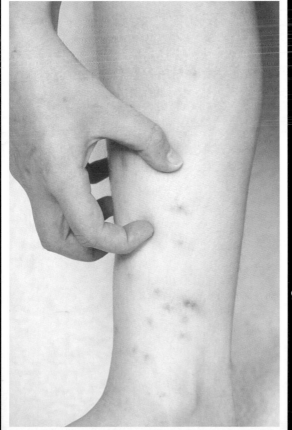

9. Scabies (Ch 8): The typical itchy rash is caused by a tiny mite and clears with treatment.

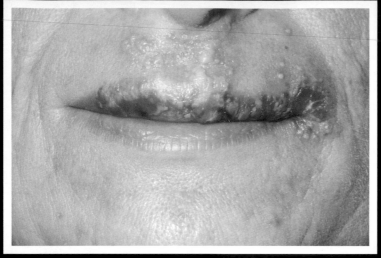

10. Cold sore (Ch 8): These tingly blisters on the lip usually disappear after 7–10 days.

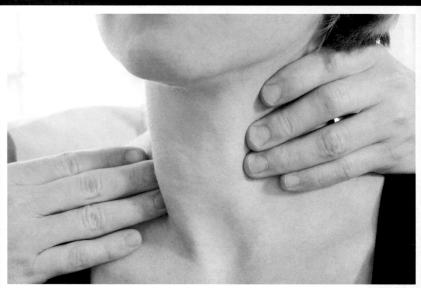

11. Swollen lymph glands (Ch 9): Swollen and painful lymph glands are often due to infection.

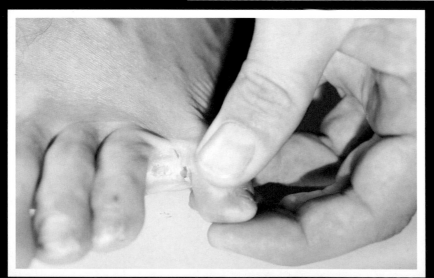

12. Athlete's foot (Ch 8): You can treat this itchy rash between the toes with anti-fungal preparations.

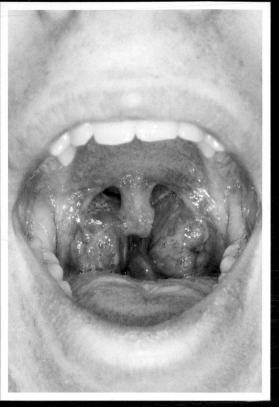

13. Tonsillitis (Ch 9): Pus on your tonsils suggests bacterial infection or sometimes glandular fever.

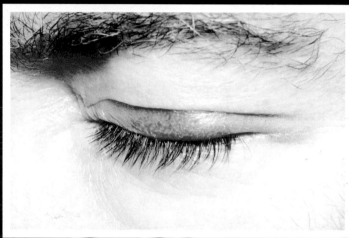

14. Blepharitis (Ch 9): In this inflammation of the eyelids vision is not usually affected.

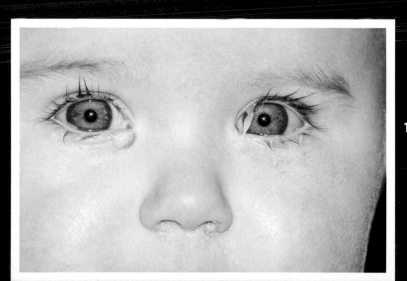

15. Conjunctivitis (Ch 9): This common eye infection often clears within a few days without treatment.

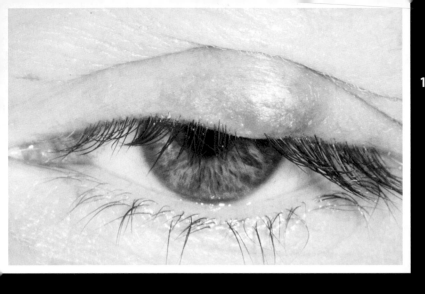

16. Stye (Ch 9): No treatment may be needed for this infection of the root of an eyelid.

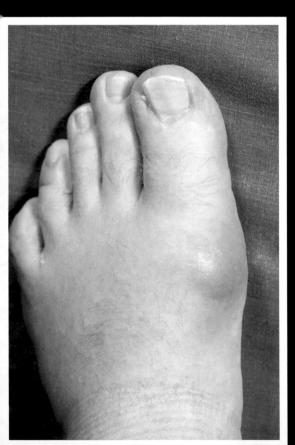

17. Gout (Ch 13): Anti-inflammatory pain killers can relieve pain from a gout attack quickly

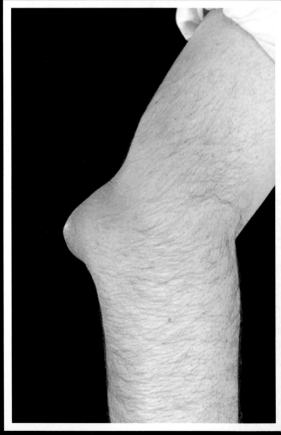

18. Bursitis (Ch 13): This inflammation and swelling behind the elbow often clears on its own

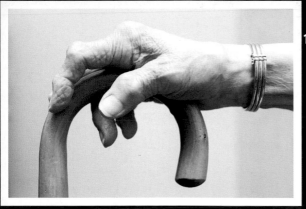

19. Rheumatoid arthritis (Ch 13):
   Inflammation, pain and swelling
   can range from mild to severe.

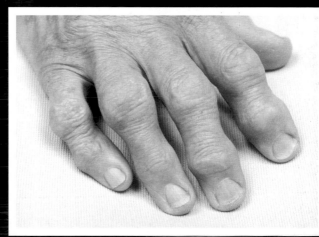

20. Osteoarthritis (Ch 13):
   Paracetamol often helps with
   relieving pain and stiffness.

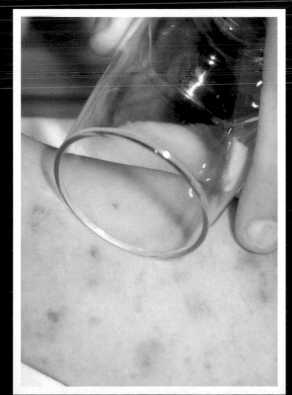

21. Meningococcal septicaemia
   (Ch 14): The tumbler test can
   help identify the typical rash.

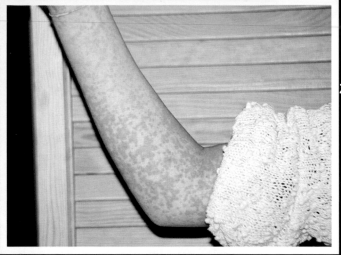

22. Measles (Ch 15): This viral infection is now rare due to MMR vaccination.

23. Impetigo (Ch 15): Antibiotics usually clear this contagious skin infection common in children.

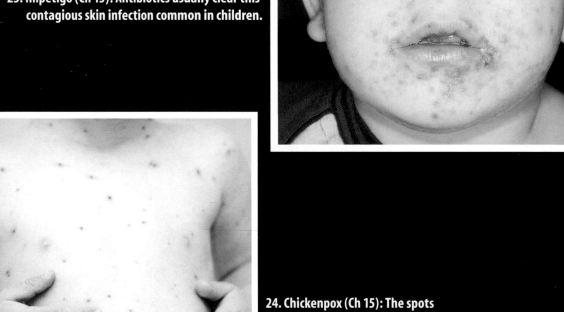

24. Chickenpox (Ch 15): The spots can be itchy but usually disappear within a week.

veins are common in older people and during pregnancy. They may lead to vein inflammation (known as *thrombophlebitis*), swelling of the lower leg or foot and skin changes (called *varicose eczema*). In most cases, varicose veins don't need any treatment, but elevating your legs, avoiding prolonged standing and wearing support stockings (available from your pharmacist) may help to relieve your symptoms. See your GP to discuss further treatment options if your symptoms are severe or don't settle.

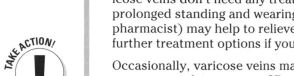

Occasionally, varicose veins may lead to leg ulcers or bleeding, in which case you need to see your GP sooner rather than later.

Possible causes of leg swelling only

If you suffer from leg swelling only (without any pain), compare your symptoms with the following conditions:

- **Fluid retention:** Retention of too much fluid may first show up as swelling around your ankles (called *oedema*) and can then – if you retain more and more fluid – move upwards into your legs. Mild ankle oedema is common and may be caused by hot weather or sitting for prolonged periods of time (for example, on a long haul flight), in which case the swelling usually settles after a day or so. Sometimes, more severe or persistent leg swelling can be due to other causes such as problems with your heart (for example, heart failure), kidneys, liver or hormonal issues. Visit your GP for further assessment and diagnosis if you're concerned.

- **Causes inside your abdomen:** Unexplained leg swelling can sometimes be an early sign of a condition inside your lower abdomen or pelvis, which in some cases may be due to cancer. The bottom line is: ask your GP for further assessment if your tummy and legs become more swollen over time for no apparent reason.

- **Medication:** Some drugs commonly cause swelling around the ankles. The biggest offenders are calcium channel blockers and steroids, so if you take these medications and suspect this side effect, see your GP for a review.

- **Underactive thyroid:** Leg swelling may sometimes be due to an underactive thyroid gland (known as *hypothyroidism*). If hypothyroidism is the cause of your swelling, you're likely to notice other symptoms as well, such as feeling tired, low mood, feeling cold all the time, constipation or dry skin. Consult your GP, as a simple blood test can confirm the diagnosis.

Possible causes of leg pain only

Here I list some causes of leg pain only – without any swelling:

✔ **Muscle strain or injury:** Muscular injuries are common after sport or unusual exercise. Simple muscular aches tend to develop after a delay of a day or two, whereas more significant muscle injuries cause instant pain. If symptoms don't improve with rest, ice and elevation, or if you experience severe pain with loss of function in your legs, see your GP for further assessment.

✔ **Peripheral vascular disease:** A reduction in blood flow to your legs because of a narrowing in one of your pelvic or leg blood vessels (called *peripheral artery disease*) often causes typical intermittent leg pain (known as *intermittent claudication*), usually in the calves. Symptoms tend to develop when walking up hill or on the flat for a certain distance, and they improve with rest.

If any of these contributory factors apply to you, you're at an increased risk of developing narrowed arteries:

• Diabetes.

• Lack of exercise.

• Obesity.

• Raised blood pressure.

• Raised cholesterol.

• Smoking.

See your GP for further assessment if you suspect any of these factors may be the cause of your leg pain.

✔ **Sciatica:** If your leg pain occurs alongside back pain, it may be due to pressure on a nerve that goes into your leg causing *sciatica* (turn to the section 'Struggling with back pain', earlier in this chapter). Consult your GP.

Being brought to your knees?

Orthopaedic surgeons love knees or, more precisely, knee joints. Their fondness is due to the fact that the knee has a brilliant design and contains a number of structures that work well together, allowing various movements in different positions, all possible because of a fascinating architecture. On the whole, knees are tough and stable – but only up to a limit. If you make them carry too much weight or push them too far, they may incur damage, resulting in pain and problems when using your knee.

If your knees are playing up, consider these possible causes (ordered from the most common to the least):

✔ **Knee injury:** If you suffer an acute and severe knee injury, go to your nearest A&E department or see your GP for further assessment, particularly if you experience any of the 'Take Action' symptoms I list later in this section. Rest, ice and raising your injured leg when you sit down are important for speeding up your recovery from minor injuries.

✔ **Injuries through overuse:** Knee problems from running or cycling are common and usually respond well to avoiding activities that make the pain worse, but continuing with other forms of exercise. Simple over-the-counter remedies help with pain relief – your pharmacist can advise you on which treatments are best for you. If your symptoms don't start to get better after a few days, or if they continue for more than one or two weeks without any sign of improvement, visit your GP.

✔ **Osteoarthritis in the knee or hip:** 'Wear and tear' of the knee becomes more common as you get older, and osteoarthritis in the hip can often emerge as referred pain in the knee. Pain may occur when you exercise or get up after resting. Your knee can also feel stiff and may be swollen. Regular paracetamol at full dose can be very effective for pain relief, but do ask your GP to have a look at your knee if this approach isn't effective for you. Depending on how severe your problem is, physiotherapy, additional medication or – sometimes – surgery may help to get you back to the next knees-up.

✔ **Other causes:** Many other conditions or events can cause knee pain, including gout, infections, tendon inflammation, inflammation of protective cushions (called *bursitis* – often referred to as *housemaid's knee* in the past) and others. See your GP if you're not sure what's going on, your symptoms are severe or they just don't get better.

Seek urgent medical help if you notice the following symptoms in connection with your knee pain:

✔ You develop an acutely hot and swollen knee with or without fever.

✔ You can't straighten your knee, and it locks in a certain position.

✔ Your knee keeps 'giving way'.

✔ Your knee pain keeps you awake or wakes you at night.

✔ You can't bear weight on the affected leg.

✔ Your pain is severe and painkillers don't keep it under control.

✔ You suffer from fever or unexplained weight loss, or you feel generally unwell.

✔ You injure your knee in a high-impact or high-speed accident.

'Bone-faced' tales. . .

Arthritis – and what to do about it – is the subject of a number of myths, which I can clarify for you:

✔ 'You can't do anything about it!': Wrong, many effective treatments are available.

✔ 'You mustn't exercise if you have it!': Wrong, gentle exercise and losing weight are beneficial.

✔ 'You can't get it if you're young!': Wrong, arthritis can also affect younger people.

✔ 'You always get better if you have an operation!': Wrong, surgery isn't always successful and is only recommended in selected cases.

✔ 'Painkillers and an operation are the only treatment options!': Wrong, various other effective treatments are available.

✔ 'You shouldn't work if you have arthritis!': Wrong, your ability to work depends on your level of functioning, and working may even be beneficial.

Getting back on your feet

Putting a foot wrong is easy, but usually doesn't hurt – at least not in a physical way. Your feet can, however, create problems for you in other ways; they can severely affect your quality of life and are a common reason for falls – particularly if you're a bit older – but foot problems are rarely serious.

Plenty of causes can be to blame for foot problems. In some cases, you can easily spot whether your problem is due to a skin or joint condition. Symptoms arising from conditions affecting your blood vessels or nerves are often trickier to suss out. See whether your problems tie in with any of these possible causes:

✔ **Achilles tendonitis:** A pain over the large tendon in the back of your ankle (called the *Achilles tendon*) suggests tissue irritation or inflammation, which is commonly caused through exercising too much (through playing tennis or long-distance running, for example), a change in your training schedule or inadequate footwear. Try rest, different shoes and over-the-counter preparations, and consult your GP if your symptoms don't settle.

However, if you experience a sharp snap and sudden pain in your Achilles tendon during exercise, or as a result of a sudden unexpected movement, your Achilles tendon may have completely or partially ruptured. Contact your GP or go to A&E.

✔ **Ankle injury:** Ankle sprains are common. For minor ankle injuries, rest your foot, cool your ankle with ice cubes or a pack of frozen peas placed within a towel and put your foot up when you sit down. Painkillers available without prescription from your pharmacist can help with relieving your symptoms. Seek medical advice, though, if you suffer from pain in your ankle straight after a high-impact fall or accident, particularly if your foot is swollen and you can't move it.

✔ **Joint problems:** Gout (which I discuss in more detail in 'Hot tips for checking out a swollen joint', earlier in this chapter) commonly affects the base of the big toe joint, causing severe pain and tenderness (see image 17 in the colour section). During an acute attack, this joint can become so sensitive that you may not be able to tolerate a blanket over it during the night. See your GP for further assessment and treatment.

✔ **Plantar fasciitis:** A stabbing pain in the base (not the sides) of your heel when put on the floor first thing in the morning, and that eases after walking, suggests *plantar fasciitis* (sometimes referred to as *policeman's heel*). A change in footwear or posture, or increased walking, can lead to plantar fasciitis, and you can relieve it by resting and taking simple painkillers. See your pharmacist or GP to discuss the treatment options if your symptoms don't improve.

✔ **Skin problems:** Itchy and sore skin between your toes can be due to *athlete's foot*, a fungal skin infection (see image 12 in the colour section). See your pharmacist for advice on which preparations to use as treatment.

This section covers just some of the numerous conditions that can cause problems with your feet. If you can't make out what the problem is after comparing your symptoms with those I list here, consult a podiatrist or your GP for a diagnosis.

To help you identify why you may be experiencing foot problems, remember that you're at higher risk of developing them when the following apply to you:

✔ You wear inadequate footwear: high heels and over-worn shoes are sometimes to blame, and they can also cause back pain.

✔ You're overweight or you suffer from diabetes, narrowed blood vessels (called *peripheral vascular disease* and described in the earlier section 'Possible causes of leg pain only'), gout or arthritis.

✔ You exercise or play sports a lot: make sure that you get proper advice on appropriate footwear from a good sports shop.

✔ You already have a structural foot condition such as flat feet.

✔ You neglect your feet! (Check out the sidebar, 'Keeping feet neat'.)

Keeping feet neat

Looking after your feet properly means that you're less likely to develop any foot problems. Always remember to dry your feet properly after washing them, and use moisturising cream if the skin is dry. Wear good-quality socks that absorb moisture well, and cut your toenails straight across and not too short, so that the corners don't cut into the skin (a problem commonly referred to as *ingrowing toenails*).

Consult your GP if any of the following apply to you:

- ✔ You can't walk properly or bear weight on the affected foot.
- ✔ You develop severe pain and bruising as a result of an injury.
- ✔ Your foot pain is due to a high-impact trauma.
- ✔ You have a painful hot swelling in your foot.
- ✔ You suffer from unexplained, additional symptoms such as fever, weight loss, or sweats or you feel generally unwell.

Part IV
Dealing with Health Problems in Specific Groups

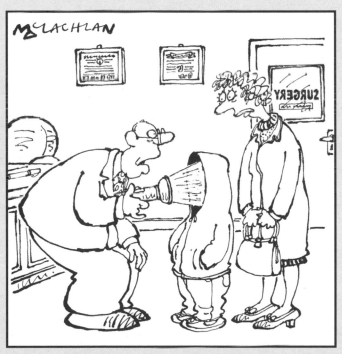

'There was no need to worry, Mrs Grimdew
—Darren's just got teenage acne.'

In this part . . .

The types of health problems that you may develop can vary depending on your age and sex, so this part breaks things down by giving guidance on dealing with medical symptoms in babies, children and adolescents. This part also sheds light on some specific women's and men's issues and covers important later-life problems.

Chapter 14

Spotting Illness in Your Newborn, Infant or Toddler

. . . .

In This Chapter

▶ Dealing with common health problems in newborn babies, infants and toddlers

▶ Knowing when your young child is really sick

. . . .

*L*ooking after a young child can be one of the most rewarding and magical experiences in life. But at times your young child – a *newborn* (from birth to four weeks of age), *infant* (from 4 weeks to 12 months of age) or *toddler* (from 12 months to 3 years of age) – is going to cry or be unhappy no matter what you do – often for no apparent reason – even if you're the best parent in the world! Especially when you're tired and exhausted after yet another sleepless night, you may worry that something must be wrong or that your child's seriously ill, and wonder what you can do.

Knowing something about spotting illness in young children can go a long way towards reducing your fears and helping you to decide what steps to take. This chapter enables you to ask yourself the right questions when your young child is unhappy or seems unwell. I also point out which clues to look out for, and provide you with some basic detective skills.

Dealing with Common Problems in Newborn Babies and Toddlers

Although this fact may be hard to swallow, your young child not being well all of the time is quite normal. In contrast to some other mammals whose offspring literally jump into this world and become independent very quickly, young human children need a lot of care and attention before they're ready to lead their own lives. At times, the first few years can be a rocky road for your newborn or toddler to travel.

Young children of course have a lot of growing to do, but their bodies also need to develop in many other ways. For example, their skin has to mature into an effective barrier that protects them from the outside world, their guts have to get used to digesting various foods and their little bodies need to develop their immune system for it to fight infections more efficiently.

Common baby problems such as skin irritations, feeding issues or coughs and colds are therefore simply signs that your baby's body is just dealing with the normal challenges of growing up. But at other times your baby or young child may develop an illness that needs a bit of additional help, or which occasionally may even be dangerous. To enable you to approach some common problems more confidently, use this section as a kind of starter pack. Most problems here aren't serious, and you can deal with many of them yourself – at least initially.

Looking at (and after!) your child's skin

In the same way that most adults don't look like supermodels, your newborn baby, although very special, is unlikely to look like those seemingly perfect babies in TV adverts or baby magazines. Minor skin blemishes are extremely common, as are various rashes. Most of these problems are completely harmless and nothing to worry about, particularly if your child is well in other respects.

In this section I give you an overview of common skin problems in babies and young children and how you can spot when something more serious may be wrong.

Bare basics about birthmarks

Most babies have at least some moles or spots, which come in various forms, colours, shapes and sizes and usually appear for no apparent reason. These marks can seem alarming to a new parent, but fortunately most are nothing to worry about, and some even disappear by themselves in time. Treatment is rarely necessary.

Here's a brief description of some of the more common birthmarks:

- ✔ **Mongolian blue spot:** This condition looks like a bluish-grey bruise and is more common in babies of races with darker skin. The spots are completely benign and go away without treatment before the day when your baby blows out two birthday candles.

- ✔ **Pigmented spots:** Brownish patches called *cafe-au-lait spots* are present on some babies. These spots are usually harmless, but if your baby has a large number of them or additional symptoms, visit your GP to rule out some potential (though very rare) underlying conditions.

✔ **Port-wine stain:** This condition usually involves a flat mark appearing on the face or limbs, sometimes covering quite a large area of skin. The mark doesn't tend to change size or colour and doesn't go away on its own. Laser therapy is effective from the age of two months onwards, but several treatments may be needed before the mark disappears completely.

✔ **Stork bite:** Also called *salmon patch*, *stork bite* is a small pink-coloured mark that may appear on the back of your baby's neck, or the forehead, eyes or lips. Most marks disappear by the time your child reaches 18 months and rarely last longer than three years. No treatment is usually necessary.

✔ **Strawberry naevus:** A bright red and slightly raised mark that may look dramatic, *strawberry naevus* is usually completely harmless. The mark can grow quite fast in the first few months of life but then tends to get smaller again over the next few years. In most cases, it disappears completely, and treatment isn't necessary unless the mark is very close to the eye and affects your child's vision.

In most cases, you discuss these problems with a midwife, hospital doctor or health visitor soon after the baby's birth, but if you're worried for any reason consult your GP.

Dry and scaly rashes

Dry skin is common in babies and young children and can be due to a number of conditions, for many of which the exact cause is unknown. Here are some of the more common ones:

✔ **Cradle cap:** In cradle cap, scales are present on the skin of your baby's head, or on parts of it. This common condition is harmless and usually goes away on its own. Using olive oil or petroleum jelly can soften the skin, which makes the scales easier to wash off.

✔ **Infantile eczema:** A rash affecting your baby's face or the inside of the elbows or knees suggests an allergic condition called infantile eczema, which often disappears as your child gets older. For mild cases, ask your pharmacist for suitable preparations to soothe and moisturise your baby's skin. If the rash affects wider parts of the body or weeps, see your GP or practice nurse to discuss more treatment options.

✔ **Seborrhoic dermatitis:** A dry and possibly inflamed scaly rash affecting wider areas of your baby's body, such as the groin, armpits, face and neck, suggests a condition called *seborrhoic dermatitis*. You don't necessarily need to treat this problem if the rash is mild; just be sure to wash and dry the affected skin folds gently. You may want to ask your pharmacist for preparations that keep the skin nice and moist. However, if the rash spreads or the skin starts to break or ooze, an infection may have set in and treatment is necessary. In this case, contact your GP surgery.

Taking care of your baby's skin

Your baby's skin is sensitive and needs looking after. Here are some tips to help you keep it healthy:

✔ Change your baby's nappy quickly when it's soiled.

✔ Don't let bath water get too hot: use a bath thermometer or test the water temperature with your elbow (the ideal bath temperature for a baby is between 36 and 38 degrees Celsius – 96.8 and 100.4 degrees Fahrenheit).

✔ Dry your baby gently but thoroughly after a bath, taking particular care of the skin folds.

✔ Let some air get to your baby's nappy area at least once a day to help avoid nappy rash.

✔ Use only mild and unperfumed soaps and bath additives.

✔ Wash your baby's hair once a week when it's grown a bit thicker, using baby shampoo.

Nappy rash

Rashes around the nappy area are common. Your baby's poo and wee contain irritant substances that can inflame the skin around your baby's genitals and anus if they're in contact with the skin for too long. For this reason, changing nappies quickly and regularly when they become soiled is important. Sometimes, though, a nappy rash can develop even when you take all the care in the world to keep your baby clean.

To minimise the risk of nappy rash, and to treat if it does strike, make sure that you gently wash away any traces of urine or faeces during each nappy change with cotton wool and lukewarm water. Afterwards, apply protective creams such as zinc and castor oil or petroleum jelly (available from your pharmacy) before putting a new nappy on your baby to help clear nappy rash. See your health visitor for advice.

Other rashes

A number of minor and more widespread rashes can affect the skin of your baby or young child. If your baby is otherwise healthy, feeds well and doesn't have a fever, such rashes are usually nothing to worry about and get better by themselves. Allow a few days, and see your health visitor or GP if the rash doesn't disappear. (For rashes that are more common in later childhood, check out Chapter 15.)

If your child develops a rash that doesn't temporarily disappear when you press on it with a glass (I describe this technique in the later sidebar, 'The tumbler test'), has a fever and is listless, drowsy or generally unwell, a rare and serious underlying illness such as *meningococcal disease* may be the cause. Head straight to the 'Recognising meningococcal disease' section later in this chapter for more details.

Vomiting and bringing up food

Many newborn babies and infants bring up some food after a feed, which can be entirely normal, particularly if they do so without effort and are otherwise well. Also, you don't need to worry when your small child throws up more forcefully once or twice without showing any signs of illness. However, small children are at increased risk of losing too much fluid and becoming dehydrated if the vomiting persists, particularly if they also have runny and frequent poos. The risk of dehydration is higher in newborn babies and in infants who don't drink enough fluid to replace the loss (the next section 'Checking for signs of dehydration' in this chapter has more information).

Persistent vomiting can be due to *gastroenteritis* – an infection of the intestines (the gut), which in the UK is commonly caused by benign viruses or other bugs that are 'doing the rounds'. Symptoms include frequent runny or watery stools (called *diarrhoea*), abdominal cramps and sometimes a fever. Usually, gastroenteritis starts to improve on its own after a few days and doesn't need any particular treatment. However, the main danger for your young child is becoming dehydrated (the next section 'Checking for signs of dehydration' has more on this problem), so you need to keep offering fluid-based feeds or water. If your child doesn't keep any fluids down and has diarrhoea as well, seek medical advice – flip to Chapter 25 for a list of useful helplines and websites or contact your GP surgery.

Persistent vomiting can in rare cases indicate a more serious underlying condition. Here are some potential causes to bear in mind:

- ✔ **Abdominal problems:** If your newborn's or infant's vomit has a green or yellowish colour and she seems to be in pain with a tender abdomen, a more serious underlying condition (such as *bowel obstruction*, which can be due to various causes) may rarely be responsible. See your GP immediately for further assessment. (Turn to the later section 'Assessing Your Unhappy or Sick Young Child' for more on how to spot serious illness.)

- ✔ **Meningitis:** Meningitis is a rare condition caused by a viral or bacterial infection in which the skin around the brain becomes inflamed. Fever and vomiting are two of the main symptoms. Flip to the 'Recognising meningococcal disease' section later in this chapter for how to spot the danger signs and what to do. If you suspect meningitis in your young child, consult your GP urgently.

- ✔ **Pyloric stenosis:** In this rare condition, the connection between your baby's stomach and intestines is too narrow. An affected baby is usually less than two months old and appears to be constantly hungry. Vomiting larger amounts than is normal for a young baby after each feed is usual and sometimes the vomit comes out with considerable force. Consult your health visitor or GP.

Checking for signs of dehydration

Dehydration is a lack of fluid in the body. Vomiting and diarrhoea can both cause dehydration and be warning symptoms that your child is in danger of lacking fluids.

Reassuringly, most children with diarrhoea and vomiting will not be dehydrated. However, do check for the following physical signs, which suggest that your young child may be suffering from dehydration and lacks fluids:

- ✔ Your child has a dry mouth. (Normally, every child has a small pool of saliva just behind the lower lip, which dries up if your child becomes dehydrated).

- ✔ Your child's soft spot (known as the *fontanelle* – an area on the top of your infant's head where the bones of the skull have not completely joined) or eyes appear sunken.

- ✔ Your child cries without tears.

- ✔ Your child appears generally unwell, lethargic or irritable.

- ✔ Your child hasn't passed urine in the past three to four hours (which you may notice because the nappies stay dry).

- ✔ Your child's skin has lost some of its elasticity.

You can treat mild dehydration by giving your child more to drink, but not giving too little or too much fluid is vital. If you're concerned that your child is dehydrated, seek advice from your health visitor or GP, or flip to Chapter 25 for a list of useful helplines and websites.

Small children with more severe dehydration are at risk of becoming seriously ill. Check out the later section on 'Assessing Your Unhappy or Sick Young Child' later in this chapter for information.

Runny stools in babies

Most breastfed babies naturally have frequent soft and aromatic (by which I mean not foul-smelling) poo, or *stools*. If, however, your child has frequent runny stools, consider the following possible causes:

- ✔ **Change in diet:** Adjusting to a changed diet, particularly when you introduce new foods, may take your newborn baby's or infant's stomach a little while – and runny stools can be the result. Don't worry if this problem happens only occasionally and settles quickly, but if it persists or the loose stools are linked to a particular food, consult your health visitor or GP.

✔ **Gastroenteritis:** Turn to the earlier section 'Vomiting and bringing up food' for further details about this common cause of diarrhoea.

✔ **Medication:** Some medicines, particularly antibiotics and those containing a sugary syrup, can cause diarrhoea. Instead of stopping the medication, speak to your GP.

✔ **Too much sugar:** Many foods, fruit juices and other drinks contain sometimes considerable amounts of sugar, which can upset your young child's stomach. To resolve the problem, always follow the instructions on drinks that you dilute and speak to your health visitor about ensuring a healthy fluid intake. Also, don't add any sugar to newborn or infant bottle preparations.

Make sure that you always wash your hands after each nappy change and before preparing baby food. Keep towels that are solely for your baby, and change them regularly. Also, sterilise all your baby's bottles regularly according to the manufacturer's instructions.

Assessing Your Unhappy or Sick Young Child

Whether you're a new or experienced parent, looking after a sick young child can be a distressing and frightening experience. Newborn babies and infants in particular can become unwell quickly, and although serious underlying diseases are rare, they nevertheless do sometimes occur. This section guides you through assessing your newborn or infant when things start to look a bit more hairy.

Coping with your crying child

Crying is a sign that your young child wants or needs attention, and this desire can be for various reasons. As you get to know your child, you discover how to interpret different types of crying and become the expert in spotting when your child's crying is different and perhaps means something more serious. When a young child's in pain, her crying usually sounds different and may go up a pitch.

If your young child doesn't stop crying despite you pulling out all the usual stops to calm her down, you may start to wonder what's going on. Here are some possible causes:

✔ **Abdominal colic:** *Abdominal colic* is a fairly common condition in which your infant cries excessively at regular intervals – coming in 'threes': on average for more than three hours a day, more than three days a week and for longer than three weeks – but is otherwise healthy. Colic often starts when your infant is around six weeks old and gets better around the age of three to four months. Experts have come up with a number of possible explanations, including painful tummy spasms or some reaction to your baby's food, but no one's really sure what causes abdominal colic. The good news is that colic is rarely dangerous and passes with time. See your health visitor for advice if you're concerned.

✔ **Benign 'natural' causes:** Your baby may cry because she's hungry, tired, thirsty, wet, too hot, too cold, needs to bring up wind, craves attention, needs a cuddle or shows sensitivity to other things that go on in the household, such as increased tension or stress. You don't need to worry if your baby's otherwise well and healthy and you don't notice any other symptoms.

A crying baby or child can be worrying for you as a parent, and fraying on your nerves. If things get too much or you want further information, phone the Cry-Sis Helpline on 08451 228669 or visit www.cry-sis.org.uk for some top tips.

If you can't find an obvious cause for your young child's crying, the next step is to check whether your child has a fever or is showing other signs of serious illness. The remaining sections of this chapter give you a basic rundown of what to watch out for when things start to look a bit dicey.

Dealing with your feverish child and spotting serious illness

At times, judging whether your young child's unwell or has a fever due to a harmless reason, or whether she may have a more serious illness, can be difficult. Deciding whether to seek help is particularly tricky when you're tired and exhausted from lack of sleep. When symptoms develop gradually, you may also become used to them and tend to ignore them.

So how can you spot serious illness and identify important possible underlying causes? Remember that your 'gut instinct' as a parent or carer is the most useful tool you have in helping you decide how to manage your young child's illness, but knowing which clues to look out for is also very helpful.

Checking your baby's temperature

Various types of thermometer are available from your pharmacy. In newborn babies under four weeks of age, use only an electronic thermometer in the armpit. However, if taking the temperature is difficult for you or you haven't got a thermometer, your perception of whether your young child has a fever is just as valid and is taken seriously by healthcare professionals. Experts no longer recommend taking the temperature in your young child's mouth, back passage or from the forehead (forehead chemical thermometers are popular but unreliable).

In young children between four weeks and five years of age, the following methods are safe to use:

✔ Chemical dot thermometer in the armpit.

✔ Electronic thermometer in the armpit.

✔ Intrared ear thermometer.

Coming to fever pitch

When your young child is ill or cries, one of the most important things to check is whether she has a *fever* – where body temperature has gone over and above 38 degrees Celsius (100.4 degrees Fahrenheit). A fever in your young child may not always be easy to spot, but whenever she is unwell, irritable, sweating or feels hot to touch, check her temperature.

Seek medical advice if your child has a fever and is less than six months old. Infections at this very young age aren't very common, and a fever can potentially indicate a more serious underlying condition.

Discovering the causes of fever in young children

Your young child may suffer from fever caused by one of the following problems:

✔ **Common cold:** Colds are usually caused by viruses and commonly show up with a fever, as well as a sore throat, a cough and a runny nose. You can use paracetamol and ibuprofen to make your child feel better, but make sure you read the instructions on the packet, as you need to give the correct dosage for your child's age. Also, try and keep the room air moist; placing a wet towel over the radiator prevents the air in a room from drying out too much. Contact your GP surgery if symptoms are severe or you're concerned.

✔ **Ear infection:** Ear infections are very common and usually occur in connection with a cold. These infections may cause your child to wake during the night, particularly where the ear looks red or your child pulls at either ear. Ear infections often get better by themselves without the need for antibiotics; paracetamol and/or ibuprofen can help to relieve any pain. If your child has a high fever that persists for more than two or three days, or if you notice pus draining from the ear canal, contact your GP surgery.

✔ **Gastroenteritis:** Tummy upsets are a common cause of fever in babies, and are often accompanied by vomiting and diarrhoea. The section 'Dealing with Common Problems in Newborn Babies and Toddlers' earlier in this chapter looks at how to assess diarrhoea and vomiting and how to recognise dehydration – and what to do about it.

✔ **Overheating:** To avoid overheating, make sure that your child has clothing and bedding that's appropriate for the season, a cot placed away from radiators and direct sunlight, and a room that isn't overly warm – a room temperature between 16 to 20 degrees Celsius (61–68 degrees Fahrenheit) is usually fine.

✔ **Throat infection:** Your infant or toddler may be refusing food if a throat infection (called *pharyngitis*, or *tonsillitis* when the tonsils are infected) is the main underlying cause. Treat symptoms with paracetamol and/or ibuprofen initially (check the instructions on the packet, as you need to give the correct dosage for your child's age); antibiotics aren't needed in many cases. Consult your GP if your child's symptoms are very severe, the fever is very high (above 39 degrees Celsius – 102 degrees Fahrenheit) or if your child's temperature doesn't come down after two to three days.

✔ **Travel-related infection:** Be sure to tell your GP if your child has recently visited a hot country; she may possibly have picked up an infection that's less common in the UK.

Approaching and assessing your feverish child

On the one hand, a fever isn't always present in every sick child, and on the other, even a prolonged, high fever doesn't necessarily mean that your young child is suffering from a serious illness. Look at symptoms in these five areas to decide whether something serious may be wrong in your young child:

✔ Breathing.

✔ Hydration.

✔ Level of activity.

✔ Signs of underlying conditions.

✔ Skin colour.

The first thing to do when your young child has a fever is to check for any immediate life-threatening signs. To help you decide whether continuing to look after your baby or young child at home is safe, or whether you need to call for medical advice, check whether your feverish child fits with one of the descriptions in the following three sections.

Being reassured in mild illness

Your feverish baby or young child is unlikely to be seriously ill if you observe the following:

- ✔ Your child's skin, lips and tongue are of normal colour.

- ✔ Your child responds to you as usual when you interact with or talk to her.

- ✔ Your child looks content and/or smiles, and stays awake or wakes up quickly as normal.

- ✔ Your child doesn't cry, or cries in the same way as normal.

- ✔ Your child's skin and eyes look as they always do, and the mouth and eyes are nice and moist.

Noticing a raised risk of serious illness

Your feverish baby or young child is more likely to be seriously ill if you notice the following:

- ✔ Your child looks unusually pale.

- ✔ Your child doesn't respond to you in a normal way.

- ✔ You have to try quite a bit harder than usual to wake your child and perhaps need to use prolonged stimulation.

- ✔ Your child is much less active than usual, doesn't look content and doesn't smile.

- ✔ Your child's nostrils flare, and her breathing appears much faster than usual (more than 60 breaths per minute if your infant's under 5 months old, more than 50 breaths per minute if your infant's between 6 and 12 months old, or more than 40 breaths per minute if she's 12 months or older).

- ✔ Your child feeds poorly and has a dry mouth, and you don't get as many wet nappies anymore.

- ✔ Your child has had a fever for five or more days.

- ✔ Your child has a swollen limb or joint, or doesn't use a limb as usual.

- ✔ Your child has a new lump somewhere on her body, which is more than 2 centimetres (just under an inch) in size.

If you notice any of these features, consult your GP, as your child needs further medical assessment.

Bringing down your child's temperature

A fever in itself isn't necessarily harmful, because it's one of the strategies your child's body uses to fight infection. With that in mind, here are some dos and don'ts about managing fevers:

✔ Don't use tepid sponging to cool your child down – experts no longer recommend this approach.

✔ Do make sure that your child isn't over- or underdressed.

✔ Do consider using paracetamol or ibuprofen if your child seems unwell or is distressed, because these medicines make your child feel better. Use ibuprofen alone if you need to bring your child's temperature down and don't routinely combine paracetamol with ibuprofen (but be cautious if your child has been diagnosed with asthma or suspected asthma). Always be sure to follow the instructions on the packet and give your child the appropriate dose.

Checking for serious illness

Contact your GP or – in an emergency – take your child to hospital quickly or call '999' if you notice any of the following signs, which can suggest potentially serious or life-threatening illness:

✔ Your child looks unwell and her skin has turned unusually pale, mottled, ashen or blue.

✔ Your child doesn't respond to you as normal.

✔ Your child can't be roused, or if you manage to do so, she doesn't stay awake.

✔ Your infant's crying is weak, high-pitched or doesn't stop.

✔ Your child grunts in an unusual way and breathes very fast (more than 60 breaths per minute).

✔ Your child's breathing appears laboured, and you notice that her chest draws in during every breath in an unusual way.

✔ Your child's skin has lost its elasticity and stays pulled up for much longer than usual when you pinch it gently between your finger and thumb.

✔ Your baby is under 3 months old and has a fever of 38 degrees Celsius (100.4 degrees Fahrenheit) or higher; or is 3–6 months old with a temperature of 39 degrees Celsius (102.2 degrees Fahrenheit) or higher.

Trust your instincts – if you suspect that your child has a serious and potentially life-threatening illness, don't hesitate to consult your GP urgently or call '999' in an emergency.

Tackling febrile fits

Fits (also called *febrile convulsions* or *seizures*) may occur when your child's temperature rises very quickly or is very high, and can be a very frightening experience for a parent. Your child's eyes may roll back, her arms and legs may shake and her body become stiff, but fits can vary a lot in the way they occur. In most cases a fit is over after a few seconds, but can last for longer.

If your child has a fit, put her on her side with the head slightly down (to prevent choking), and don't shake her. Try to bring her temperature down by taking off some clothes if the room is warm. When your child is awake again, give paracetamol or ibuprofen (read the instructions on the packet, as you need to give the correct dosage for your child's age). Contact your GP – particularly if your child has had a fit for the first time.

Consult your doctor urgently or call '999' if you notice the following:

✔ Your child doesn't get better quickly after a fit.

✔ Your child's fit lasts for more than five minutes.

✔ Your child has a series of fits, with gaps in between.

✔ Your child finds breathing difficult.

✔ Your child wasn't fully conscious just before the fit and isn't back to normal one hour afterwards.

The Patient UK website provides an excellent information leaflet on febrile convulsions if you want to find out more – visit www.patient.co.uk for further details.

Recognising meningococcal disease

'Could it be meningococcal disease or meningitis?' is one of the most common questions that parents have when their young child is ill or has a fever. *Meningitis* and *meningococcal disease* are serious conditions that can make your child ill at any time, and are alarming because babies and young children become unwell so quickly, with sometimes devastating consequences. Meningococcal disease can cause meningitis, blood poisoning (known as *septicaemia*) or both. However, do remember that they're very rare, that the majority of young children who do get them survive and that if your child has a fever she's much more likely to be suffering from a benign condition such as a virus infection.

Meningitis

Viruses and bacteria are usually responsible for *meningitis* – a rare inflammation of the skin surrounding your child's brain and nerves in the back bone. When brought on by a virus, meningitis is rarely life-threatening, but it can still make your child very unwell. The good news is that a complete recovery is most likely afterwards.

The low-down on meningococcus

A bug called *meningococcus* is the one that most commonly causes bacterial meningitis in the UK and causes so much worry for parents. In addition to causing meningitis, meningococcal bacteria can also get into your child's bloodstream and cause blood poisoning, which is known as *septicaemia*. The umbrella term for these two conditions is *meningococcal disease*.

The bugs that cause meningococcal disease are passed around by coughing, sneezing and intimate kissing, and often live in the back of people's throats – including your baby's –

without causing any trouble. In fact, most people come into contact with or even host these bugs at some stage without noticing or getting ill. These bugs may even be good for humans, in that they help to strengthen the immune system.

However, babies and young children are at higher risk because their immune system isn't yet fully developed. If your baby's or child's immune defences aren't quite strong enough or the bug is a particularly nasty one, meningococcal disease can develop.

Bacterial meningitis, however, is the dangerous form, but is far less common than viral meningitis. It can be fatal unless treated quickly. Your child's still likely to recover from bacterial meningitis if she receives treatment, but sadly some babies and young children suffer permanent brain or other damage, or even die from the infection. Effective vaccines are available to prevent some forms of meningitis – but not all.

Meningococcal septicaemia

A number of different germs can cause blood poisoning, but the condition is especially dangerous when caused by meningococcus bacteria (called *meningococcal septicaemia*), which may occur together with meningitis or on its own. In general, meningococcal septicaemia is more dangerous and life-threatening than meningitis, but fortunately is very rare (see image 21 in the colour section).

As with meningitis, spotting meningococcal septicaemia isn't always easy, but the main sign to look out for is a rash (go to the photo section in this book to see what it may look like). The key feature of the rash in meningococcal disease is that it doesn't temporarily disappear when you apply pressure (take a look at the later 'The tumbler test' sidebar). The rash may start as tiny pinpricks anywhere on your child's body before spreading quickly and changing into lesions that look like fresh bruises. Spotting the rash is more difficult when your child has darker skin, and so check the paler areas of the skin such as the palms of the hands, soles of the feet, the mouth and under the eyelids. For further information visit the Meningitis Trust website www.meningitis-trust.org.

Spotting meningococcal disease in the early stages isn't easy because symptoms and signs can be very similar to other, more benign illnesses such as viral infections. Be on the lookout for these common signs and symptoms of meningitis in babies and toddlers:

✔ Your child has a high fever, with or without extreme shivering.

✔ Your child displays an abnormal dislike of being handled.

✔ Your child's soft spot (the soft area on the top of the scalp in young children where the skull bones have not quite fused) is unusually tense or bulging.

✔ Your child has unusually cold hands or feet.

✔ Your child develops an unusual rash – particularly if this doesn't go away when you press on it with a glass (check out the sidebar 'The tumbler test' and image 21 in the colour section).

✔ Your child uncharacteristically refuses food or is vomiting.

✔ Your child's skin is unusually pale and blotchy.

✔ Your child has developed a staring and blank expression.

✔ Your child is unusually drowsy or difficult to wake.

✔ Your child seems to have a stiff neck or an arching of the back.

✔ Your child moans in an unusual way or cries in an abnormally high pitch.

✔ Your child has a fit.

✔ Your child's body is floppy or seems lifeless.

These symptoms and signs may appear in any order, but they aren't necessarily all present and your child usually – though not always – gets worse quickly over a few hours. Trust your instincts – if you suspect meningitis or septicaemia, get medical help immediately. Don't wait until your child gets a rash.

TECHNICAL STUFF

The tumbler test

If your young child has a rash, use the *tumbler test* to check whether the rash *blanches* (fades on pressure). Press the bottom or the side of a glass firmly against your child's skin (see image 21 in the colour section). If the rash disappears, meningococcal disease is unlikely.

Treat a fever with a rash that *doesn't* fade under pressure as a medical emergency, because meningococcal septicaemia may be the underlying cause. Seek medical advice immediately and call '999' if your child is very unwell or gets worse very quickly. This illness really is one of those few situations when getting help quickly can make the difference between life and death. However, don't wait for the rash to occur if your child is obviously very ill – the rash may appear late or not at all. Reassuringly, the vast majority of children who develop a rash don't have meningococcal disease.

Chapter 15

Assessing Illness in Your Pre-School Child

In This Chapter

▶ Approaching general health problems

▶ Checking out symptoms around your child's head

▶ Dealing with common chest troubles

▶ Looking at symptoms 'down below'

As your child grows out of the newborn and infant stage and develops into a toddler and pre-school child, a host of new health problems may emerge. As is true for illnesses in general, most of these potential problems are benign and get better by themselves.

During the pre-school years you may become concerned about the way that your children are growing, developing or behaving, or you may start to worry that something's wrong with their eyesight or hearing. Coughs and colds may appear so frequently that they have you tearing your hair out in frustration and leave you feeling exasperated.

In this chapter I cover some of the most common and important health problems that pre-school children can develop. Obviously, some conditions can occur at any age, and so if you can't find what you're looking for here, take a look at Chapters 14 and 16 – or indeed at the chapters covering 'adult' health problems – as well.

Assessing General Health Problems

Here, I look at some general health problems that commonly cause parental concerns and anxieties, such as fainting and rashes.

Dealing with faints and fits

If your child suddenly faints or becomes drowsy, being alarmed and worried is the natural response. Don't panic, though – although such episodes can be frightening for you as a parent, as long as your child gets back to normal within a minute or so and is breathing normally, the chances are that the event was a one-off and that he has no serious underlying health problem. Nevertheless, you're going to want to know what caused the fainting.

Simple faints

Fainting – where someone suddenly and temporarily loses consciousness – is usually due to an unexpected and short-lived drop in blood pressure. Your child may faint because he feels hungry or anxious, as a reaction to an unpleasant sight – blood or needles are common culprits – or because of pain. Children usually look pale prior to fainting and may complain of dizziness (this is commonly described as *feeling faint*).

Here's what you can do to help if your child feels faint or has fainted:

- ✔ **Body position:** If possible, lie your child down with his legs slightly raised. Alternatively, sit your child down and ask him to lean forward with his head between his knees, but be aware that this position may not be enough to make your child feel better. Lying down is always preferable. If your child starts to feel better, don't allow him to get straight up; wait a few more minutes.

- ✔ **Food and drink:** If your child hasn't eaten enough and the fainting or feeling faint may be due to hunger, a sweet drink and a light snack usually work wonders. Wait until your child is no longer unconscious or very drowsy after a faint before giving anything to eat or drink.

- ✔ **Medication:** If your child feels faint or has fainted because of sudden pain, give some paracetamol or ibuprofen, assuming that he's conscious. (Make sure you read the instructions on the packet, as you need to give the correct dosage for your child's age.)

If your child is otherwise well, comes round after a minute at the most and doesn't have any other health problems or symptoms, you normally don't need to worry. However, consider seeking medical advice if fainting episodes recur or if you have any additional concerns about your child's health.

Fever fits and faints

Fitting (or *febrile convulsion*) – when convulsions affect your child's whole body – and fainting can occur as a result of fever (a body temperature of 38 degrees Celsius, or 100.4 degrees Fahrenheit, or higher), particularly if the temperature has risen quickly. Consider a fever fit if your child has an underlying illness such as an unspecific viral or ear infection.

The following signs are typical of fever fits:

- ✔ Fits may last from a few seconds to a couple of minutes, or even longer.
- ✔ Fits may cause your child to become stiff, or his arms and legs may shake uncontrollably. Your child can also become 'blue in the face': that is, he develops a bluish discolouration to his skin and tongue, which in fits is due to a temporary lack of oxygen in the blood.

Take the following actions if your child has a fever fit:

- ✔ Lie your child in the *recovery position* during the fit – on his side with his head in line with his body or even slightly lower (turn to Chapter 24 for more detailed instructions).
- ✔ Avoid putting anything in your child's mouth or shaking your child.
- ✔ Give paracetamol or ibuprofen (read the instructions, as you need to give the correct dosage for your child's age) to bring the fever down, and to make him feel better as soon as the fit is over and he's recovered.
- ✔ Remove blankets and clothing layers if your child's overly wrapped up.

Particularly if this fit is your child's first, contact your GP immediately. In the vast majority of cases, though, fever fits aren't due to a serious underlying cause and your child is likely to make a full recovery with no lasting damage. Your child will probably be a bit drowsy after the fit, but will usually get back to normal within an hour or so.

Occasionally, a fever fit may be due to a more serious underlying illness. Call your GP or an ambulance straight away if you notice these signs in your child:

- ✔ Your child's fitting or jerky movements last for more than five minutes.
- ✔ Your child doesn't recover quickly after the fit has passed.
- ✔ Your child gets another seizure quickly after the first one.
- ✔ Your child appears unwell or finds breathing difficult.
- ✔ Your child wasn't fully awake before the fit started or isn't fully conscious an hour after the fit.
- ✔ Your child may have a more serious underlying illness such as meningitis or a chest infection (turn to Chapter 14 on how to spot serious illnesses in younger children).

A fever fit isn't due to epilepsy and doesn't usually cause any long-term problems (many parents worry about brain damage) unless it lasts for longer than half an hour or so. Research shows that children who have fever fits do just as well later in life in terms of their general health and achievements as those who don't.

Epileptic fits

During an *epileptic fit* (also known as a *seizure*), the brain fires electrical impulses at a much higher rate than normal. Repeated epileptic fits are referred to as *epilepsy*. Nobody really knows why some children or adults develop epilepsy. Symptoms may vary depending on how severe the condition is and which part of the brain is mainly affected.

In essence, two main forms of epilepsy exist:

- ✔ **Grand mal:** In *grand mal epilepsy*, sufferers fall to the ground without warning and can get injured as a result. They may take several minutes to come round again, during which time they may jerk uncontrollably. Usually, your child falls asleep or feels very sleepy afterwards.

- ✔ **Petit mal:** Although in attacks due to *petit mal epilepsy* people become unconscious, they don't fall to the ground. Attacks don't normally last for longer than 10–15 seconds, during which your child may stare blankly, stop talking and not respond to you talking. Children often grow out of petit mal epilepsy after puberty.

During an epileptic fit, take the following action:

- ✔ Place your child on his side as soon as possible, with his head slightly extended to avoid choking on any vomit and to prevent injury (known as the *recovery position* – turn to Chapter 24 for further information).

- ✔ Resist the temptation to try and restrain your child from moving.

- ✔ Avoid putting anything into your child's mouth.

- ✔ Move any nearby objects that may lead to injury out of the way.

- ✔ Allow your child to sleep after an attack.

See your doctor if you suspect that your child may suffer from epilepsy. Your GP is likely to refer your child to a specialist for further assessment and drug therapy and advise you about special precautions you need to take with regard to activities such as cycling and swimming.

Understanding drowsiness and confusion

Anyone – your child included – can feel somewhat drowsy and confused when not getting enough sleep or after just waking up. However, sudden and unexpected sleepiness is an important symptom that you need to take seriously. Children commonly become sleepy or a little drowsy when they become unwell – perhaps due to a cold or minor viral infection – but sometimes excessive drowsiness or sleepiness can be caused by something more serious, for which your child may need medical treatment.

Infectious causes of drowsiness

Many viral and other illnesses such as the cold or an ear infection can make your child sleepy. These illnesses aren't usually serious, and giving paracetamol or ibuprofen often helps make your child more alert again. (Make sure you read the instructions on the packet, as you need to give the correct dosage for your child's age.)

Another possible cause of drowsiness is *gastroenteritis* (a tummy bug). You can tell if your child has the infection by the runny stools, which may or may not be accompanied by vomiting. Drowsiness may also result from your child losing too much fluid (called *dehydration* – flip to Chapter 14 for more info). Unless your child responds quickly to you offering plenty of fluids, seek medical advice – refer to Chapter 25 for a list of useful helplines and websites, or contact your GP surgery.

Sometimes, a more serious illness may be causing your child's drowsiness, and so seek medical advice immediately if he's unusually drowsy or sleepy and you notice one or more of the following signs:

- ✔ Fever over 38 degrees Celsius (100.4 degrees Fahrenheit).

- ✔ Very unwell appearance. Your child looks unusually pale or dusky, doesn't respond to you as normal or breathes much faster than normal (Chapter 14 has more information on how to recognise signs of serious illness).

- ✔ Vomiting, but no diarrhoea.

- ✔ Headache, the inability to tolerate the light, a rash that doesn't go away on pressure or the inability to bend the head forward. All these symptoms may be signs of *meningococcal disease* (a rare but important cause of *meningitis*, which I describe in detail in Chapter 14).

Drowsiness due to medication

Certain drugs – particularly some *antihistamines*, which are commonly given for hay fever and other allergies – have the potential to make your child slightly drowsy. If you've given your child a new drug, as prescribed by a doctor or one that you obtain without prescription, carefully check the drug information on the bottle or the enclosed information leaflet to see if drowsiness is a potential side effect. If your child is otherwise well, you usually don't need to worry – he should get better quickly when the effect of the drug in question has worn off.

Seek medical advice immediately if your child becomes drowsy and you notice any of the following symptoms after your child takes any new medication, because they may indicate a drug allergy:

- ✔ A new unexplained rash.

- ✔ A sudden and unexplained wheeze.

- ✔ Your child appears unwell. For example, he takes on an unusual skin colour, doesn't respond as normal and breathes faster than usual (refer to Chapter 14 for more info on spotting serious illness in children).

Drowsiness as a result of poisoning

Pre-school-age children are very curious and love to explore the world around them. As well as trying to touch objects that catch their attention, they also like to put things into their mouths. For this reason, accidental poisoning is a common reason for pre-school-age children attending Accident & Emergency (A&E) departments, and so always consider this possibility if your child suddenly becomes drowsy for no apparent reason.

You may suspect poisoning if your child vomits for no apparent reason, if you notice any unusual fluids, tablets, berries or other plant material in or around his mouth or if you find any empty or open containers of potentially poisonous substances lying around where they shouldn't be.

If you suspect that your child may have ingested something harmful, such as cleaning solutions, poisonous berries, alcohol or medication prescribed for someone else, take the following action:

- ✔ Don't try to induce vomiting.

- ✔ Lie your child down on his side (the _recovery position_ – turn to Chapter 24 for instructions).

- ✔ If your child continues to vomit, place him face down on your lap, because this position helps to prevent choking and inhalation of the poisonous substance.

Seek medical advice as soon as possible, even if your child appears completely well. You can help the health professionals by telling them what your child has swallowed, when and in what quantity (particularly in the case of medicines), if indeed you know. Take any relevant containers or plant samples along to the hospital or your GP – they can contain very useful information for the doctors when deciding on the appropriate treatment.

Drowsiness in diabetes

On rare occasions, some other underlying condition such as too much sugar in the blood (known as _diabetes mellitus_) may cause drowsiness. Consider this condition if your child has been increasingly tired all the time, drinks much more than you feel is normal or keeps passing a lot of urine. Diabetes is more likely if such symptoms develop gradually and get worse over time. Contact your GP surgery – a simple blood test helps to confirm the diagnosis.

Head injuries causing drowsiness

Occasionally, drowsiness may result from a head injury. See 'Heading off head injuries in children' later in this chapter, for tips on what to look out for.

Spotting the spots

Rashes and skin problems are very common in children, but some rashes show up in such a way that even health professionals sometimes struggle to make an exact diagnosis. The really important thing as a parent is to decide whether your child's rash is likely to point towards a serious underlying illness or not.

The first thing to establish when you're faced with a new rash in your toddler is whether your child has a fever or not. You don't need to worry too much if:

- ✔ Your child doesn't have a fever (Chapter 14 shows you how to check).

- ✔ Your child's rash *blanches* (goes away) on pressure – do the 'tumbler test' by pressing a glass against the rash (see Chapter 14).

- ✔ Your child is otherwise well.

To see what the rashes I cover here look like, check out the photo section.

Rashes with a fever

Fever – where your child has a temperature of 38 degrees Celsius (100.4 degrees Fahrenheit) or above – is usually a sign of some form of infection (usually due to viruses or bacteria). If you suspect that your child has a fever, consider these conditions:

- ✔ **Chickenpox:** This viral infection is *very* contagious, but harmless in most cases. Your child develops itchy spots – you can almost see them appearing one by one – which then turn into fluid-filled blisters (see image 24 in the colour section). Usually, the child has only a mild illness, although older children and adults can become more unwell.

   Giving paracetamol regularly can make your child feel better (read the instructions so you give the correct dosage for your child's age) and calamine lotion can help reduce any itching. Encourage your child not to scratch – although this is easier said than done – because scratching can lead to scarring (though on the whole this risk is small). Your child is no longer infectious after all the lesions have dried up.

- ✔ **Drug reactions:** If your child has taken any medicines in the past week, consider the possibility of a rash being caused by a drug – antibiotics in particular, which doctors commonly use to treat infections. Any fever may be due to an underlying infection, but can sometimes be caused by the reaction to the drug itself. Stop taking any suspected drugs and consult your GP.

✔ **Roseola infantum:** This viral infection usually affects children aged under three. Typically, the rash appears after your child has had a high fever for a few days and shows as a flat light-red rash on the trunk together with swollen lymph glands in the neck. Recovery takes about a week, and this condition is entirely harmless.

Most children in the UK take part in the typical immunisation schedule, so childhood infectious diseases such as measles, mumps and rubella (or *MMR* for short) have become rare. However, not all parents get their children vaccinated, so in places these infections have become more widespread. Further possible causes of your child's rash and fever are therefore:

✔ **Measles:** Your child usually has a runny nose, a cough and red, blood-shot eyes. Flat and dull red spots tend to appear first on the face before the rash spreads to areas behind the ear and eventually your child's trunk (see image 22 in the colour section).

✔ **Mumps:** This infection can be easy to recognise because of tender and swollen glands on one or both sides of the face and a sore throat.

✔ **Rubella:** The fever in rubella, or German measles, tends to be only mild. Typically, the glands in the back of your child's neck are very swollen, while flat pinkish spots appear on the face and trunk. The neck swellings led doctors of the past to claim that they were able to diagnose this rash in the dark – and appear very clever!

These childhood infections on the whole tend to be mild, and your child is likely to get better without any specific treatment – which, by the way, is only available for relieving symptoms and managing complications rather than treating the infections themselves. Consult your GP for confirmation of the diagnosis and advice on suitable treatment. However, these illnesses do increase the risk of additional bacterial infections of the ears or lungs, and complications such as inflammation of the brain, although rare, are possible.

Look out for the following symptoms and signs in your child, which may indicate complications and prompt you to seek medical advice immediately from your GP, or turn to Chapter 25 for a list of useful helplines and websites:

✔ Drowsiness or sleepiness.

✔ Earache, or severe headache.

✔ Fast or laboured breathing.

✔ Intolerance of bright light.

✔ Refusal to drink and possible dehydration.

✔ Vomiting more than once.

Also take a look at Chapter 14, which has additional details on how to spot serious illness in children.

Rashes without a fever

A number of skin conditions can cause rashes or skin lesions without a fever. You can easily identify some of these conditions, whereas others can be a bit more tricky to diagnose. Here's a quick rundown of some common ones:

- ✔ **Eczema:** Infantile *atopic eczema* – a red, itchy and dry skin condition – is common and often runs in families (Chapter 8 has more details on eczema). Many children with atopic eczema, which is due to a form of allergy, also have asthma and hay fever. The rash often affects the wrists, hands, inside of the elbows and the back of the knees, but other body areas may also be involved. If your child has only mild symptoms, ask your pharmacist about moisturising creams and ointments. If these simple measures fail to improve your toddler's skin, however, see your GP or practice nurse for confirmation of the diagnosis and advice on treatment options.

- ✔ **Impetigo:** This infection produces one or more blistery patches – usually on the face – which dry up resulting in a yellowish crust (see image 23 in the colour section). The lesions may heal up quickly; if not, see your GP or practice nurse who may prescribe antibiotic creams or – in more severe or prolonged cases – oral antibiotics. Impetigo is infectious, so don't share towels with your child.

- ✔ **Insect bites:** Flea bites and other insect bites are common. Usually, they show up as a small number of spots, which often appear in a line, within a small area. Ask your pharmacist for advice on suitable treatments.

  You can find additional information on identifying and managing insect bites on the Patient UK website at www.patient.co.uk/health/Insect-Stings-and-Bites.htm.

- ✔ **Scabies:** Scabies is a common parasitic infection that your child may pick up from other youngsters. The rash usually affects the whole body, but infected-looking spots or small 'burrows' may appear between the fingers. See your pharmacist, minor illness nurse or GP for advice on treatment, which usually consists of applying an insecticide to your child's body. Unfortunately, scabies is contagious, and so other members of your household also need treatment (Chapter 8 contains more details).

- ✔ **Tinea:** Tinea is a fungal infection that may affect moister areas of the skin such as the bottom, armpits, groins and genitalia. Treatment is with antifungal creams, which are available from your pharmacist, or which you can get on prescription from your GP surgery.

Diagnosing Problems Around Your Child's Head

Problems affecting children's heads are extremely common. In this section I focus on those problems that you may find difficult to deal with, or which tend to cause a lot of worries among parents.

Heading off head injuries in children

Because so many nerves supply the skin on the human head, injuries there tend to hurt a lot – with the result that people become quite protective of their heads. Children, though, are naturally prone to bumping their heads. They fall over, run into things or throw toys and other items at each other.

Children's skulls are still growing, and aren't quite as strong as an adult's, but minor head injuries are unlikely to cause any damage. Don't worry if:

- ✔ Your child is completely well after a head injury.

- ✔ You can't see any cut or damage to the skull.

- ✔ Your child doesn't have a headache, hasn't passed out and carries on as normal.

However, do be aware of the following types of head injuries, which can potentially lead to more serious problems:

- ✔ A fall onto the head from a height.

- ✔ An object falling onto the head from a height.

- ✔ A high-speed or high-impact head injury, such as a fall from a bicycle at speed or from a climbing frame.

- ✔ A hit from a heavy or fast-flying object.

Your child is likely to cry and be distressed after a head injury, but will usually settle down quickly. Giving paracetamol or ibuprofen can help to provide pain relief, particularly if your child's head suffered minor bruising (read the instructions, so that you give the correct dosage for your child). Letting your child sleep afterwards does no harm, but check his breathing every hour or so for a while and ensure that his sleeping position looks normal. If you're concerned, check that you can wake your child. A grumpy response is fine – only worry when you can't rouse your child. Seek medical advice – see Chapter 25 for some useful helplines and websites, or contact your GP – when you have any worries, particularly if any symptoms persist for more than a week or two and don't start to improve.

On rare occasions, even what appears to have been a minor head injury can damage the blood vessels surrounding the brain or indeed the brain itself, and unless your child receives urgent treatment, longer-lasting damage may result. Such symptoms of brain damage or bleeding inside the skull can occur immediately or after a delay of hours, days – or very rarely – weeks after the original injury.

Look out for the following warning signs (which I've ordered starting with the most common and least serious signs) in your child, which may indicate a possibly more serious head injury, and seek medical advice immediately:

✔ Vomiting twice or more.

✔ Headache that gradually gets worse: a mild headache after a head injury, though, is common and nothing to worry about.

✔ Inability to walk properly, unusual dizziness or fitting.

✔ Unusual drowsiness when you'd expect your child to be wide awake (although some tiredness is quite normal after a head injury).

✔ Confusion, or acting strangely.

✔ Clear fluid or blood leaking from your child's ear or nose.

✔ Complaints of visual problems such as double vision or blurring.

✔ Not properly moving a body part such as an arm or a leg.

✔ Sudden inability to hear or understand you or to speak properly.

✔ Unusual breathing – too fast or only very slowly.

Eyeing up eye and vision problems

Redness and itching of the eyes are common in young children. You can often treat these symptoms at home initially without seeing a health professional.

Spotting eye inflammation and infection

Some common eye problems due to infection or inflammation include:

✔ **Blepharitis:** In *blepharitis* the eyelid margins rather than the eye itself are inflamed (which may or may not be due to an underlying infection). The eyelid skin may be scaly, and your child may complain of itchy eyes (see image 14 in the colour section). Blepharitis is more common in children who also suffer from *dandruff* (a scaly and itchy scalp) and isn't usually contagious. Eyelid hygiene is the most important part of treatment (you can find more advice on the Patient UK website, www. patient.co.uk/health/Blepharitis.htm). See your GP for advice if your child's symptoms don't settle.

✔ **Conjunctivitis:** *Conjunctivitis* is an infection or inflammation of the eye lining and the inside of the eyelids, which appear red and inflamed. Typically, the eyelids stick together because of a discharge (see image 15 in the colour section). Try to wipe this discharge off gently with boiled and then cooled-down water and a clean ball of cotton wool. Avoid spreading the infection by using a separate towel for your child. In severe infections or if symptoms persist after a few days, visit your practice nurse or GP who may prescribe antibiotic eye drops or gel.

As a possible cause, also consider a reaction to chemicals (such as chlorine in swimming pools, or soap) or an allergic reaction to pollen (as in hay fever) if your child's eyes appear red and inflamed.

✔ **Stye:** *Styes* are non-infectious small boils within the eyelid at the base of an eyelash (see image 16 in the colour section). In most cases no treatment is necessary, because the stye pops, discharges pus or just disappears. If the stye bursts, just gently wipe away the pus with moist cotton wool, using a fresh cotton wool ball each time you wipe. Seek medical advice if the stye doesn't go away, gets bigger with time or if the eye itself becomes painful and red.

Dealing with eye injuries

Injuries, unless they're very minor, are the main danger to the eye, and seeking medical advice immediately is essential. Common injuries include:

✔ **Blows to the eye:** Children often throw things at each other, and so blows to the eyes are common but in many cases not serious. Use a clean pad or small flannel to cover the affected eye, and seek medical advice if the pain doesn't settle quickly or if other problems show.

✔ **Chemical injury:** Immediately flush the affected eye with plenty of water. Doing so may be tricky with a screaming child, and you may need to get help from someone else. Tilt your child's head back and sideways with the affected eye down, part the eyelids with your thumb and index finger, and rinse the eye with lots of water. When you think that you've removed all the chemical substance, cover your child's eye lightly with a clean pad or small flannel and seek medical advice immediately.

✔ **Cuts to the eyelid or eye itself:** These cuts may occur due to injury with a sharp object. Put a clean pad onto the affected eye and cover the other eye as well before getting medical help.

For further details of how to manage eye injuries, turn to Chapter 5.

Looking at vision problems

If you or someone else (for example, a school teacher) suspects that your child's vision is deteriorating, arrange a routine eye test with your optician to test out your concerns and pick up any vision problems. Any sudden loss of vision is quite rare in children and requires immediate medical attention.

Not playing with fire: Preventing childhood injuries

Children under five are at particular risk from accidents, most of which happen in and around the home. Making your home safer for youngsters isn't that hard, and so consider the following:

✔ **Averting the possibility of drowning:** Never leave a child under five alone in the bath, and don't rely on older children to supervise younger ones. Garden ponds are hazardous for smaller children.

✔ **Avoiding burns and cuts:** Keep kettles and toasters out of reach and your children away from your oven, your barbecue and from food that's just come out of the microwave. Use the back rings of your cooker and be careful with hot drinks if youngsters are playing nearby – never pass them over a child's head or leave them where your child can easily reach them. Keep knives and other sharp objects such as scissors or razors out of reach.

✔ **Limiting mobility and access:** Fit and use stair safety gates, fireguards and child locks for your appliances. Use a five-point harness when your child is sitting in a highchair.

✔ **Preventing fire:** Fit fire alarms in your home and make sure that your children don't have access to matches or firelighters.

✔ **Reducing the risk of accidental poisoning:** Lock away medicines, alcohol, cleaning fluids or other dangerous substances well out of reach of your children. Make sure that your kids don't have access to weed killers or fertilisers in a garage or shed.

✔ **Reducing the risk of choking:** Keep small objects away from small children and don't feed them peanuts. Cut grapes in half for children before they eat them.

Children need to discover how to handle risks, but taking these simple steps is all about preventing potentially *serious* injuries. Remember, though, that even if your own home is child-safe, other people's houses may not be.

To become confident in preventing and managing children's accidents, I recommend attending a first aid course. Details of courses are available on the British Red Cross www.redcross.org.uk or St Johns Ambulance www.sja.org.uk websites. You can find further information on preventing childhood accidents on the Child Accident Prevention Trust website at www.capt.org.uk.

Common vision problems in children include:

✔ **Refraction errors:** These errors, which may run in families, include *short-sightedness* (difficulties with seeing faraway objects), *long-sightedness* (problems with focusing on nearby objects) and *astigmatism*, in which the front of the eye is unevenly curved, leading to slightly distorted vision. See your optician if you suspect any of these errors.

✔ **Squint:** *Squinting* occurs when one of your child's eyes seems to go its own way so that the eyes don't work together properly, giving your child a cross-eyed appearance. Squinting can be normal in babies under three months of age, and is usually nothing to worry about. However, see your optician or GP for assessment if you notice squinting in your older child.

Chapter 9 contains even more information on tackling eye problems.

Hearing about ear and hearing problems

Ear problems are extremely common in young children, with the main symptoms being earache and loss of hearing.

Approaching ear pain or discomfort

Ear pain can be very distressing for your child and is a common reason for children suddenly waking at night. Infections, which tend to occur suddenly and often as a result of a cold, are often the cause of ear pain, but other problems can also be to blame:

- **Ear wax:** Some youngsters have problems with excessive ear wax, which may be caused by narrow ear canals or frequent exposure of the ears to water, although often no specific underlying cause exists. Ear wax can block the outer ear canal and occasionally lead to inflammation or infection. Regularly using softening ear drops such as olive oil – available from your pharmacist in a dropper bottle – can help. If this approach fails, you may need to arrange for your child's ear to be cleared using suction or other methods – contact your GP surgery.

- **Foreign body:** Young children are notorious for putting objects into any cavity they can find – ears and noses are very popular! Anything goes – from peas and berries to small toys. Unless you can easily get hold of the object, don't remove it yourself but leave the job to a health professional, to avoid causing any damage to the ear canal.

- **Infection of the middle ear:** This condition, also known as *otitis media*, can result from an infection that spreads from your child's throat to the ear via a ventilation canal called the *eustachian tube*. Your child often has an accompanying fever and feels unwell. Giving paracetamol or ibuprofen can help to make your child feel better (read the instructions as you need to give the correct dosage for your child's age). If the pain suddenly improves and you then notice a thick discharge from your child's ear, the eardrum has likely ruptured. See your GP, who's likely to prescribe antibiotics to help the rupture to heal after a few weeks.

- **Infection of the outer ear:** This condition, also known as *otitis externa*, can occur if your child's ear has been exposed to a lot of water (for example, from swimming). Your child's ear is itchy, with any pain getting worse when you pull gently at the earlobe; you may also notice a discharge. Your practice nurse or GP can prescribe antibiotic and anti-inflammatory ear drops if appropriate, after assessment.

✔ **Insects:** Sometimes, small insects can make their way into your child's outer ear (I'm squirming as I write this!). Try floating the little invader out with a bit of tepid water. Alternatively, get your child to lie on his back in a bath with his ears under water while you gently pull the earlobe of the affected ear upwards and backwards to straighten the ear canal. If this tactic fails, seek help from your GP or the local A&E department.

✔ **Pressure trauma:** If your child suffers from ear pain during flights in an aircraft, *barotrauma* – due to a mismatch in pressures between the middle and outer ear – may be responsible. Barotrauma is especially likely when your child has a cold or blocked nose, in which case avoiding air travel may be best. You can give paracetamol to relieve any pain.

To prevent barotrauma, give babies a bottle or breastfeed during take-off and landing. Older children are usually happy to suck on a sweet for the same effect! Symptoms often improve quickly in a few hours or days, but see your GP if symptoms don't settle or you're worried for other reasons.

Hearing problems

Hearing difficulties in your child can develop gradually, and you may not spot them straight away. Useful pointers that your child's hearing isn't as good as it should be include the following:

✔ Your child regularly turns up the television or stereo volume.

✔ Your child often asks you to repeat what you just said.

✔ Your child's hearing causes other people to comment that it may be impaired – remember that you may be used to his poor hearing.

All the painful ear conditions that I look at in the preceding section 'Approaching ear pain or discomfort' can cause problems with hearing. Other possible causes are as follows:

✔ **Glue ear:** The term *glue ear* describes the build-up of what appears to be sticky fluid behind the eardrum – usually due to problems with ear ventilation because of a poorly functioning *eustachian tube* (which connects your child's middle ear with his throat). So if hearing loss persists, visit your GP for diagnosis and further assessment. To improve drainage of the affected ear, doctors sometimes recommend a simple operation in which a small cut is made in the eardrum and a tiny plastic tube called a *grommet* is inserted, which then falls out naturally after a few months, allowing the eardrum to heal again.

✔ **Infections:** In rare cases, childhood infectious diseases such as mumps, measles or meningitis can cause hearing loss. Read the 'Spotting the spots' section earlier in this chapter for information on how to identify these illnesses, and consult your GP for further assessment.

✔ **Loud music:** Many children have personal music players and listen to music through headphones. Listening at medium volumes usually poses no risk to your child's hearing, but permanent hearing damage can occur if your child regularly listens to loud music. As a rough guide, your child needs to turn down the volume when you can hear the music in the room through your child's headphones.

✔ **Pregnancy-related or inborn hearing defects:** Children of women who contract *rubella* during pregnancy can develop deafness. Other congenital hearing defects may run in families but are rare. Consult your health visitor or GP if you're concerned that your child may be affected.

If your child has hearing problems, his speech development may become affected, and so seeking medical advice is important if you're concerned about your child's hearing.

Looking at Coughing and Breathing Problems

All children develop coughs and colds. Although many parents naturally worry about ongoing coughs that don't seem to settle, coughs and colds usually get better eventually without much treatment. Unless your child appears unwell or his breathing is affected, you don't normally have to worry. You also don't need to fear that a cough due to the common cold will cause any lasting damage to your child's lungs. However, you may occasionally be faced with a more serious underlying problem that requires medical help.

Consider the following causes if your child is coughing:

✔ **Common cold:** The cold is a common viral infection. Your child may also have a fever and a runny nose and may have picked up the illness from someone in the family. Simple colds usually settle by themselves; apart from giving paracetamol or ibuprofen to make your child feel better (check the instructions first, as you need to give the correct dosage for your child's age), you don't need to give any other specific treatment.

✔ **Influenza:** The flu and other flu-like illnesses (caused by influenza or similar viruses) may also cause a cough, but your child is likely to feel more unwell compared to the common cold. Rest and regular fluid intake are important, and your child usually starts to feel better after a few days.

If your child also develops breathing problems or noisy breathing, consider the following possible causes:

✔ **Inhaled foreign body:** If a cough comes on very suddenly in your otherwise well child, he may have inhaled a foreign body such as a peanut or other small object. If the cough doesn't settle quickly and your child is short of breath, consult your GP or go to the nearest A&E. Your child may need assessment and removal of the foreign body in hospital.

✔ **Asthma:** *Asthma* is an inflammatory condition leading to narrowing of the airways, which may cause coughing and difficulty breathing – particularly at night – in your child. Asthma can vary in severity, ranging from very mild symptoms to severe wheezing and shortness of breath. If you suspect that your child has asthma, visit your GP for further assessment and help with management. For further information about asthma, check out the Asthma UK website at `www.asthma.org.uk`.

A number of substances can trigger an *asthma attack*, in which breathing symptoms quickly become more severe. Seek immediate medical advice.

✔ **Chest infection:** Viral or bacterial infections (perhaps following on from the common cold) may occasionally spread from the throat or windpipe to your child's chest. Your child is likely to have a fever and breathe faster than usual. See your GP, because your child may need antibiotics.

Breathing problems can sometimes be serious. Seek medical advice if you notice any of the following in your child:

✔ Severe cough lasting for longer than two to three weeks.

✔ Lips, tongue and skin taking on a blue colour.

✔ Not eating or drinking.

✔ Unusual drowsiness or lethargy, and looking unusually unwell.

✔ Very fast, difficult or noisy breathing.

Delving into Problems 'Down Below'

This section looks at some health problems in the 'lower department' that are relatively common in pre-school children. (Check out Chapter 14 for information on diarrhoea, and you can read up on issues around abdominal pain, urinary problems and bed-wetting in Chapter 16.)

Coping with constipation

Constipation – where passing stools is difficult or where they become particularly hard – can be painful for your child. Consider whether any of the following potential causes may apply to your child:

- ✔ **Anal tear:** Passing hard stools can sometimes lead to a small tear or split in your child's anus, which can cause pain and minor bleeding when going to the toilet. Your child may try to hold stools for fear of pain, which exacerbates the problem. Take your child to your GP for further assessment and treatment.

- ✔ **Changes in diet:** Children's bowel functions can change markedly due to new diets, for example when visiting people or on holiday. Ensure that your child drinks a lot and eats plenty of fruit and vegetables. Things usually and quickly return to normal without any further treatment.

- ✔ **Loss of fluid:** Your child may become constipated due to loss of fluid, perhaps because of vomiting, diarrhoea, fever or hot weather, or because he's just not drinking enough. Make sure that you give your child plenty to drink. His stools are then likely to get back to normal soon.

- ✔ **Stool holding:** Children can become anxious – and obnoxious! – about opening their bowels, particularly when you're perhaps trying a bit too hard with the toilet training. Give lots of praise and try to relax while ensuring that your child takes in plenty of fibre and fluids.

Other rare causes of constipation can be responsible, so consult your health visitor, pharmacist or GP for advice on possible courses of action when your child's stools are very hard, passing stools is painful or you're concerned for other reasons. If your child also has abdominal pain, check out Chapter 16.

Not all children open their bowels every day. Some youngsters 'do a poo' several times a day, whereas others may go once or twice a week. As long as stools aren't too hard and your child isn't uncomfortable getting them out, you don't need to worry or do anything. A temporary change in your child's bowel movements because of a fever, stress, or variations in diet is normal.

Tackling genital problems in boys

Any swelling or pain in your little boy's genitals can be serious, so don't lose any time and take a closer look. Some conditions need *urgent* assessment and treatment by a doctor, whereas others are relatively harmless.

Problems affecting the tip of the penis and foreskin

Problems affecting the penis and foreskin are fairly common, with itching and pain being important symptoms. Consider the causes in the following list:

- ✔ **Balanitis:** *Balanitis* is a common and fairly harmless condition caused by inflammation or infection of the tip of your boy's penis and foreskin, which becomes sore and perhaps slightly swollen. The condition is easily treatable with creams from your pharmacist or GP.

✔ **Overtight foreskin:** The *foreskin* (the bit of skin that covers the tip of the penis) is normally quite tight during a boy's first few years and can't be pulled back over the tip of the penis. As your boy grows older, the chances are that the foreskin becomes looser with time. See your GP for further assessment if you think this problem is causing inflammation or pain, particularly during erections. An overly tight foreskin is called *phimosis*, and an operation to widen the foreskin (known as *preputioplasty*) or – in extreme cases – remove it completely (called *circumcision*) may in certain circumstances be appropriate.

✔ **Urine infection:** If your boy only has pain in his penis when he passes urine, he may be suffering from a urine infection. See your GP.

Problems with your boy's testicles

Take any pain or swelling in your boy's testicles seriously, as you may need to act quickly. If he has a problem, consider the following possible causes:

✔ **Cysts:** A fluid-filled and often pea-sized sac called an *epididymal cyst* may develop in the tubes attached to the back of your boy's testicles (you can't usually see an epididymal cyst but you may be able to feel it). These cysts are usually harmless, but consult your doctor for assessment.

✔ **Hernia:** If your boy has a painless swelling in his groin or close to the skinned bag that contains his testicles, it may be due to a *hernia*, which occurs when parts of the inside of the abdomen push through a weak spot in the abdominal muscle wall (flip to Chapter 11 for more info on hernias). Consult your GP for an assessment.

✔ **Injury to a testicle:** If your boy has testicle pain that doesn't go away within a few minutes, due to an injury, seek medical advice so that any serious damage to his genitals can be excluded.

✔ **Torsion of the testis:** Sudden onset of severe pain on one side of your boy's scrotum – particularly if accompanied by nausea, vomiting and lower tummy pain – may be due to a testicle twisting around itself. This problem can happen anytime (even during sleep) for no apparent reason, and no way of preventing it exists. If you suspect a torsion in your boy, consult a doctor or take him to A&E straight away – no matter what time of day – because your boy is in danger of losing his testicle unless he receives treatment quickly.

Dealing with genital problems in girls

Itching and irritation are the most common problems in a young girl's genital area. Consider the following:

✔ **Thrush:** *Thrush* is a fungal infection, which commonly occurs after your girl has taken antibiotics, or when she suffers from diabetes or for no obvious reason at all. Typically, your girl has redness and itching in her genital area together with a thick creamy-white discharge from the vagina. See your GP for assessment.

✔ **Vulvovaginitis:** Soaps, inadequate hygiene or sometimes *threadworms* (these infect the gut, and their main symptom is itching around the anus – see your pharmacist for advice) may cause inflammation and irritation of the genitalia, which is called *vulvovaginitis*. You don't normally see any discharge from the vagina, and itching can be severe. Avoid soaps and bath additives, and ask your child to always wipe her bottom from the front to the back. Also use cotton underwear rather than synthetic fabrics, and make sure that your girl changes her underwear daily or more frequently, particularly if her underpants become damp or soiled during the day. If the problem doesn't settle with the above measures, speak to your pharmacist or GP.

Chapter 16

Identifying Health Problems in Your School-Age Children

*H*aving run the gauntlet of seemingly never-ending coughs, colds and other infections during their pre-school years, children on the whole tend to enjoy better health and are ill less frequently upon reaching school age. Health problems that children may encounter at this age rarely or never occur in babies or toddlers, so are likely to be different to their previous illnesses. (For common medical conditions that start in earlier life but can persist into school-age, such as *eczema* or *asthma,* turn to Chapters 14 and 15.)

In this chapter I focus on the symptoms and conditions that commonly cause anxiety for parents, and I aim to help you become more confident in assessing illness in your older child. Although serious health problems are rare in children, spotting important symptoms and signs early increases your child's chances of faster treatment and cure.

Moving Up to Common Head and Limb Problems

As children grow older, symptoms such as headaches and problems with their limbs become more common. Although problems in these areas are mostly benign and go away by themselves, many parents find them worrying and aren't quite sure what to do for fear of dealing with a potentially serious underlying cause. This section aims to help.

Heading off headaches

Headaches in children are common, and in most cases you can spot the underlying cause if you know what to look for. Occasional headaches with no other symptoms are usually nothing to worry about and can be due to emotional tension or simple reasons such as hunger.

Here are some other common causes for headache:

- ✔ **Eye problems:** Sometimes vision problems can cause headaches, but probably not as commonly as you may think. These headaches are usually mild and related to activities such as watching television or reading. Take your child to an optician for an eye test if you suspect visual problems.

- ✔ **Head injury:** Mild headache after a head injury is common, but the pain usually gets gradually better rather than worse. Check out the section on 'head injuries' in Chapter 15 for further information.

- ✔ **Meningitis:** Although rare, meningitis is one of the main concerns for most parents. You can find more information about meningitis in Chapter 14, but here's a list of important additional features of meningitis to look out for (which can differ slightly from those in younger children):

  - A fever over 38 degrees Celsius (100.4 degrees Fahrenheit).

  - Vomiting without diarrhoea.

  - Unusual drowsiness or fits.

  - Your child doesn't tolerate bright light.

  - Your child complains of a sore neck and doesn't like to bend her neck forward.

  - A rash that doesn't disappear on pressure (see image 21 in the colour section).

- ✔ **Migraine:** If your child has recurrent headaches together with other symptoms such as nausea, vomiting, visual problems or tummy aches without a fever (known as *abdominal migraine*), migraine is a possibility. Check out Chapter 9 for more about migraine, and see your GP for further assessment and advice on the treatment options.

- ✔ **Viral infections:** Colds or other viral infections often cause headache, which tends to be relatively mild. Air pockets in the bones of your child's face may also become inflamed or infected (which is known as *sinusitis*), causing facial pain. These conditions often settle on their own but may need treatment with decongestants or antibiotics when symptoms persist for more than a few days. Consult your pharmacist, practice nurse or GP.

Handling hip problems in children

Children love to run around and play, and often get into the occasional bit of rough and tumble. Thanks to their liveliness, hip pain in children often occurs due to overuse, but some potentially serious underlying causes can require urgent hospital assessment. So unless you're sure that your child's hip symptoms are due to a benign cause, seek medical advice.

Your child's hip pain may be caused by one of the following conditions, all of which need further medical assessment. I list them starting with the more commonly occurring conditions:

- **Irritable hip:** Also called *transient synovitis*, this condition may start suddenly preceded by a viral infection. Apart from the hip pain, your child doesn't feel unwell.

- **Perthe's disease:** This condition, in which the blood supply to the ball of the hip joint is disturbed, mostly affects boys between five and ten years old; accompanying knee pain and limping are common.

- **Slipped cartilage:** Especially in overweight boys between 10 and 15 years of age, the cartilage connecting the growing parts near the hip joint may slip, causing hip pain that often goes into the groin and knee.

- **Joint infection:** On rare occasions, the hip joint can become infected. Your child is likely to have another underlying infection, a fever and feel unwell, and usually is unable to walk; any movement in the hip is extremely painful.

- **Arthritis:** Joint inflammation may occur with or after viral infections or as part of a condition called *juvenile chronic arthritis*, which is the most common persistent form of arthritis in childhood.

The following additional symptoms indicate that your child's hip pain may have a serious cause:

- Constant pain even at rest or at night.

- Fever and a feeling of being unwell.

- History of high-speed or high-impact injury.

- Inability to walk or bear weight on the affected leg.

- Limping for more than a couple of days for no apparent reason.

- Severe pain which doesn't improve within hours.

Don't delay in consulting your GP if any of these features are present – your child may need urgent treatment in hospital.

Addressing knee problems in children

If your child develops knee problems, the pain is most likely to be due to an acute injury or overuse and usually settles quickly by itself without the need for any treatment. As long as your child can walk and jump, can move the knee without problems, is otherwise well and the knee is getting better with time, you don't need to worry too much.

Knowing a little about the following conditions helps you to decide what to do when your child has knee problems:

✔ **Injury:** Knee pain due to sports injuries or from a fall is common in children. Unless any of the red flag symptoms that I describe a little further on in this section are present, you can usually safely wait and see whether the pain gets better by itself. Paracetamol (check the instructions on the packet, as you need to give the correct dosage for your child's age) or other preparations available over-the-counter may help relieve any discomfort in the meantime – consult your pharmacist.

✔ **Overuse:** Injuries due to running around too much, hiking or engaging in new activities such as roller-skating are common. In older children, a condition known as *Osgood-Schlatter disease* is common, in which overuse causes inflammation at the top of the shin bone. Stopping these activities until the pain settles is usually enough, but the pain may take a couple of months to fade. Ibuprofen, taken as a tablet or put directly onto the knee as a gel, may help (check the instructions so that you give the correct dosage for your child's age). Your pharmacist can recommend suitable pain relief, but consult your GP if you're concerned.

✔ **Unusual knee shape:** *Knock knees* and *bow legs* may sometimes cause long-standing knee pain. See your GP for assessment if the pain is bothersome and doesn't settle with rest and over-the-counter medication.

Sometimes, knee pain may be due to what health professionals call *referred* pain from the hip or spine. If your child has knee pain, check whether she also has the following red flag symptoms or signs, which need to prompt you to seek medical advice immediately:

✔ A feeling of being unwell, fever or vomiting.

✔ A knee that keeps giving way.

✔ A limp for no apparent reason or that doesn't improve.

✔ An additional pain in the hip.

✔ An inability to bear weight fully on the affected leg.

✔ An inability to move the leg properly, and the knee is fixed in a certain position (called *locking*).

✔ A pain that's severe, constant and doesn't get better at rest or at night.

Looking at Tummy and Urinary Troubles

Any parent whose school-age child doesn't have tummy pain at least once can count themselves extremely lucky! Although stomach pain is a common symptom, thankfully, most tummy problems are minor and not due to any serious underlying cause. Knowing some of the symptoms and signs that may indicate a more serious problem helps you to manage your child more confidently, and in this section I explain what symptoms to look out for, and what they may mean. (You can read more about stomach problems and urinary conditions in Chapters 11 and 12.)

Attacking abdominal pain

Plenty of conditions can cause stomach pain in your child. Only a handful or so are relatively common or important to know about. Here are some common causes of abdominal pain in school-age children, starting with the more frequently occurring ones:

- **Emotional causes:** Often, abdominal pain has no obvious physical cause, and stress and emotional problems may be to blame. Emotional causes often bring on relatively mild recurrent tummy aches that can be present for weeks or months with pain that tends to come and go, but with no other physical symptoms. Consult your GP if you're concerned.

- **Gastroenteritis:** This tummy bug may also bring on diarrhoea and/or vomiting, and your child may have a mild fever. Read Chapter 14 for more information.

- **Urinary tract infection:** See the following 'Coping with urinary problems and bed-wetting' section.

- **Infections:** Almost any kind of infection can cause abdominal pain in children, so if your child has a cold or flu-like symptoms, this problem may be the reason for the stomach ache. Ask your pharmacist for suitable over-the-counter preparations to help ease your child's symptoms.

- **Testicular torsion:** If your son develops abdominal pain suddenly and in addition has a very tender and perhaps swollen testicle, seek medical help immediately. Your boy's testicle may have twisted around itself, cutting off the blood supply to the testicle, and unless operated on within a few hours, the testicle may 'die' and become useless. Therefore, don't hesitate to call for medical help immediately.

- **Appendicitis:** The *appendix* is a small finger-like pouch attached to the large bowel. For reasons that aren't well understood, the appendix can become inflamed and infected – a condition called *appendicitis*. Because the appendix may then burst, your child usually needs an operation (called an *appendicectomy*) to remove it before it causes a potentially serious infection called *peritonitis* inside your child's tummy.

Appendicitis may be difficult to spot – particularly in the early stages – and symptoms vary from child to child. Here are some important additional clues to look out for:

- A raised body temperature of 37.3 degrees Celsius (99 degrees Fahrenheit) or more (note that this is *lower* than the usual definition of fever in children – refer to Chapter 14).

- Continuous stomach pain for a few hours, or pain that gets worse quickly, particularly if accompanied by lack of appetite, nausea and vomiting.

- Dislike of anyone touching the tummy or pressing even lightly on the right lower abdomen.

- Pain that typically starts in the middle of the stomach near the belly button, before shifting to the lower right area of the abdomen.

- Preference for laying very still without moving and pain that gets worse on walking.

- Worsening pain when you ask your child to suck in her tummy and pop it out as far as possible.

If you suspect appendicitis, call your GP or take your child to the nearest Accident & Emergency (A&E) department. Chapter 11 has more on appendicitis.

For mild abdominal pain that shows up without any danger signs, rest, paracetamol and perhaps a well-padded and wrapped hot water bottle may be all that your child needs. But if you notice any red flag symptoms or are concerned, call for medical help immediately.

Coping with urinary problems and bed-wetting

Children are all different as regards passing urine – some seem to 'go' all the time, whereas others have little problem lasting for hours without needing to go to the toilet. Small children in particular usually have to go quite often and may not be able to give you much warning (you may be used to hearing 'I really really need to go!'), whereas older children become much better at controlling their bladder. Obviously, if your child drinks often she's going to produce more urine and need to go to the loo more than if you continuously need to remind her to drink.

Common urinary problems

The most common urinary symptoms in children are as follows:

- ✔ Complaining of pain or a burning sensation when passing urine.
- ✔ Passing urine more frequently.
- ✔ Wetting the bed after having been 'dry' for a while (see the following 'Bed-wetting' section).

If your child develops urinary problems, consider these possible causes, starting with the more common ones:

- ✔ **Urinary tract infection:** If your child complains of burning or stinging when passing urine, goes to the toilet much more frequently and has cloudy or even smelly urine, she's likely to have a *urinary tract infection*. Your child may also be feverish and feel slightly unwell, and may have some pain or discomfort in the middle of the lower abdomen over the bladder area. Starting to wet the bed at night again after being 'dry' for a while is another important sign. This infection is much more common in girls than in boys.

- ✔ **Emotional problems:** Many people go to the toilet more often when stressed, and children are no exception. If your child is going through a difficult period consider the possibility of underlying psychological stress as a reason for needing to go to the toilet frequently. However, emotional problems never cause pain or discomfort on passing urine, and so if the problem doesn't pass quickly or you're concerned, consult your GP to make sure that no other underlying medical condition is present.

- ✔ **Diabetes:** On rare occasions, passing urine more frequently or in larger volumes may be a sign of *diabetes mellitus* – a condition in which your child has too much sugar in her blood because of a lack of the hormone *insulin*. This condition is fairly rare in children, but getting your child checked is important when her urinary symptoms don't settle and no other obvious underlying cause is present, particularly if she also complains of tiredness and has been drinking much more than usual.

Unless your child's urinary problems are mild and settle quickly and completely by themselves, or when you're not sure what the problem may be, see your GP who's likely to test your child's urine and check for underlying conditions. Check out Chapter 12 for more details on urinary problems.

Bed-wetting

Most children are 'dry' at night at around the age of seven, and both children and their parents get distressed when bed-wetting (also known as *nocturnal enuresis*) persists into school-age. A number of reasons may be responsible, some of which you may be able to address and influence yourself.

Contrary to common belief, physical conditions only rarely cause bed-wetting, and emotional or so-called *functional* reasons – those without an underlying disease – are much more common.

Here's a quick guide to help you spot some of the causes of bed-wetting, starting with the common ones:

- **Constipation:** If your child is complaining about having hard stools and has infrequent bowel movements, constipation may be the underlying problem – hard stool in the back passage may be putting pressure on the bladder (called *faecal impaction*). Turn to Chapter 11 for more information on constipation and bowel problems.

- **Emotional factors:** Some children start wetting their bed again in times of emotional distress, for example, when their parents go through a divorce, someone close to them or their pet dies, or they are being bullied at school. Where emotional factors are the cause of the problem, the bed-wetting usually improves after a week or two.

- **Urinary tract infection:** A urine infection is a common cause of bed-wetting in a child who has been dry at night before. See the preceding 'Common urinary problems' section.

- **Lack of arousal from sleep:** Your child may just not wake up when her bladder gets full – she may sleep through even if the bed is wet. In this case your child may benefit from what's called an *enuresis alarm* (for further information check out the ERIC (Education and Resources for Improving Childhood Continence) website, www.eric.org.uk.

- **Increased urine production at night:** When increased urine production at night is the cause, your child usually doesn't show any urinary symptoms during the day, but may wet the bed early in the night with large wet patches. Excess drinking in the evening can bring this problem on, and so try restricting your child's fluid intake before bedtime. If this tactic fails, your child may respond to treatment with a drug called desmopressin or other medication.

- **Overactive bladder:** Children with an overactive or small bladder often also show urinary symptoms during the day.

- **Physical causes:** On rare occasions, an obstruction in the 'plumbing' or other rarer medical conditions can cause bed-wetting.

Try to speak openly with your child about the problem and find out what she thinks about it. And don't worry – most children grow out of wetting their beds and become 'dry'. Their bladders grow bigger and can hold more urine, and the muscles that 'seal' the bladder get stronger with age. Children's sleep also becomes lighter as they get older, and they become more sensitive to the urge to go to the toilet at night or in the early hours of the morning.

If your own attempts to fix the problem fail and you're still concerned, consult your school nurse or GP for further assessment and to talk about the management options, of which many are available. Seeing a health professional with your child is especially important if:

- ✔ You suspect a physical underlying cause.
- ✔ Your child (or you!) suffers severe emotional distress.
- ✔ Your child still wets the bed as an adolescent.
- ✔ Your child wets herself during the daytime.

Many parents worry about the negative social and emotional effects of bedwetting on their child. Nocturnal enuresis can affect whole families due to feelings of shame and embarrassment, which may become apparent when your child goes on a school trip or gets invited to a sleepover. You and your child may find that building up the courage to consult a health professional is difficult, or you may never have thought of speaking to someone before.

For your and your child's sake, don't be afraid to seek advice if you're worried. A number of strategies and treatments are available, including timing your child's fluid intake, periodically waking your child at night, moisture alarms, hypnosis, star charts, and retention and control training. For more information on treatment options and how to introduce them, take a look at *Children's Health For Dummies* by Nicci Talbot, Katy Holland and Dr Sarah Jarvis (Wiley), which contains a lot of practical advice. Also check out the ERIC website (www.eric.org.uk) which has lots of additional information.

Looking at Behavioural Problems

Children all behave differently, and telling normal behaviour from abnormal behaviour isn't always easy. Here's a list of some of the potential causes that may be to blame when you feel that your child has behaviour problems:

- ✔ Attention deficit hyperactivity disorder, or ADHD (check out the 'Dealing with hyperactivity' section later in this chapter).
- ✔ Autism, or autism spectrum disorder, including a condition called Asperger syndrome (see 'Understanding autism', later in this chapter).
- ✔ Deafness (see Chapter 15).
- ✔ Depression (see Chapters 17 and 21).
- ✔ Emotional problems (see Chapter 17).
- ✔ Epilepsy (see Chapter 15).
- ✔ Learning disability (see 'Meeting common behavioural problems' later in this chapter).
- ✔ Obsessive compulsive disorder, or OCD (see Chapter 22).

Making a diagnosis of a behavioural problem can be difficult even for experienced GPs, who sometimes need to seek the advice of specialists. If you're concerned about your child's behaviour, the information in the next few pages helps you decide whether your child may benefit from further assessment.

Meeting common behavioural problems

As your child grows, ensuring that she develops normal hearing, vision and intelligence is important. Developing slower or more quickly than normal can cause behavioural problems, particularly at school. If your child is slower with learning certain reading or writing skills than her peers, or has problems with language, a condition called *dyslexia* may be responsible, and behavioural problems may develop as a result – though this has nothing to do with her level of intelligence. Likewise, if your child is particularly gifted, boredom and lack of stimulation in the classroom may sometimes lead to unhappiness, frustration and therefore disruptive behaviour. Most teachers are quite good at spotting this problem, but higher than average intelligence being the main underlying cause may not always be apparent.

Other causes like depression or anxiety may also be responsible for your child's behavioural problems. Or she may just behave at the outer ranges of what most people consider to be 'normal' or 'acceptable' behaviour, which varies depending on circumstances and the social and cultural environment.

If you're concerned, speak to your child's teachers, the school nurse or your GP, who can help you judge whether to wait and see how your child progresses, or whether further action may be necessary. You can find further information on mental health problems in Chapter 17.

Dealing with hyperactivity

About 5 in every 100 children in the UK suffer from *Attention Deficit Hyperactivity Disorder*, or ADHD – a condition in which children are restless, act impulsively or have difficulty sustaining attention. Of course, children all do these things at times to a lesser degree, but in ADHD the behaviour is more exaggerated.

ADHD may appear as one of three types:

- **Combination type:** A combination of both inattention and hyperactive-impulsive types.

- **Hyperactive-impulsive type:** Your child may be very fidgety and run around in situations where sitting still is more appropriate. Quiet play may be an 'alien concept' for your child, and to your 'delight' she may talk endlessly! Children of this type may also have difficulty waiting their turn, and often interrupt others.

✔ **Inattention type:** Your child may find concentrating and paying attention difficult. She may not seem to listen properly, be easily distracted and may not follow instructions (realistically, no child responds or listens all the time, but I mean 'not following instructions' in an 'abnormal' kind of way). As a result, your child may appear forgetful and keep losing things.

As a result of such behaviours, your child may suffer developmental problems, intellectually and socially. Experts aren't sure what causes the condition, but they think that problems during pregnancy, familial factors, birth complications and severe emotional or physical neglect may all increase the chance that a child may develop ADHD.

Whatever people may say or think, your parenting skills, emotional stress within the family and watching television certainly don't cause ADHD, although these factors may possibly aggravate certain behaviours.

In a child who suffers from ADHD, the features are present in more than one setting or environment, for example, both at home and at school. The impulsiveness, restlessness and lack of attention can significantly affect school performance and your child's relationships with others, so that the overall effect on your child's life can be considerable.

Because any child with ADHD has a higher chance of developing depression and behavioural problems than other children, early recognition of the condition and treatment are important. If you're concerned, consult your school nurse, teacher or GP who can advise you whether your child may have a problem and what needs to be done about it, if anything. When your child's behaviour is outside of what you or your child's teachers would describe as normal, your child may require assistance at school to improve behaviour.

In some cases, your child may need assessment by a specialist, who can exclude physical causes such as hearing problems, epilepsy or an overactive thyroid gland that may be affecting your child's behaviour. Such an assessment is also useful for making sure that your child doesn't have any additional issues such as low self-esteem, anxiety or depression. To confirm an ADHD diagnosis, your child needs to fulfil strict criteria, and symptoms have to have been present for at least six months.

Various treatment options are available, which include support in terms of behavioural strategies as well as drug treatment. For further information about the condition, check out the website of the charity ADHD Information Services at www.addiss.co.uk.

Understanding autism

Autism is a condition in which children and adults have problems with everyday social interactions, which can affect communication with and relating to other people. The exact causes of autism are unknown, but experts believe that both genetic and environmental factors play a role.

You may suspect autism when your child is as young as 18 months or so, but symptoms often become apparent only much later. Look at the following areas to decide whether your child is showing any signs of autism:

- **Behaviour:** Children with autism throw tantrums more often than you'd expect, and you may notice odd movement patterns in them. Your child may also show little interest in people.

- **Communication:** Children and adults with autism find that making sense of the world around them and joining in with everyday conversations and chitchat is difficult. Your child's likely to be slower in terms of language development, can appear deaf and have difficulty talking with others, and may not respond in a way that you'd expect when you talk to her.

- **Co-ordination:** Children with autism find acquiring common skills such as handwriting or using cutlery difficult.

- **Imagination:** Children with autism typically struggle with imaginative play, such as 'pretend' games (for example, peek-a-boo and hide-and seek); they're more likely to focus on trivial and minor things around them. For example, instead of playing with a toy car, your child may be fascinated by and only pay attention to the car's wheels. Looking back, your child may not have enjoyed being swung or bounced on a knee as a toddler. Another typical feature is that children with autism don't come to their parents to show them objects or things that they've created.

- **Routines:** Repetitive behaviours are common in autistic children, who often feel uncomfortable without routines and resist changes to their regular activities. To a degree this behaviour is normal in young children but non-autistic children become more relaxed as they get older.

- **Social communication:** Children with autism often talk *at* others rather than *with* them and tend to find appreciating thoughts and feelings in other people difficult.

- **Social interaction:** Children with autism may appear indifferent to other people, especially to other children, and rarely initiate contact with others. When they do interact with other children, it may often appear 'odd' or repetitive, and they may behave inappropriately without being concerned about the reactions that this behaviour may provoke. Poor eye contact during conversations is typical, 'social smiling' is rare and children may prefer to play alone rather than with others.

Recognising autism in your child early on enables her to get the support and care she needs, to avoid problems at school and to help prevent depression as she gets older. Then, identifying the main problems in your child's life helps you as well as teachers and support staff to explore and develop imaginative solutions. For these reasons, and because autism can have a negative effect on your child and your family as a whole, recognising the condition and getting help is very important. Your school nurse or GP can refer your child for further specialist assessment. In addition, The National Autistic Society has lots of information available on their website www.autism.org.uk.

Perusing General Health Issues

In this section I cover two conditions. The first – obesity – is increasingly common and of concern to health professionals because children may become ill and are more likely to die from this condition and its consequences than from the second one – cancer. Cancer is rare, but dangerous: the thought of it can worry anyone. The concern is often unjustified, but spotting signs of cancer early can make all the difference.

Overcoming obesity

Obesity – when too much body fat affects health or wellbeing – in childhood has become increasingly common in the UK. Apart from risks to physical health, obesity in children may lead to psychological and social problems and to a greater likelihood of being obese in adulthood.

Calculating the *body mass index*, or *BMI* (see Chapter 7), can help in diagnosing obesity so contact your GP practice if you think that your child may be too heavy for her height and age. Alternatively, you can calculate your child's BMI yourself and find out if she's a healthy weight by using the calculator on the MEND (*Mind, Exercise, Nutrition – Do it*) website at www.mendcentral. org/aboutobesity/bmicalculator. You can also find lots of additional information on healthy ways of living for your whole family in the websites I list in Chapter 25.

If you're concerned that your child is overweight or obese, consider the following causes:

- ✔ **Dietary habits:** Eating too much of the wrong types of food (including 'ready-made' meals, some of which contain a lot more calories, fat and sugar than freshly prepared food), drinking lots of sugary drinks, having out-of-control eating habits and bingeing on food are common causes of childhood obesity. Having dedicated mealtimes instead of always eating in front of the TV, where people tend to eat more, is one way of changing your dietary habits.

- **Genetic causes:** If your child is obese for no apparent reason, particularly if she's under the age of two and is also quite short, a genetic familial trait may in rare cases be responsible. Learning difficulties, unusual body appearance and vision or hearing problems are additional signs. Consult your GP if you suspect genetic causes.

- **Hormonal conditions:** If your child suddenly and rapidly gains weight, particularly if her height and weight were normal before, consider hormonal causes. Ask your GP for an assessment.

- **Lack of exercise:** Obesity is almost always a mismatch between intake (the amount and type of food and drink that your child eats) and output (moving around), and if your child is more couch potato than fitness fanatic, lack of exercise can be the cause. You can do a lot to encourage exercise in your children, though, including:

  - Engaging non-competitive family exercise. Kicking a ball around or playing frisbee, hide-and-seek or tag, for example, are great ways to get your kids moving.

  - Putting your kids' favourite music on and dancing together.

  - Considering walking to school – or part of the journey – together instead of taking the car.

  - Going outside to play or walk with your children after a meal instead of lounging in front of the television.

For more ways to keep children healthy, check out *Nutrition For Dummies, Raising Happy Children For Dummies* and *Children's Health For Dummies*.

If you're concerned that your child may be overweight, contact your school nurse or GP surgery. These health professionals can properly measure and assess your child's height and weight, and also help if you and your child are being negatively affected by obesity – perhaps due to tensions within the household or bullying at school. Seeking help sooner rather than later can help to avoid longer-term problems such as depression or low self-esteem. Muscle and joint problems are also common in obese children, particularly in the back, hips, knees and feet. Various other health conditions can develop in your obese child, and weight reduction can go a long way to prevent these problems from happening.

The NHS Choices website (www.nhs.uk) has video footage of how to measure your child's height and weight and the National Obesity Forum website at www.nationalobesityforum.org.uk has information about and steps you can take to tackle obesity. Your school nurse or GP can offer help and advice, too.

Getting the low-down on calories

Food contains *calories* – the currency of energy – which people burn off when they move, exercise or think. Even when you're not doing anything, your body burns off calories just to keep you alive. In essence, when you take in more calories than you burn off (fatty and sweet foods and drinks in particular tend to contain a lot of calories), your body stores them as fat.

Although a certain amount of fat in your tissues is fine, too much can lead to health problems.

Plenty of ways exist to make children's diets healthier – turn to Chapter 25 for a list of websites where you can find useful information and resources.

Removing the worry about cancer

When a child falls ill for no apparent reason or develops 'odd' symptoms, some parents worry that *cancer* – where cells in the body start growing 'out of control' – may be to blame. The possibility that your child may have cancer can creep into your mind, because cancer is potentially serious or perhaps because you know someone whose child has been affected by it. You've probably also seen stories on TV or read about youngsters with cancer in newspapers and magazines.

Reassuringly, cancer in children is rare, and the vast majority of health problems in children aren't due to cancer.

Cancer is a serious diagnosis, however, with implications for the whole family and people close to you, as well as the affected child. It can make your child very ill and, although highly advanced treatments are available, cancer can lead to premature death. Many different types of cancer can occur, but most are very rare. The main types of cancer in children and adolescents include:

- ✔ Bone cancer.
- ✔ Brain tumour.
- ✔ Cancer of soft tissues.
- ✔ Leukaemia (cancer of the blood).
- ✔ Lymphoma (cancer of the lymph tissue).

The main features of cancer – in adults as well as children – are symptoms that tend to develop gradually and that you can't explain otherwise, and health problems that may be 'unusual' and unlike anything that you've noticed before in your child. Because symptoms tend to develop slowly, spotting cancer can be quite difficult, even for health professionals. To help, here's a list of some danger signs. Consult your GP for further assessment, to rule out the possibility of cancer, if you're in doubt or if your child:

- Complains of an ongoing and worsening headache, which may be accompanied by vomiting, limb weakness or other 'odd' symptoms such as problems with vision, concentration or performing simple tasks.

- Complains of unexplained constant bone pains that aren't due to injury.

- Develops lumps and bumps anywhere on her body that get bigger with time or don't disappear – and that you can't explain.

- Feels increasingly unwell and tired for more than a couple of weeks or so, for which you can find no other explanation (remember, though, that tiredness is rarely due to cancer).

- Loses weight for no apparent reason.

- Starts to look very pale without apparent reason (many kids look pale and 'off colour' at times due to simple viral or other infections, which is normal – in these cases, the colour returns when the illness is over).

- Suffers from bad regular night sweats that soak her pyjamas and mild, unexplained fevers that aren't due to a cold or other minor infection.

- Suffers from unexplained 'nervous' symptoms such as numbness, tingling, limb weakness, new squinting, seizures, 'strange' behaviour or any other symptoms that gradually appear and refuse to go away, or become worse with time.

- Suffers from unexplained shortness of breath.

Chapter 17

Dealing With Teenage Health Troubles

....

In This Chapter

▶ Looking at common teenage health problems

▶ Approaching more serious emotional and physical issues

....

Most *teenagers* – that is, young people between childhood and adult-hood (roughly and on average between the ages of 13 and 17) – are fit and well, and ready to get out and explore the world. If you belong to this age group, the chances are that you readily take on the challenges of looking after your own health and taking on new responsibilities when it comes to managing your own medical problems.

If you suffer from a common chronic medical condition such as asthma or diabetes, not surprisingly and for good reason you may resent or even rebel against being ill because it makes you feel different from your friends. As a result, your health may suffer.

Various – physical and mental – health problems occur more frequently in adolescence. *Acne*, for example – a common skin condition leading to spots on the face and other parts of the body – affects many young people at a time when they least need it, because of their increased awareness of their bodies and physical appearance. Eating disorders such as anorexia nervosa and bulimia also tend to start during adolescence. Although such disorders aren't particularly common, they can have an enormous impact on young people's lives and lead to sometimes serious or even life-threatening health problems.

This chapter aims to give you some answers and guidance about health prob-lems that typically occur during adolescence, and when you should consider seeking professional help.

Performing Your Own 'Teenage Health Check'

If you're a teenager and are worried that you may be suffering from emotional or physical problems but you're not quite sure what's going on, the first step towards tackling these is to identify the relevant issues. Go through this checklist to consider whether you:

- ✔ Have an ongoing medical condition (such as asthma or diabetes), which has become more difficult for you to manage.

- ✔ Are engaging in risk-taking behaviour (specifically, behaviour that can have serious health consequences: I talk more about this problem in the 'Recognising More Serious Mental and Physical Health Problems' section later in this chapter).

- ✔ Have problems at home.

- ✔ Have 'issues' at school – in terms of learning or with teachers or fellow pupils.

- ✔ May have an eating disorder.

- ✔ Don't get enough exercise.

- ✔ Are engaged in alcohol or drug misuse.

- ✔ Are involved in crime.

- ✔ May have mental health problems, which can include acts of self-harm or even suicidal ideas.

- ✔ May have sexual problems or be at risk of sexually transmitted infections.

Sometimes, you may be able to suspect health problems just by looking at your body or into the mirror, and so here are some clues that you may find useful (I expand on all these aspects throughout the rest of this chapter):

- ✔ **Being overweight:** Obesity is becoming increasingly common and can lead to numerous health problems in the future (you can read up on childhood obesity in Chapter 16). To find out what would be a normal weight for your height and age you can calculate your ideal body mass index, or BMI on the NHS Choices website, www.nhs.uk (flip to Chapter 7 for more on weight issues).

- ✔ **Being underweight:** Any evidence that you may be too thin or too light may suggest an eating disorder or less rarely a more serious underlying illness. However, you may not perceive yourself to be underweight, but other people may have made comments in this respect.

✔ **Mood:** Talking in a low voice, finding it difficult to maintain eye contact with other people, sudden changes in your behaviour and increased withdrawal or tearfulness for longer than you or other people close to you think normal are pointers that you may be unhappy or depressed (check out Chapter 21 for more information on depression).

✔ **Skin:** Acne is common, and you may be self-conscious about your spots and suffer considerably. Maybe you have cuts on your forearm from self-harming behaviour.

If any of these possibilities ring bells with you, this chapter aims to help you with approaching the topic and dealing with it yourself – or with the help of other people, such as your friends, parents, teachers or your school nurse. If you struggle, consider seeking advice from your GP, particularly if you're worried about any medical problems.

You may be reluctant to see a health professional because you fear that anything you say or discuss may 'leak out' to other people, such as your parents. But be reassured that all health professionals treat everything you say and discuss according to strict rules of confidentiality. The ideal situation is to see your GP or other health professionals together with your parents, but any health professional will be very happy to see you by yourself if you prefer. Even if taking the first step may be difficult for you, sometimes speaking to someone who isn't directly involved in any way can be much easier, particularly where sensitive issues are concerned.

For more information, you may want to check out the excellent youthhealthtalk website at www.youthhealthtalk.org, which provides lots of information and stories from teenagers with potentially very similar health problems to you, which you may find reassuring and encouraging.

Dealing With Acne

A change in sex hormones during adolescence not only leads to the development of physical sexual characteristics, but also to skin changes – greasy skin and spots in particular. *Acne* is the main skin condition that affects young people and can cause a lot of unhappiness.

Many teenagers suffer from acne to some degree. In most cases the condition is mild and a number of effective treatments are available, which – although they may not always make your spots disappear completely – can improve your skin considerably.

When your spots are painful, tender and unsightly, or they affect larger parts of the body, treatment is best to prevent scarring. Acne typically affects your face, but you may also develop spots on your back and chest.

In acne, various types of spots may be present – sometimes all at the same time. The most common ones are as follows, starting with the less severe ones:

- ✔ **Blackheads:** Small black spots called *blackheads* may occur on or around your nose or chin. Blackheads alone don't usually cause any longer-term problems and may not need treatment at all, but if they cover wider areas or bother you in terms of your appearance, various creams, lotions and gels may help. Your pharmacist or GP can advise on suitable preparations. Try not to squeeze blackheads by hand, because this action may lead to infection and possible scarring.

- ✔ **Pustules:** *Pustules* tend to be a bit larger than blackheads, are usually slightly raised and may have a white centre. Their appearance suggests that some mild underlying infection may exist within a spot, which – if extensive or severe – may require slightly more aggressive treatment, including *topical* (this means you apply them as a cream or gel directly to your skin) or oral antibiotics available on prescription from your GP.

- ✔ **Cysts:** Inflamed and tender lumps suggest *cysts*, which can lead to scarring. Arrange further assessment with your GP, because appropriate stronger treatment can prevent scars from developing. If you need more intensive treatment, your GP can explain the options to you and may offer to refer you to a skin specialist (known as a *dermatologist*) if necessary.

You can take several measures to manage mild acne:

- ✔ Don't wash too much – gently washing the face with lukewarm water once or twice a day is enough. Strong or abrasive soaps, excessive scrubbing, very hot water and using rough flannels can all make your skin worse rather than better. Contrary to popular belief, antiseptic washes don't do much good.

- ✔ Use only preparations that your pharmacist or doctor recommends, which may include non-perfumed creams and lotions.

You can do a lot to treat acne and prevent scarring, and so facing up to the problem and seeking medical help when simple over-the-counter treatments don't help is important and can really make your skin look much better. Unfortunately, no 'quick fix' for acne is available, and treatment may last for several weeks, months or sometimes years.

Setting the record straight about acne

Many people hold false beliefs about acne. For example, no evidence exists that certain foods, such as chocolate, or stress cause this skin condition – and you can't catch acne from another person. Don't believe a word when people say that acne may be due to poor hygiene – exactly the opposite is true, in that frequent washing can make acne worse. Don't think that medical treatment doesn't work – it does, but only if you adhere to the treatment; and avoid wasting money on sunbeds – nothing suggests that they're effective in improving acne.

Recognising More Serious Mental and Physical Health Problems

Serious medical conditions are rare in adolescence, but certain conditions which often start at the end of childhood can lead to sometimes more serious physical – and mental – consequences. Teenage health concerns may sometimes seem trivial, but more severe health problems aren't always immediately apparent. If you, your friends or your parents are worried about your health, don't hesitate to contact your GP surgery for advice. General practice teams are very aware of health issues in young people – some GP surgeries even run confidential Adolescent Health walk-in clinics. Finding out what's available in your patch is a good idea – most practices provide this information on their website.

Understanding eating disorders and weight problems

Eating disorders are fairly common in young people. The main conditions include *anorexia nervosa*, *bulimia* and *binge eating*, which are often triggered by life events such as bereavement, parents divorcing, bullying at school or major illness.

Bulimia is around five times more common than anorexia and tends to start around the age of 18 or 19. The majority of sufferers – around 90 per cent, in fact – are female. Both conditions can severely affect quality of life and cause severe health problems, which is why taking them seriously is so important. However, many teenagers with eating disorders often don't recognise that they may have one, and usually the people around them are the ones to voice their concern.

Anorexia nervosa

Anorexia nervosa is a psychological condition, which can lead to sometimes serious physical problems. Around 1 in 250 women and 1 in 2,000 men suffer from anorexia nervosa at some point, which usually develops around the age of 16 or 17. In anorexia, teenagers can have an intense fear of gaining weight, even when their body weight is normal or already lower than normal for their age. Young people with anorexia have a disturbed experience of their body shape or weight that may affect their self-image excessively and lead to constant worries about body weight. If you suffer from anorexia, you may start to worry only when symptoms develop, and it may take a long time before you find the need – or the courage – to talk about your concerns with your friends, parents or a health professional.

Any of the following warning signs can indicate that you may be suffering from anorexia, starting with the 'typical' ones:

- ✔ You have what others may perceive as an excessive pre-occupation with food, eating and mealtimes.

- ✔ You suffer from low mood, withdraw from some or all of your usual activities and have low energy levels.

- ✔ You suffer period problems and absent periods (although these symptoms are unreliable guides).

- ✔ You persistently lose weight, which you may find difficult to acknowledge or perhaps even try to hide from others – for example by wearing wide and baggy clothes. (Remember that maintaining a stable weight during your teenage years is equivalent to weight loss in an adult, so weight loss at this age is a serious matter.)

- ✔ Preference for eating alone.

- ✔ You develop ritualistic patterns of eating and other 'compulsive' activities.

- ✔ You feel cold a lot of the time.

- ✔ You exercise a lot (with the aim of losing weight).

- ✔ You feel sick a lot of the time.

- ✔ You become constipated and find it difficult to open your bowels (due to reduced food intake and malnutrition), or you get runny stools from using laxatives.

Additionally, a number of physical signs may be present in anorexia, such as:

- ✔ Your puberty is delayed compared to many of your friends. If you're female, this can mean that you're late in starting to have your periods compared to your friends.

- ✔ Your glands at both sides of your face near the angle of the jaw swell up (known as *parotid swelling*), which can be a result of not eating enough or not eating healthily enough.

- ✔ Your skin becomes less elastic due to not drinking enough (known as *dehydration*).

- ✔ Your skin looks pale due to *anaemia* (lack of blood) as a result of a poor diet.

- ✔ If you're a woman, your breasts shrink.

- ✔ Your hair becomes thin, and you grow soft hair (also known as *lanugo hair*) on your face and body.

Anorexia nervosa can cause numerous and often severe health problems; in rare cases it can even be fatal. Here's a list of some main complications of anorexia:

- ✔ Serious heart problems.

- ✔ Increased risk of infections.

- ✔ Kidney problems including kidney failure.

- ✔ Lack of blood (anaemia).

- ✔ Low blood pressure and feeling faint.

- ✔ Low blood sugar.

- ✔ Low potassium in the blood (which can lead to problems with heart rhythm and can be caused by laxatives and other medication).

- ✔ Weak bones (or *osteoporosis*).

For these reasons, if you suspect that you may suffer from anorexia, try to answer the following questions:

- ✔ **How much would you like to weigh?** If you aim for a weight that is below what's regarded as a 'healthy' weight (refer to Chapter 7 on how to calculate this for your height and age), you're at risk of anorexia.

- ✔ **How do you feel about your weight?** Having a normal weight but being unhappy about it makes you more prone to developing anorexia.

✔ **Are you happy with your body?** Being unhappy with the way you look is a typical symptom of anorexia.

✔ **Do you believe yourself to be fat when others say that you're too thin?** This may suggest that your body image – rightly or wrongly – is different from others around you, which is a common symptom of anorexia.

✔ **Do you get a sense of achievement when you're losing weight?** This in itself isn't a problem, and only becomes one if you keep going even after reaching a 'healthy' weight.

If you suspect that you may suffer from anorexia, try to speak about your concerns with people whom you trust, such as your friends, your parents, your school nurse or your GP. If the diagnosis is confirmed, your GP may advise further referral to a specialist with an interest in eating disorders if appropriate and if you agree. In rare and severe cases, hospital admission may sometimes be necessary to prevent you from starving to death.

You can find out more about anorexia on the NHS Choices website (www. nhs.uk), from *beat* – the Eating Disorders Association – on 08456 341414 or their website www.b-eat.co.uk, or on the Patient UK website (www. patient.co.uk).

Bulimia

Many people became aware of this condition after the fact emerged that Princess Diana's 'secret disease' for many years was bulimia, until she sought treatment. Bulimia is far more common than anorexia, and 90 per cent of people with bulimia are women in whom this usually develops around the age of 18 or 19 – but this condition can also start much later in life. In *bulimia*, you indulge in binge eating, and then try hard to prevent gaining weight afterwards by, for example, using laxatives, vomiting or fasting – which can have psychological, physical and social consequences. Typical for this condition is that you may feel completely out of control with regard to your eating patterns.

Certain clues can indicate that you may suffer from bulimia:

✔ You binge on food and then make yourself throw up afterwards.

✔ You use laxatives as a means of trying to empty your bowels.

If you are bulimic, your body weight is usually normal, but you may develop other physical signs, such as:

✔ Bloodshot eyes as a result of vomiting.

✔ Poor teeth (*dental caries*) due to the acid within vomit.

✔ Thick skin or small wounds on the back of your hand from self-induced vomiting.

In mild cases, the condition may be short-term or intermittent, but if you're in the least bit concerned, try to talk to someone you trust and arrange an appointment with your GP for further assessment. For further information check out the NHS Choices website at www.nhs.uk/Conditions/ Bulimia/Pages/Introduction.aspx or the *beat* (the Eating Disorders Association) website at www.b-eat.co.uk (you can also call them on 08456 341414). The Patient UK website (www.patient.co.uk) provides patient information leaflets on bulimia and self-help for eating disorders.

Binge eating

People who binge eat consume large amounts of food – usually in private – even if they're not hungry. Feelings of guilt or disgust at having eaten so much usually follows the bingeing, which can indicate underlying psychological problems such as anxiety or depression (turn to the next section 'Diagnosing depression and self-harm' and Chapter 21 for more info on these). But don't worry, over-indulging in your favourite foods once in a while is not an eating disorder.

Although binge eating can affect anyone, it's more common in women than in men and usually starts during adolescence or in early adulthood.

Binge eating can become a problem if you:

- ✔ Lose control over how much you eat.
- ✔ Live a life that is dominated by food.
- ✔ Have to make yourself sick at times because of feeling too full.
- ✔ Are visibly putting on weight.

Check out the Patient UK website, which has a useful Patient Information Leaflet at www.patient.co.uk/health/Eating-Disorders-A-Self-Help-Guide.htm. Further help and advice is available from *beat* (the Eating Disorders Association) on 08456 341414 or via their website at www.b-eat.co.uk. Consult your GP for further assessment and help if you're worried about your physical or mental health.

Diagnosing depression and self-harm

I probably don't need to tell you that mood swings tend to become more frequent in adolescence – and this is quite normal. However, if mood problems start to affect your life in a major way, depression and in severe cases self-harming may occur. Self-cutting or even overdoses of medication such as paracetamol are therefore relatively common among teenagers. Research suggests that perhaps as many as around 10 per cent of teenagers may self-harm at some stage.

Distinguishing between being moody and depression can be difficult, as can knowing how to respond. You can easily feel out of your depth as regards to dealing with more severe emotional problems, and so if you find this aspect difficult, don't worry – you're not alone. Self-harming behaviour can be very unsettling for you as well as people close to you.

In this section I focus on issues around self-harm in teenagers, and I also briefly touch on how to spot signs of depression. You can find more about mental health problems, including depression and alcohol and drug misuse, in Part V.

Depression

Mood swings are so common in teenagers that spotting signs of actual *depression* – which occurs when you have a persistently low mood together with other symptoms, and neither you nor people close to you can get you out of this situation – can be difficult. More than just normal 'ups and downs' may be at play if you:

- ✔ Feel guilty or hopeless for most of the time.

- ✔ Lose your appetite and your clothes become looser, suggesting weight loss.

- ✔ Are more tired than usual and have little energy.

- ✔ Sleep much more than usual or you think would be normal – or you sleep much less and wake early in the morning.

- ✔ Become more anxious and don't like to go out anymore.

- ✔ Don't seem to get much enjoyment out of life.

Depression may require further assessment and treatment. Turn to Chapter 21 for more information.

Self-harming

Some apparently normal teenagers may cut themselves to help them deal with emotional suffering. If you feel this way, remember that you're not alone. Research shows that as many as 6 per cent of children who are around 15 years old have harmed themselves at least once. Self-harm is more common in teenage girls, usually between the ages of 15 to 19 years, although even younger children may self-harm.

If you're in a state of particular distress, you're at higher risk of harming yourself in one of several ways:

- ✔ **Attempted suicide:** Suicide among teenagers is rare, but suicidal ideas are always worrying. Talk to someone you trust if you have suicidal thoughts and seek professional help.

- ✔ **Self-cutting:** Common objects used for self-cutting include razor blades, pins, needles, glass or scissors.

- ✔ **Self-poisoning:** See the following 'Overdoses' section.

Although self-harm and attempted suicide can be uncomfortable to deal with and are probably things you'd rather not talk to other people about, knowing a little about potential warning signs and what to do can go a long way to prevent a lot of suffering.

You're at an increased risk of self-harming if any of these situations apply to you:

- ✔ You get into trouble at school with other pupils or teachers and you're severely distressed by this fact.

- ✔ You have suffered a traumatic relationship break-up.

- ✔ You develop persistent thoughts of suicide and self-harm.

- ✔ You have attempted suicide in the past.

- ✔ You talk or write about harming yourself.

- ✔ You have written a suicide note that you want others to find.

- ✔ You suffer from depression, anxiety or other mental illness, or from alcohol problems (turn to Part V for more info).

- ✔ You keep thinking and saying how hopeless life seems to be and you don't get much enjoyment out of life.

- ✔ You feel that you have little support from your friends or family members.

If you identify with any of the above situations, consult your GP who can discuss with you the best way forward. Remember that your GP will be happy to see you by yourself, although it's usually preferable (though not essential) to have a parent or carer with you.

Overdoses

Every medicine, whether prescription or over-the-counter, comes with instructions that give you the recommended dose. An *overdose* is when you take more than this amount. Overdoses can be accidental, most often through carelessness or because you forget that you've already taken your dose that day, but these are usually minor. Intentional overdoses with the intent of deliberate self-harm as a response to emotional trauma in your life can be altogether more serious – and life-threatening.

If you have taken an accidental or intentional overdose, get immediately to the nearest Accident & Emergency (A&E) department or call '999'. Obviously, you need to act very fast – you may become ill very quickly even when you still feel well. Try to have the following information ready for the emergency medical team ('999' call handlers tell you exactly what to do while you wait):

✔ The type of substance you took.

✔ The strength of the substance: take the packet or bottle along if possible.

✔ The quantity you took and whether you

- Vomited afterwards.

- Have taken alcohol or other drugs (both prescribed medication as well as illicit drugs) as well.

Most teenagers who take an overdose do so as a 'cry for help', without actually wanting to kill themselves. Ironically, they're often unaware of the harm that, for example, paracetamol can do, and how dangerous an overdose can be.

When you have suicidal thoughts, you're at higher risk of committing suicide. Seek professional help if:

✔ You've suffered from severe emotional problems for more than a month, and this situation doesn't seem to improve.

✔ You keep making plans to harm yourself – or you've made preparations.

✔ You've written a suicide note.

✔ You feel hopeless about the future and are convinced that things aren't going to get much better.

Take suicidal thoughts and threats of or actual self-harm seriously and seek medical help and advice sooner rather than later if you're at all concerned. Although rare in teenagers, suicide is the worst thing that can happen to you and your parents, your wider family and other people close to you. Being able to recognise the warning signs may help to save you from serious harm.

For further help – particularly in a crisis – you can call the Samaritans on 08457 909090 or visit their website (www.samaritans.org). You can get additional information and support from the National Self Harm Network (visit their website www.nshn.co.uk or phone 0800 6226000), YouthNet UK at www.thesite.org or MIND (visit their website – www.mind.org.uk – or phone 0845 7660163).

TIP

Sex, drugs and . . . alcohol

The teenage years can be tricky ones for you. You may find that you're tempted to experiment with drinking alcohol or using drugs – and you may start sexual activities. You can benefit from being aware of some of the risks involved, which can help you make informed decisions about whether you want to engage in activities that are new to you:

✔ **Alcohol:** Despite restrictions on the sale of alcohol to under-age people, many teenagers find ways to get access to alcoholic drinks. Although occasional consumption of small amounts of alcohol is unlikely to do much damage, you should try to avoid drinking alcohol if you're under-age. *Binge drinking* – when you consume a lot of alcohol in one session – as well as regular high alcohol consumption can cause severe health problems over time. Among many teenage groups a 'culture of drinking' exists in the UK, and you may struggle not to be one of the crowd. Consider addressing this problem openly with your peers and discuss possible strategies with your parents, your school nurse, like-minded friends or your GP. The charity Drinkaware (www.drinkaware.co.uk) provides help with regard to alcohol-related problems in under 18s.

✔ **Drugs:** As you get older, you may get access to and feel tempted to experiment with drugs such as cannabis or 'harder' drugs such as heroin. Taking drugs can lead to serious physical and mental health problems – and they can kill. Lots of reliable information is available – ideally get

the low-down *before* you put yourself at risk. For further information, telephone the charity FRANK (on 0800 776600) or visit the website (www.talktofrank.com).

✔ **Sexual health:** When hormones start to kick in, you'll have a natural drive to engage in sexual activities, and so being aware of the risks of accidental pregnancy as well as sexually transmitted infection is important. The UK has a high rate of unwanted teenage pregnancies, and so sex education is now firmly embedded in the national curriculum. 'Safer sex' (by using condoms) and contraception are important issues to think about. The charity Brook is geared towards people aged under 25 and has lots of useful further information (0808 8021234; www.brook.org.uk).

✔ **Smoking:** Many teenagers try out smoking cigarettes at some stage. This experiment doesn't mean that you'll become a smoker, but getting addicted to nicotine is easy, so try to make sure you're aware of the risks (and costs) of smoking. The Patient UK website has a great information leaflet on Smoking Facts available at www.patient.co.uk. If you already smoke, consider stopping – lots of help is available from the NHS (for further information check out smokefree.nhs.uk).

You can also find further information on these topics in this book. Check out Chapters 18 and 19 for more details of sexually transmitted infections and Chapter 23 for information on alcohol and drug problems.

Chapter 18

Understanding Women's Troubles

· ·

· ·

*P*roblems with periods, fertility, sex, pregnancy and childbirth are incredibly common, and yet many women find talking about them difficult. Symptoms of abnormal vaginal bleeding, for example, can be very frightening, and you may feel that you're the only one who's affected by the problem.

Knowing what's normal and what isn't can also be hard. Many couples trying for a baby, for instance, don't know that for a year or so to pass until the woman conceives is quite normal. Knowledge about what's normal and when to consider seeking medical advice can therefore come in handy, because you're then able to reassure yourself or receive treatment, if needed.

Women's health is a large topic. Instead of giving you too much detail, in this chapter I provide an initial overview of likely causes of some of the main symptoms. I let you know when you're able to deal with some of the health problems yourself, and when to seek medical advice from your GP, so I hope you become confident in distinguishing between the two options.

Bleeding Nightmares: Menstrual Problems

Problems with menstrual periods are incredibly common. Most menstrual symptoms are benign and usually don't last for very long, but many women suffer from painful, heavy or irregular periods on a regular basis. As a rule,

when these problems start to interfere too much with your life or you suspect that something else may be wrong, the best thing to do is consult your
GP for an assessment.

Keeping the floods at bay: Heavy periods

Most women's periods last for about five days or so, with a peak in terms
of blood loss around day three, but quite a bit of variation exists between
women. Tampons or normal sanitary towels are usually enough to soak up
the blood that you lose. If your periods last for much longer or have recently
become heavier, however, or your normal sanitary aids aren't sufficient to
cope with your blood loss, you may be suffering from what health professionals call *menorrhagia*. If this situation is the case, see your GP for help with the
diagnosis and further management.

To give you an idea as to what may be the problem, here's a selection of possible causes:

- **Coil:** The coil is a *intrauterine contraceptive device* or *IUD*. Heavy menstrual bleeding can be a side effect when you've had the coil inserted.
  Don't worry too much if your bleeding isn't *that* heavy, but if you're
  bothered by it or worried, see your GP for further assessment.

- **Endometriosis:** Doctors are unsure of the precise cause, but endometriosis is probably due to womb-lining tissue spreading outside your
  womb. The condition can start at any time between 20 and 40 years of
  age – or sometimes earlier. Apart from being heavy, your periods are
  likely to be more painful, too.

- **Fibroids:** Benign muscular growths called *fibroids* inside your womb can
  gradually cause heavier and sometimes more painful periods. Fibroids
  tend to be more common in women over 35 years of age.

- **Medication:** Treatment with blood-thinning medication (known as *anti-
  coagulation*) can easily lead to heavier and more prolonged periods.

- **Miscarriage:** If you're sexually active, one heavy but late period can
  potentially be due to an early miscarriage. When this event happens, the
  period is also likely to be more painful than usual. If you suspect that
  you may have had a miscarriage, visit your GP.

- **Thick lining of the womb:** You may have a thicker lining of the womb
  than usual, which can mean that you always have heavy periods.
  Although this is not usually a big problem, over time you may lose more
  blood than your body can replace, leading to *anaemia*. Features of anaemia include tiredness and a pale complexion, and if you suspect that you
  have it, consult your GP for further assessment and treatment.

✔ **Underactive thyroid:** Heavy periods may be a symptom of an underactive thyroid gland (also known as *hypothyroidism*), in which case you're likely to have other symptoms as well such as being tired, weight gain, hair loss, constipation and feeling cold all the time. The condition is easily diagnosed with a blood test, and treatment is simple.

Other rarer causes can also be responsible for your heavy bleeding. However, you may be surprised to discover that doctors don't find a cause in as many as 1 in 2 women. Your GP may refer you to a specialist for further investigation and treatment if appropriate, and if you feel tired your GP may also arrange a simple blood test to find out whether you're anaemic or your thyroid gland isn't producing enough hormones.

Sometimes, other and potentially more serious underlying causes can be present, which indicate that you need to consult your doctor. These symptoms include the following:

✔ You begin having heavy periods when you're 40 years or older.

✔ You look very pale and feel tired all the time, which suggests anaemia.

✔ You also have persistent bleeding between periods.

✔ You've had an abnormal *smear test* (as part of screening for cervical cancer) in the past.

✔ You have pressure symptoms in your lower abdomen or genital area.

✔ You suffer from abdominal pain in between your periods.

If the bleeding is continuous, very heavy (like 'flooding') and you feel unwell or faint, seek medical advice immediately. Various treatments are available for heavy periods, and certain 'coils' can make your periods lighter (such as the Mirena intrauterine system).

Managing painful periods

A certain amount of pain or discomfort (health professionals call this *dysmenorrhoea*) at the time of your monthly periods is normal. This discomfort may take the form of a cramp-like pain in the middle of your lower abdomen. Symptoms are usually mild and in most women they don't interfere with day-to-day life.

If you find that your period pains have always been bad, get worse or stop you from getting on with your daily life, consider the following possible causes, starting with the most common one:

✔ **Primary dysmenorrhoea:** If you've always suffered from painful periods you probably have what's called *primary dysmenorrhoea* ('primary' here just means that you've had the problem right from the start and for no obvious reason). Younger women in their late teens and early twenties most commonly have this condition, but it may continue for much longer. Sometimes dysmenorrhoea may improve after you've had a baby.

Although no obvious reason usually exists for the painful periods, experts think that the problem is likely due to hormonal reasons. Over-the-counter painkillers or a well-wrapped hot water bottle held to your tummy may help, but your GP can prescribe stronger medication if necessary. Some women prefer to go on 'the pill' (unless good reasons exist why they shouldn't), which tends to make periods lighter and is useful as reliable contraception. Again, talk to your GP about this option.

✔ **Pelvic inflammatory disease:** This disease is an infection of tissues low down inside your stomach – particularly the tubes attached to your womb. This condition is more likely if you also have pain in between your periods and you suffer from vaginal discharge. Consult your GP, who may take swabs from your vagina to try and confirm the diagnosis and prescribe antibiotics and painkillers as appropriate.

In addition, the coil, fibroids or endometriosis (see the preceding section 'Keeping the floods at bay: Heavy periods' for more details) can cause painful as well as heavy periods.

As a guide, consult your GP if you're worried, have additional symptoms such as abdominal pain, or you just don't know what's going on.

Discovering more about absent periods

Most young girls get their first period between the ages of 10 and 14, although some don't start menstruating until a couple of years later. Periods are normally a bit irregular in the first few years before settling into a regular cycle in most women, and the number of days between menstrual periods varies from woman to woman, ranging from about 24–36 days.

Amenorrhoea, or periods that never start or suddenly stop, can occur for a variety of reasons:

✔ **Menopause:** If you're around the age of 50, your periods may come to a natural end. Check out the 'Managing menopausal problems' section later in this chapter for more information.

✔ **Polycystic Ovary Syndrome (PCOS):** *PCOS* is one of the most common hormonal conditions affecting women in their fertile years. The main symptoms are irregular or absent periods, weight gain and increased

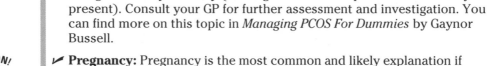

hair growth on your body (although these developments aren't always present). Consult your GP for further assessment and investigation. You can find more on this topic in *Managing PCOS For Dummies* by Gaynor Bussell.

✔ **Pregnancy:** Pregnancy is the most common and likely explanation if you normally have regular periods and are sexually active – particularly if you haven't used any contraception. The easiest way of finding out whether you're pregnant is to contact your local family planning clinic or do a home pregnancy test, which you can buy from your pharmacist over-the-counter. These tests are very reliable and you get a positive result from the date of your missed period if you're pregnant.

✔ **Primary amenorrhoea:** *Primary amenorrhoea* is a condition in which you've never had a period in your life, and is quite normal up to the age of 14 or so. If you haven't had a period by your 16th birthday, or if you get regular cyclic pain every few weeks without any bleeding, you may want to check in with your doctor.

✔ **Stopping contraception:** If you stop taking the combined oral contraceptive pill, your periods may take a while to return to normal or may even stop altogether, although usually for not much longer than three months.

✔ **Stress and similar factors:** Emotional and physical stresses (such as long-distance running or other heavy and regular exercise) can lead to lighter or absent periods.

✔ **Using certain contraception:** If you take the progesterone-only pill, your periods may also become irregular or stop completely. Consult your family planning clinic, GP or practice nurse if you're concerned and not sure what to do.

If your symptoms don't fit with any of these conditions, other causes – some of which are quite rare – may be responsible. In addition to your absent periods, be alert to the following warning signs that need to prompt you to seek medical advice from your GP:

✔ You notice new hair growth on your face or body.

✔ You haven't reached puberty and are 15 years or older.

✔ You're over 16 years old and haven't had a period.

✔ You suffer from weight loss, tiredness, fever, feeling unwell or have lost your appetite.

✔ You don't think that any of the conditions I list in this section are likely as the potential underlying cause.

Coping with irregular vaginal bleeding

Irregular vaginal bleeding is bleeding that occurs between your 'regular' periods – even if these may themselves be slightly irregular – or in other words, bleeding that's unusual or outside what's 'normal' for you. Check out the following list of possible causes to see whether any of your symptoms fit:

- ✔ **Cervix abnormalities and cervical cancer:** Vaginal bleeding that occurs after or during sexual intercourse or after the menopause may be caused by minor cell abnormalities of the neck of your womb (called the *cervix*). See your GP for further assessment, because you may require further testing to exclude rare but more serious causes such as *cervical cancer*.

  Just under 3,000 women are diagnosed with cervical cancer in the UK each year. Some women with cervical cancer also notice an offensive smelling vaginal discharge and pain or discomfort during sex. As with most cancers, the earlier cervical cancer is diagnosed the better, because treatment is generally then more successful.

- ✔ **Contraception:** Bleeding between periods may also be a side effect of contraceptive methods such as the oral contraceptive pill or the coil (or IUD). You may also bleed if you miss a couple of pills, or if you've had severe diarrhoea or vomiting, which can reduce the absorption of the pill. Bleeding may also occur if you've recently taken the morning after pill. Usually, you don't need to worry, but talk to your family planning clinic or your GP, who may be able to suggest alternative types of contraception.

- ✔ **Ectopic pregnancy:** If you've been sexually active within the past 12 weeks and have missed a period before, call your GP straight away. Your bleeding can potentially be due to a complication of early pregnancy called *ectopic pregnancy* (turn to the section 'Handling pregnancy problems' later in this chapter for further info), when the pregnancy is outside your womb in one of your *fallopian tubes* – with the risk of rupture. Additional abdominal pain makes this condition even more likely. If your GP confirms your suspicions, you're likely to need further tests and possibly an operation in hospital. The main danger is that an ectopic pregnancy can lead to a ruptured blood vessel, which is a medical emergency. If you suddenly develop abdominal pain and feel very weak or collapse, call '999' immediately (also check out the later section, 'Handling pregnancy problems').

- ✔ **Pregnancy:** If you think you may be pregnant, do a pregnancy test (home tests available from the pharmacy are very accurate) or arrange a pregnancy test via a local family planning clinic or your GP surgery. Bleeding in early pregnancy is common and doesn't always mean that you have a problem, but if you're pregnant and bleeding, you need to consult your GP immediately for further assessment.

✔ **Vaginal and womb disorders:** If you're over the age of 40 and more than six months have passed since your last period, your bleeding may be due to a minor problem inside your vagina, but can also come from abnormalities inside your womb. In rare cases, *endometrial cancer* (a cancer of the lining of your womb) may be causing the bleeding. Always consult your doctor if you experience unusual or unscheduled vaginal bleeding after the age of 40.

Telling exactly what's causing your vaginal bleeding is difficult in most cases, and so if you're in any doubt consult your GP.

Talking Sex

Sexual problems are more common than you may think. Some people have high expectations as to what may be considered normal, but in other cases underlying medical problems cause difficulties with sexual relationships.

In this section I give you an overview of the more common sexual problems that can cause a lot of concern in many women (as well as their partners). If you'd like to read up about sexual health problems in more detail, take a look at the charity Relate's website at www.relate.org.uk, which has a lot of useful information.

Experiencing pain during or after sex

Pain during sexual intercourse (also called *dyspareunia*) can be a real turn-off, and plenty of causes may be responsible. Longstanding problems with pain or discomfort during or after sex can severely affect your sex life and your relationship, and so consulting your GP is worthwhile if your symptoms persist or you're not sure what's going on.

Consider that your pain may be from these common reasons, starting with the common ones:

✔ **Dry vagina:** A dry and tight vagina that makes penetration difficult may be due to anxiety or tension around sexual activities, but can also occur for no obvious reason. Problems due to a dry vagina are common in later life, particularly after the menopause or when couples don't have enough time alone and sex becomes a bit rushed. Talking about this issue with your partner and using a lubricating gel may help. If the problem persists, consult your GP who can rule out an underlying physical cause and may suggest referral for sex counselling if appropriate.

✔ **Vaginal soreness:** Your vagina may become sore if you've had sex again for the first time after a break, or if you've had a long sex session – this type of soreness usually settles quickly. Your vagina is also likely to feel sore for a few weeks after delivery of a baby, and so waiting until everything has healed is best before you start having intercourse again, particularly if you've had stitches. When you do, using lots of lubricating jelly can help – especially if you feel a bit anxious initially. See your doctor if you still experience pain six weeks after delivery, you also suffer from vaginal discharge (turn to the 'Dealing with vaginal discharge' section later in this chapter) or you're worried for any other reason.

✔ **Endometriosis:** In endometriosis, tissue that's normally found only inside your womb spreads to surrounding tissues. Pain during intercourse is a common feature of endometriosis. Typically – but not always – symptoms due to endometriosis tend to be worse around the time of your periods. See your GP for further assessment.

✔ **Ovarian or cervical causes:** If you have no problems with your periods and you've only recently started having pain during intercourse, a *cyst* (a small and benign fluid-filled sac) in your ovary may be the cause. Inflammation of the *cervix* (the neck of your womb) can also cause painful intercourse. However, if you've always had deep pain during intercourse, particularly a pain that occurs only in certain positions, your symptoms may be caused by pressure on your ovary. If you're concerned or have any additional symptoms such as abdominal pain and bloating, urinary symptoms, tiredness, bowel problems or weight loss, always see your GP for further assessment and to rule out a more serious cause such as ovarian cancer (which becomes more common in older age).

Losing interest in sex

Each person is different as regards sexual desires, and saying what's normal and what isn't is quite difficult. Some women feel the desire to have sex (also called *libido*) every day (or even more than once a day), whereas others are quite happy with once a week, once a month or less.

The main reason for women seeking medical advice is when the desire for sex suddenly or for no apparent reason disappears, or if the lack of sex drive causes friction in the partnership. Both physical and psychological causes may be involved – sometimes together, and so seeking advice from your GP or a sexual health counsellor is worthwhile when you're worried.

Check this list to see whether any of these causes (starting with the commoner ones) may apply to you, but be aware that many others exist, too:

- ✔ **Pain on intercourse:** Pain during or after sex can be very off-putting and adversely affect your libido (read the preceding section, 'Experiencing pain during or after sex').

- ✔ **Pregnancy and having a baby:** Pregnancy and looking after a baby or small child is hard work – and sex may be the last thing on your mind, particularly if you're very tired or have other health problems. Make sure that you let your partner know how you feel, and perhaps consider having sex at times when you're more likely to feel like it, instead of when you're bound to be tired. If you think any medical issues are also in the way, consult your GP.

- ✔ **Sexual and general relationship problems:** If you or your partner have any 'issues' or difficulties as regards sex (for example, premature ejaculation in your partner or you'd like to achieve orgasm but find it difficult), losing interest is easy – which can be true for both of you. Not feeling generally happy in your relationship can negatively affect your sex life as well.

  Talking openly about these issues – which can admittedly be quite difficult and feel daunting – can take a lot of the pressure off. However, if you don't make progress, seek professional advice from your GP or a sex counsellor. And don't worry – sexual problems are incredibly common and you're not the only one who experiences difficulties.

- ✔ **Anxiety and depression:** Sexual desire is closely related to how you feel in general. Feeling anxious or tense for whatever reason can easily dampen your enthusiasm for sex. Stress at home or at work, fear of becoming pregnant or any other worries or concerns that are on your mind may all play a role, too. Flip to Chapter 21, which has loads more information on dealing with anxiety, stress and depression.

- ✔ **Medication:** Certain drugs such as the oral contraceptive pill, antidepressants, blood pressure lowering medication and others may all affect sex drive in both men and women. Check the drug information sheet and consult your GP when you feel your reduced libido may be due to a drug side effect.

- ✔ **Hormonal abnormalities:** If your partner says, 'it's your hormones, darling', he may even be right – for once! Some hormonal problems, such as an underactive thyroid gland, can occasionally lead to a reduced interest in sex. If this situation is the case, you're likely also to have some problems with your periods in that your bleeds may be absent or very heavy, as well as other symptoms such as constipation, feeling tired or cold all the time, or lack of energy, to name just a few. See your GP who is likely to arrange a simple blood test if necessary.

If you lose interest in sex, see your GP for an assessment and further help if you can relate to any of the following situations:

- ✔ You have severe relationship problems that are putting your partnership at risk.
- ✔ You feel depressed, particularly if you've had a baby recently.
- ✔ You think you may have an undiagnosed physical illness.
- ✔ Your partner is violent towards you.

Although you're likely to be able to improve your sex life (depending on the cause of your reduced libido), this improvement may take some time – it's best not to expect a quick fix or miracle cure.

Dealing with vaginal discharge

A certain amount of discharge from your vagina is normal, and you probably already have a good idea of what's usual for you, depending on what stage you're at in your menstrual cycle. But when you get a larger amount of discharge that has an offensive smell, or you have additional symptoms such as a burning sensation or itching around your vagina, or pain during sex, you may be suffering from an infection that needs treatment or from some other underlying cause.

Check the following list to see if any of these conditions (starting with the commoner ones) may apply to you:

- ✔ **Contraception:** An increase in vaginal discharge is common when you start taking the oral contraceptive pill or you have the coil (IUD) inserted. See your GP if you're bothered by the discharge or have any other concerns.

- ✔ **Pregnancy:** An increase in vaginal discharge is normal when you're pregnant.

- ✔ **Vaginal thrush:** *Thrush* is a benign yeast infection that can cause considerable itching and a whitish discharge, which can look a bit like cottage cheese. Being pregnant, wearing tight underwear made of synthetic fabrics that prevent ventilation, taking antibiotics or washing yourself frequently down below with perfumed products such as vaginal deodorants all make developing vaginal thrush more likely. Your pharmacist can suggest a number of effective over-the-counter treatments, but see your GP if the symptoms persist.

- ✔ **Various other vaginal infections:** Other vaginal infections – some of which can be transmitted sexually – can cause discharge. A profuse and fishy smelling discharge without itching or soreness may be due to what's called *bacterial vaginosis*, which isn't passed on during sex.

Sexually transmitted infections causing discharge include *chlamydia*, *gonorrhoea* and *trichomonas* infection – but you may not get any discharge at all. See your practice nurse or GP, who may take a sample from your vaginal secretions to check for an infection.

✔ **Foreign body:** A forgotten tampon or diaphragm in your vagina can easily lead to increased vaginal secretions. Just remove it and see what happens. If the discharge doesn't settle within a few days, visit your GP – just in case the item has led to an infection that needs treatment.

✔ **Cervical problems:** Raw areas on the neck of your womb (called the *cervix*) may occasionally cause vaginal discharge. In rare cases, cancer of the cervix can also cause vaginal discharge or bleeding. If you suspect this condition, see your GP for further assessment.

If you use any treatment for vaginal infections, remember that certain creams or gels can weaken condoms and other contraceptive devices such as some female diaphragms and caps made of latex. Anything made of polyurethane is still safe to use. Also, be aware that some antibiotics can interact with the combined oral contraceptive pill and some patches. Always tell your doctor if you're pregnant – or think that you may be – or if you're currently breastfeeding, because these situations affect the types of treatments that you're able to take safely.

If you have any further concerns but can't find the answer here, check out the Family Planning Association website at www.fpa.org.uk, which has lots of additional information.

Safer sex

Health professionals keep pressing home the message about *safe sex*, and with good reason – safer sex methods provide the best protection against sexually transmitted infections – particularly when you're with a new partner. Undiagnosed and untreated infections can cause considerable long-term problems (for example, with fertility). Using condoms every time you have vaginal or anal sex with a new partner offers you the best protection. Also be sure to avoid sharing sex toys with other people – but if you do, make sure that you wash them or cover them with a condom prior to using them again.

For a recap on how to use condoms correctly and for plenty of other useful information, check out the Family Planning Association website at www.fpa.org.uk. Get checked at your local sexual health clinic (you can usually find details easily in the Yellow Pages and on the Internet) or contact your GP surgery if you think you suffer from a sexually transmitted infection or are at risk.

Looking at Women's Common Concerns

In this section I deal with conditions that many women ignore or suffer for a while before seeking help. I don't cover every aspect of these conditions, but I highlight the main issues and give you some idea when to seek additional help and treatment.

Preparing for pre-menstrual syndrome (PMS)

Pre-menstrual syndrome, or *PMS*, is the name given to the various symptoms that many women suffer prior to their periods. These symptoms may include feeling irritable or even aggressive, headaches, tiredness and feeling bloated, and they may go on for years. This situation can be hard on you if you're affected as well as for everybody else around you, and so here are a few things you can try to alleviate the problem:

- **Keeping fit and healthy:** Try to look after yourself and make sure that you get enough sleep. Coping with symptoms of pre-menstrual syndrome should be easier when you're physically well, and so squeezing some exercise into your day-to-day life where possible and eating healthily, may help you to cope with your symptoms much better.

- **Maintaining a menstrual diary:** Writing down the days of your period and trying to predict your next 'off period' can help with planning ahead – you may want to try and keep your timetable as free as possible on those days or pre-warn other family members.

- **Talking:** Discuss the problem with other people around you at a time when you're feeling well – they'll then be much more understanding and more likely to support you when you're feeling down again.

If all these efforts fail, speak to your pharmacist – a number of over-the-counter preparations are available to you that you may find helpful. If you still struggle, see your GP for further assessment, to ensure that no other underlying cause for your symptoms is present and to discuss various further treatment options.

Keeping abreast of breast problems

Breasts are made up mainly of fatty tissue and glands that produce milk when you've had a baby, and can vary quite considerably in form, shape and size as well as in the way they feel. For example, some women always have 'lumpy' breasts. If you have periods, your breasts also slightly change depending on which stage in your menstrual cycle you're at, and your breasts may occasionally become tender or change shape.

Common breast concerns

Here's a summary of some common causes of breast tenderness and pain. If you're worried about yours, check whether any of these causes may apply to you:

- ✔ **Contraception:** Your breasts may become tender when you use certain types of oral contraceptive pill. See your practice nurse or GP who may be able to prescribe you an alternative preparation.

- ✔ **Fibroadenosis:** Some women have naturally 'lumpy' breasts – a condition known as *fibroadenosis*. This condition is nothing to worry about, although your breasts may become tender at times, particularly around your periods. If your breasts have always been this way, don't worry – but consult your GP if your breasts change in any way from what's normal for you or you're concerned.

- ✔ **Hormonal causes:** Breast pain is common just before a period and is usually nothing to worry about, particularly if you've always suffered from this problem. Try simple over-the-counter painkillers when you have severe discomfort and consult your pharmacist or GP for other treatment options if you need something stronger. If you also have other symptoms prior to your periods, read the preceding section 'Preparing for pre-menstrual syndrome (PMS)'.

- ✔ **Pregnancy:** Your breasts and nipples are likely to become a bit tender when you're pregnant, so consider doing a pregnancy test (available from your pharmacist) if being pregnant is a possibility. You're also likely to feel tired, but the main clue to suggest that you may be pregnant is that you miss a period.

Breast lumps and breast cancer

Breast cancer – where a cancer is confined to the breast or the surrounding areas such as the lymph nodes under the arms – is the most common cancer affecting women. The problem with breast cancer – as indeed with many other cancers – is that it can spread to other areas of your body (known as *invasive* breast cancer). Various forms of breast cancer exist – some more serious than others – and it can have many causes, including gene abnormalities and raised hormone levels in the blood. You're at an increased risk of developing breast cancer the older you get, or if close relatives of yours suffer from breast cancer.

Reassuringly, 9 out of 10 breast lumps are benign, which means they aren't due to cancer. However, any new lump in your breast raises the possibility of breast cancer, and so consulting your GP is always a good idea.

If you do develop breast cancer and it's detected and treated early, a good chance exists that you're going to achieve a complete cure, which is why taking new breast lumps seriously is so important. Women over the age of 50 in the UK are offered regular X-ray checks (called a *mammography*) to try and detect cancer early on. Women under 50 aren't currently offered a mammography – cancer in younger women is rarer and more difficult to detect through mammography because of denser breast tissue before they go through the menopause (you can read about the menopause in the 'Managing menopausal problems' section later in this chapter).

Check your breasts regularly (see the 'Breast awareness' sidebar) and look out for changes that may possibly signify breast cancer, such as:

- ✔ A change in the shape or size of your breast.

- ✔ A lump or thickened tissue in one of your breasts (changes that happen at the same time in both breasts are unlikely to be due to cancer), particularly when the lump persists after you have your period.

- ✔ A change in the skin of your breast, such as dimpling.

- ✔ A blood-stained discharge from one of your nipples.

- ✔ A new rash on your nipple or the skin around it.

- ✔ A new swelling or lump in your armpit (particularly if this lump is *not* tender – benign skin infections can sometimes cause tender lumps).

These symptoms and signs don't necessarily mean that you have cancer, but do indicate that you need to see your GP straight away. If you want to find out more, look at the CancerHelp UK website at www.cancerhelp.org.uk.

Breast awareness

To be able to detect any changes in your breasts, become familiar with the way your breasts look and feel at different times – you can do this under the shower or when you get dressed, whatever you find easiest – so that you know what's normal for you. Know what changes to look for (see the earlier 'Breast lumps and breast cancer' section) and report any changes without delay to your GP. Make sure you attend breast screening sessions if you're 50 years or over.

For further information explore the NHS Cancer Screening Programmes website at www.cancerscreening.nhs.uk/breast screen/breastawareness.html.

Tackling lower abdominal pain

Deep lower abdominal pain (also called *pelvic pain*) is common in women. In Chapter 11 you can read about the general causes of abdominal pain. This section deals mainly with causes of abdominal pain that are relevant just to women, assuming that you're *not* pregnant (for pregnancy-related causes of abdominal pain turn to the 'Checking Out Fertility and Pregnancy Concerns' section later in this chapter).

Chronic pain in your lower abdomen can have many potential causes:

✔ **Bowel problems:** Conditions commonly causing chronic lower abdominal pain are *diverticular disease*, in which little pouches form inside your large bowel that becomes infected or inflamed, and *irritable bowel syndrome* – a common gut disorder of unknown cause with recurrent symptoms of abdominal pain, bloating and bouts of diarrhoea and/or constipation.

✔ **Endometriosis:** Period abnormalities are common in this disorder, which you can read more about in 'Keeping the floods at bay: Heavy periods' section earlier in this chapter.

✔ **Fibroids:** Fibroids are benign, non-cancerous swellings in your womb (check out the earlier section, 'Coping with irregular vaginal bleeding').

✔ **Ovarian cyst:** These fluid-filled sacs can appear in one of your ovaries, commonly causing persistent or intermittent lower abdominal pain (see also the 'Experiencing pain during or after sex' section earlier in this chapter).

✔ **Pelvic inflammatory disease:** A sexually transmitted infection can cause this condition.

✔ **Pelvic venous congestion:** Congestion of some blood vessels in your lower abdomen may cause pelvic pain around the time of your periods.

This list gives just a brief overview – numerous other potential causes can also bring on pain in your lower abdomen. Pain in this area can be quite tricky to suss out and leaving the initial diagnosis to your GP makes sense. If your GP can't make a diagnosis from an initial assessment, she may send you for further investigation or even refer you to hospital for additional tests.

Managing menopausal problems

When your ovaries stop producing the hormone *oestrogen* at the end of your reproductive years (usually around the age of 50), you enter the *menopause*, or 'the change'. Strictly speaking, the menopause is the date of your last period, but most people use the term to refer to the time around your last period, which may last for a few years.

The drop in hormone levels can cause a host of symptoms, both psychological and physical, and so many women find that the menopause isn't the easiest time in their lives, which hardly seems fair: after coping with monthly periods and perhaps childbirth, even the end of your reproductive years may not come easy. Saying that, the situation isn't all doom and gloom – many women 'sail' through the menopause without any major problems.

Here's a list of some common menopausal symptoms:

- A burning sensation and itching in your genital area.
- Changes to your skin.
- Changes to your periods, which eventually stop altogether.
- Dryness and persistent discomfort in your vagina.
- General irritation, anxiety, forgetfulness and symptoms of depression.
- Hot flushes and night sweats.
- Loss of libido.
- Migraines.
- Pain during sexual intercourse because of lack of lubrication.

Many women find talking about some of these symptoms difficult, and suffer in silence. If you suffer from any such symptoms, you feel you're entering the menopause early (called *premature menopause*) or you have any other concerns, do see your GP because various treatments are available that can improve or get rid of your symptoms. Options include topical hormone preparations and oral hormone replacement therapy (HRT). You may need continued treatment for quite a while for it to be effective.

After the menopause you're also more likely to develop thinning of your bones (known as *osteoporosis*) – you can find further details and a short video explaining osteoporosis on the NHS Choices website at www.nhs.uk/conditions/osteoporosis/pages/introduction.aspx.

It's your hormones – or lack thereof. . .

The use of HRT has been a hot topic in the media in recent years. Some concerns about HRT are justified, but sometimes they get exaggerated, for example with regard to increased risks of certain cancers, thrombosis, heart disease or stroke.

As with any medical treatment, the most important thing is that you're fully informed about the benefits and potential harm of your treatment, on which you can then base your decision as to whether you want to proceed with it, or not. Although good evidence exists that the risks of taking HRT are real, the risk is often relatively small. For many women, the benefits of using HRT in the short term to treat menopausal symptoms often outweigh the potential risks.

Your GP can discuss all the relevant issues with you, but if you want to read up about this topic beforehand, check out the Patient UK website at www.patient.uk, which has a useful patient information leaflet on the subject.

Checking Out Fertility and Pregnancy Concerns

Difficulties conceiving and pregnancy-related problems are common. In this section I give you a broad overview of these topics and some sources of additional information, but speak to your GP or midwife – if you're currently pregnant – if you need further help and advice.

Finding out about fertility problems

If you've been trying for a baby for a year or so and you haven't been able to conceive, you're not alone. For a woman to take a year or so to conceive is quite normal, but sometimes an underlying physical cause – in the man or the woman – can make conceiving more difficult, and in rare cases impossible. Lots of reasons may be responsible, and so in this section I offer an overview of the common ones. (You can find more information on the topic in *Pregnancy For Dummies* by Sarah Jarvis, Joanne Stone, Keith Eddleman and Mary Duenwald).

Consider whether any of these causes of failure to conceive may apply to you:

- ✔ **Blocked tubes:** If you've ever suffered from a pelvic infection (such as infection of your fallopian tubes, which is called *salpingitis*), your tubes may be blocked, impeding an egg from travelling from your ovaries to your womb. Sometimes, a previous *ectopic pregnancy* outside your womb or a termination of pregnancy may also play a role. See your GP for further assessment and to discuss the management options.

- ✔ **Hormone problems:** Irregular or infrequent periods suggest that you may suffer from a hormone imbalance, which may affect your fertility. A condition called *polycystic ovary syndrome*, or *PCOS*, is the most common hormone disorder affecting women in their reproductive years and often presents with fertility problems. Check out *Managing PCOS For Dummies* by Gaynor Bussell and consult your GP for advice if you have PCOS and are having a hard time conceiving.

- ✔ **Long-term illness:** Some chronic illnesses such as diabetes, thyroid gland disorders or chronic infections can affect your fertility. See your GP for further advice if you suffer from any of these illnesses and you're trying without success for a baby.

- ✔ **Stress:** Sometimes, couples can get into a real rut (pun not intended!) about trying for a baby. Instead of enjoying sex, intercourse may become a matter of routine when sex is dictated by the diary rather than because you both feel in the mood. Try to take your time even if your reason for having sex is for you to become pregnant – your partner is likely to have an increased volume of ejaculate when he's more aroused, and your sexual organs may become more receptive if you take it slowly, don't rush and are more stimulated. Other 'stresses' in your life, such as worries about your job or money, may also adversely affect your fertility.

Generally speaking, if you've been pregnant in the past and particularly when you've had one or more babies, the chances of any medical causes are less compared to when you've never been pregnant, although you may still want to get checked out by your doctor. If appropriate, your GP can arrange further investigation and refer you to a fertility expert.

If you want to read up about this topic, check out the Patient UK (`www.patient.co.uk`) or the NHS Choices website at `www.nhs.uk/conditions/infertility/pages/introduction.aspx`, which have additional useful information about infertility.

Handling pregnancy problems

For the majority of women, pregnancy is an exciting and longed-for experience. Although you may feel tired and exhausted at times, the chances are that you're going to enjoy your pregnancy. Unfortunately, for some women the opposite can be true – being pregnant can seem like an ongoing struggle.

If you're pregnant, you're likely to have already seen your GP and/or midwife, and you've probably already been given information about common pregnancy problems. Therefore, I cover here only those issues that can be tricky to deal with, because they're not always obvious and are potentially serious for you or for your baby – or both. Thankfully, not many of these conditions exist, but the ones in this section are worth knowing about.

Ectopic pregnancy

When you're pregnant, your baby normally grows right inside your womb. But in an *ectopic pregnancy*, for various reasons your fertilised egg doesn't reach your womb. Instead, it implants outside the womb, commonly in one of your fallopian tubes, and because the tube doesn't have enough room for the baby to grow you may develop abdominal pain.

The main complication of an ectopic pregnancy is a rupture of a blood vessel, which can lead to severe bleeding into your abdomen and make you very unwell very quickly, and so urgent assessment is essential.

Seek medical advice if any of the following symptoms apply to you:

- ✔ You're about six weeks or so pregnant and suddenly develop lower abdominal pain, particularly if this pain affects one side only.

- ✔ You lose dark blood (which may look like prune juice) from your vagina.

- ✔ You feel faint or have collapsed – call '999' straight away.

These symptoms don't necessarily mean that you have an ectopic pregnancy – plenty of other potential causes can be to blame – they just mean that you need to seek medical help urgently for further assessment just to make sure.

For further information, check out the Ectopic Pregnancy Foundation website at www.ectopicpregnancy.co.uk.

Pre-eclampsia

Pre-eclampsia can occur during pregnancy due to problems with your *placenta* – the organ that links your baby's blood supply with your own. This condition is a common complication of pregnancy and can lead to abnormally raised blood pressure (known as *hypertension*), abnormal protein in your urine (called *proteinuria*) and fluid retention (or *oedema*), and the condition can lead to growth problems in your baby (experts call this *intrauterine growth retardation*). Pre-eclampsia may occur when you're more than 20 weeks pregnant. Because this condition can harm your baby as well as yourself, get yourself checked out by your midwife or GP if you notice any of the following symptoms, particularly if you also notice reduced movements in your unborn baby:

- You develop a new and perhaps severe headache.
- You suffer from blurred vision or other visual problems.
- You get pain or discomfort in your upper abdomen.
- You develop swollen ankles or hands, or a puffy face.
- You vomit and don't feel well.

In pre-eclampsia, you also have high blood pressure and protein in your urine, which is one of the reasons why your midwife and GP may check these levels as a matter of routine.

Bleeding in pregnancy

Vaginal bleeding in pregnancy is common and occurs in about 1 in 4 pregnant women. In most cases the cause of the bleeding is benign, but contacting your midwife or GP urgently for further assessment is important, just to get checked out and to ensure that you have no other serious underlying problem, particularly if you also suffer from abdominal pain.

Shortness of breath in pregnancy

After you're more than 28 weeks pregnant, shortness of breath on exertion is quite usual. If, however, you get breathless on very mild exertion or without any exertion (particularly in the earlier stages of pregnancy), consult your GP without delay to exclude other underlying causes.

Other pregnancy-related problems

You may have a host of other questions and concerns about your pregnancy – don't hesitate to speak to your midwife or GP, who can answer your queries. If you want to read up about pregnancy-related issues first, however, the Patient UK website at www.patient.co.uk has some excellent patient information leaflets. Also refer to *Pregnancy For Dummies* by Sarah Jarvis, Joanne Stone, Keith Eddleman and Mary Duenwald, which has a lot of info on this topic.

Chapter 19

Looking at Men's Issues

· ·

· ·

*M*any men aren't keen on going to the doctors and put off seeking medi-cal advice until a health problem starts to interfere with their life – in terms of work, family life, sports or socialising: in addition, busy lives mean that making time to see a health professional can be difficult. Some men feel embarrassed or ashamed about admitting to having health problems, or just dislike talking about medical matters. Other issues, such as a fear of getting a serious diagnosis and not wanting to cause a fuss, lead many men to put off seeing their GP because they feel that keeping a stiff upper lip is important, hoping that the problem may go away on its own.

Although certain conditions do go away in their own time, in other instances you really need to seek medical help sooner rather than later. If you ignore certain medical problems for too long, they creep up on you eventually – and you only make the problem more serious, both for you and those close to you who may also be affected. I regularly see male patients who left visiting the doctor far too late – when earlier assessment and treatment may have prevented serious health problems (for example, with regard to certain male cancers and symptoms such as chest pain or unexplained weight loss).

All this advice is relevant to most chapters in this book – I just repeat it here in case this chapter is the only one that grabs you. I hope to be able to reas-sure you about some of the more common health concerns – and to prompt you into action just in case you may have a potentially serious underlying condition.

Looking Under the Bonnet: Problems With the Family Jewels

Minor penis problems are incredibly common, and yet many men take weeks, months or sometimes years to summon up the courage to speak to a health professional about their concerns. Which is a shame, because in most cases the worry and anxiety that you may have some abnormality, or that you're somehow different, can be avoided. Reassuringly, most penis conditions are minor and may not even need treatment. In this section I let you know when to seek medical help and when you can deal with the problem yourself.

Solving problems with your penis

Physical problems – things to do with appearance – with regard to your penis can cause a huge amount of concern, particularly if you belong to a younger age group. Many penile problems such as minor skin changes are often entirely benign and part of what you can consider as 'normal'. I sometimes sense the sigh of relief and reassurance of anxious men that follows my careful explanation of this fact! (Problems with penis function – for example with erections and premature ejaculation – feature in the 'Checking Out the Engine: Sexual Problems' section later in this chapter. If you want to find out more about urinary problems in men, check out Chapter 12.)

If you're worried about the look of your penis or you've developed a new problem, compare your symptoms with the following descriptions, starting with the more common ones:

✔ **Balanitis or thrush:** If the tip of your penis (the glans) is red and inflamed you're likely to be suffering from an irritation of the skin, known as *balanitis*. You're more likely to develop balanitis if you suffer from diabetes or take oral antibiotics. (Chapter 20 has much more info on diabetes.)

Balanitis can be caused by an infection with a fungus (called *candidiasis* or *thrush*), irritation from tight clothes or from your own penis secretions, which may accumulate under your foreskin unless you wash them away regularly. The infection may lead to a burning or stinging sensation at the tip of your penis when you pass urine. Make sure that you pull your foreskin back every time you wash your penis, and don't use soap until the problem settles. See your pharmacist for some antifungal cream such as *clotrimazole*, which is available over-the-counter without prescription. If your symptoms don't settle, see your GP for further assessment.

✔ **Friction soreness:** A sore penis after sexual activities is a common problem. Usually, this soreness is due to your penis rubbing inside or against your partner's body, but can also be a reaction to the material used in condoms. Your symptoms usually settle quickly by themselves, but try using a different brand of condom if you suspect this problem is the cause. To help prevent soreness, make sure that you both take your time to get aroused enough before attempting penetration. Alternatively, use plenty of lubricating jelly, which can work wonders.

✔ **Sexually transmitted infection:** If you've had unprotected sexual intercourse and have developed sores, blisters or ulcers on your penis, you may have a _sexually transmitted infection_, or _STI_ for short. Avoid sexual intercourse until you identify the underlying problem. (You can find out more in the 'Spotting sexually transmitted infections' section later in this chapter.)

✔ **Tight foreskin:** If you can't pull back your foreskin over your glans when your penis is erect – or, worse, when it's not – you're likely to be suffering from an overly tight foreskin (known as _phimosis_). Don't try to pull the foreskin back with force – you won't succeed and may cause a tear. Consult your GP who may consider giving you topical steroid creams (usually _hydrocortisone_) to soften your foreskin. If this approach fails, the problem can often be corrected by a small surgical procedure in which the foreskin is widened (known as _preputioplasty_) or removed (called _circumcision_), depending on how tight your foreskin is and other factors, such as the presence of scarring.

✔ **Genital warts:** You may be suffering from genital warts if you notice hard, wart-like lumps on the skin of your penis. These lumps are caused by a virus infection, can grow quite fast and may be transmitted through sexual contact. See your GP or go to a sexual health clinic for further assessment and treatment – don't treat this condition yourself because you may cause damage to the sensitive skin on your penis.

✔ **Penis cancer:** Cancer of the penis (also known as _penile carcinoma_) is a rare tumour – usually in older men – that can occur anywhere on the penis, but most commonly affects the tip. Initially you may notice a burning or itching sensation under your foreskin before you see or feel an ulcer or lump that doesn't go away. See your GP urgently if you suspect penile cancer – the earlier you receive treatment the better.

Many other conditions can affect your penis, so if you're concerned make an appointment with a local sexual health clinic to get your problem checked out, or see your GP. And don't be too embarrassed: these issues are day-to-day stuff for your GP and other health professionals – and no worse for them than 'looking under the bonnet' is for a mechanic. Honestly.

Coping with scrotal and testicular problems

Your testicles (also called *testes* or, more informally, 'balls') are the glands hanging between your legs that produce your sperm. They hang 'outside' your body, in a sac called the *scrotum*, because your sperm matures better at lower temperatures. To make sure that you try to avoid damage to your 'bits', the testicles have a lot of nerves, so that you automatically try to protect them to avoid pain.

The most common symptoms with regard to testicles are pain and swelling. If you get severe or ongoing problems like these with your testicles, you almost always need to see your GP for further assessment. Delaying for too long puts you at risk of becoming infertile, or worse, losing a testicle. In the case of testicular cancer, early treatment quite literally saves lives.

If you suffer from problems with your testicles, compare your symptoms with these descriptions of selected conditions to see whether you need to act quickly, starting with the more common ones:

- ✔ **Epididymal cyst:** Fluid-filled cysts in a tubular organ attached to your testicle (called the *epididymis* – where your semen is stored and matures) are usually small (often not more than the size of a pea) painless lumps that grow slowly and that you can feel rather than see. These cysts are harmless, and nobody really knows for sure why they occur. By feeling the lump carefully, you may be able to make out whether it's attached to or part of your testicle, or separate from it. Sometimes, you may notice more than one cyst at the same time, either on one or both sides. Consult your doctor to confirm the diagnosis.

- ✔ **Hydrocele:** Fluid may accumulate between the different layers of tissue covering your testicles, which is called *hydrocele* – a swelling in your enlarged scrotum that develops gradually and feels a bit like a balloon filled with water. This condition is common, harmless, not painful and becomes more common the older you get – but can appear at any age. You may not need treatment, but consult your GP for further assessment.

- ✔ **Varicocele:** Intermittent pain or a 'heaviness' in your testicle, particularly after prolonged standing or exercise, may be due to congested veins in your scrotum called *varicocele*, which may feel and look like a 'bag of worms'. See your GP for further assessment.

- ✔ **Orchitis and epdidymo-orchitis:** *Orchitis* is an infection of the testicle, which becomes tender and swollen, and is commonly due to mumps (if you've been vaccinated against mumps with the *MMR immunisation*, orchitis is unlikely). In *epididymo-orchitis* the infection spreads to the epididymis. Common causes are a sexually transmitted *chlamydia* infection in younger men or prostate enlargement if you're older. See your GP for diagnosis. If confirmed, you need treatment with antibiotics.

✔ **Testicular torsion:** Occasionally, a testicle may suddenly twist around itself inside your scrotum, which is called *testicular torsion*. This condition is more common in younger men and can happen at any time – even during sleep. Your testicle becomes exquisitely tender to touch, and the pain comes on fast, is usually severe and may spread into your groin and lower abdomen – which is why you may misdiagnose this problem as appendicitis. You may feel sick or vomit, and you're likely to feel faint as well. Call your doctor or go to the nearest Accident & Emergency (A&E) department immediately, because you need urgent treatment in hospital.

✔ **Testicular cancer:** Most swellings in your scrotum aren't due to *testicular cancer*, but any new lump has the potential to be. Testicular cancer is very treatable and has an excellent prognosis when caught early. For this reason, check your testicles regularly – say, once a month or so – under the shower and feel for any changes, particularly lumps. Consult your GP without delay if you notice any of the following:

- A new lump in one of your testicles, which may or may not be painful (this lump can be as small as a pea or larger).

- A heavy feeling in your scrotum, a dull ache in the affected testicle or pain in your lower abdomen, in addition to a new testicular lump.

Many other conditions can also affect your testicles, and as a rule getting things checked out by a health professional promptly is the best idea, instead of waiting too long. If you want to discover more about testicular cancer, check out the CancerHelp UK website at www.cancerhelp.org.uk, which has lots of additional useful information.

Checking Out the Engine: Sexual Problems

Sexual problems are extremely common and can be distressing for both partners. For men, erection problems (also known as *erectile dysfunction*, or *impotence*), premature ejaculation and reduced sex drive top the list. The good news is that a lot of help and treatments are available – the bad news is that you can't always get a 'quick fix' for the problem.

Tackling problems with erections

Occasionally being unable to have a full erection – or perhaps not a lasting one – even if you feel aroused, is normal. However, you – or your partner – may start to worry when this problem happens more and more often. Some men may achieve an erection only when they masturbate, or only with one partner but not another. The type of sex can also play a role – for example, you may have no problems with oral sex, but can't get or maintain an erection when you're trying to have vaginal or anal intercourse.

When you have problems with erections, the first – and usually best – thing to do is to speak openly with your partner about it. You may find that she (or he) isn't too concerned, because you can still enjoy sex together in many other ways, such as oral sex or mutual masturbation. You may find that both of you become much more relaxed after you talk openly – which in itself may be enough to get you back on track.

However, if you develop problems with erections, consider whether any of the following possible causes may apply to you:

- **Anxiety and depression:** These common conditions (which you can read about in more detail in Chapter 21) often affect erections in a negative way. Reassuringly, effective treatments are available for anxiety and depression, so the chances are good that your erections will become stronger again when you get better. Saying that, taking medication for the treatment of anxiety or depression may in itself sometimes affect your sexual function slightly. But don't worry, this effect is often short-lived and mild, and it should certainly not put you off taking antidepressant medication.

- **Chronic illness:** Some chronic medical conditions and their treatments can cause erection problems. For example, if you suffer from diabetes, back problems, multiple sclerosis, prostate problems, heart disease, or you've had surgery to your back, you may have difficulty (or find it impossible) to achieve erections. Erection problems can occasionally also be a side effect of medication used to treat long-term conditions such as high blood pressure.

- **Intermittent erectile dysfunction:** Being unable to have an erection whenever you want to is absolutely normal. Simply not being in the mood for sex, perhaps because you've had a long day and are tired, or when you're mentally exhausted or stressed for any other reason, can be enough to prevent you from getting an erection. As long as this problem doesn't affect your confidence or cause anxiety, you've no reason to worry, particularly if the problem only occurs intermittently without causing friction in your relationship.

- **Lack of sexual desire:** You can find more information on this common problem in the later section 'Losing interest in sex'.

- **Nervousness:** If you have problems with your erection only when you're starting a new relationship, performance anxiety may be the underlying cause (also check out the following section, 'Dealing with premature ejaculation'). As long as the problem settles and doesn't affect you or your relationship, you have no need to worry.

If you're concerned that any of these conditions apply to you and the problem doesn't settle, consult your GP who can assess you thoroughly, arrange further investigations if needed and discuss the various treatment options. Medication and other treatments as well as behavioural approaches such as sex counselling can all be very effective. Remember that a physical cause for your erections is less likely if you wake sometimes with a hard penis.

Just a quick word about sex counselling: for many men talking about sex to a complete stranger is an alien concept, but talking to a stranger is exactly the point. After you overcome your initial fear and reluctance, talking to someone trained in this field may be much easier than you think simply because you don't know each other. Consider calling Relate on 0300 1001234 or visit the website at www.relate.org.uk, where you can find lots more relevant information, or speak to your GP about other locally available services.

Many treatments and therapies for erection problems are advertised in shops and on the Internet. When you're suffering from erectile problems you may be tempted to give in and place an order, but just a word of caution: not all medication sold this way comes from a reliable and trustworthy source. So if you want to make sure that you're getting reliably manufactured preparations, obtain these via your GP and pharmacist instead of ordering them yourself.

Dealing with premature ejaculation

Coming too quickly happens to almost every man at some stage – and to some men more often than others. However, ejaculating with little stimulation, having little or no voluntary control or coming earlier than you or your partner want to, particularly if you or your partner – or both – find this distressing, is called *premature ejaculation*. To give you a rough time frame, if you always or nearly always ejaculate within one minute of penetration and can't delay it voluntarily, experts classify this problem as premature ejaculation.

Two main forms exist:

- ✔ **Lifelong premature ejaculation**, where the problem starts from the word 'go' with the first sexual experience.
- ✔ **Acquired premature ejaculation**, when the problem occurs only in later life.

Premature ejaculation is probably the most common male sexual problem, but counts as a problem only if it affects your sexual relationship and you or your partner – or both of you – feel frustrated. As a reaction, you may both become more anxious or stressed about attempting intercourse, which in fact can make the problem even worse.

Reassuringly, premature ejaculation isn't normally due to any underlying disease or condition – in fact, it's much more frequently due to one or more of the following factors:

- **Inexperience:** You're bound to find controlling your orgasm difficult when you start your first sexual relationship(s). This problem often improves with time.

- **New partner:** You're more likely to ejaculate prematurely when you're starting a sexual relationship with a new partner. Quite often, when your relationship matures and the initial anxiety and excitement starts to wear off, you may find that premature ejaculation becomes much less of a problem.

- **Past sexual experiences:** Premature ejaculation may be a problem for you if you 'learned' to come quickly in your early sexual encounters, perhaps because of fear of being discovered or because you masturbated frequently and in a rushed sort of way. Maybe you felt guilty about masturbating and trained yourself to ejaculate quickly.

- **Performance anxiety:** Concerns that you're unable to satisfy your partner may lead to premature ejaculation.

Many self-help and other treatment options are available. However, you're most likely to achieve and maintain lasting benefits from talking to your GP and perhaps a sex counsellor about this issue, because they're able to advise you on the most appropriate course of action. Here's a selection of possible treatments that may work for you:

- **Behavioural techniques:** Various behavioural techniques to find out how to control or strengthen important muscles in your pelvis exist that you may find helpful, including the *squeeze technique*, *stop and start*, *desensitisation* and *pelvic floor exercises*.

- **Condoms:** Some men with a very sensitive tip of their penis (or *glans*) find that using condoms makes them last longer.

- **Talk to your partner:** Discussing the problem openly with your partner is often a good first move – it's likely to help reduce your anxiety and may be therapeutic in itself. While talking, try to find out what other types of stimulation your partner enjoys.

- **Try to take your time and relax:** A reasonably good chance exists that you may be able to 'unlearn' your sexual response, and gradually increase the time you take to climax, if you and your partner try not to rush when you have sex. However, this approach can take time to bear fruit – sometimes weeks or even months.

This section is just a quick run-through of the causes and what you can do to help yourself. If you want further information and advice on the treatment options, including details of the behavioural techniques I mention, contact your GP for a referral to a local psychosexual counsellor, speak to a trained Relate consultant on 0300 1001234; or visit the Relate website at www. relate.org.uk.

Losing interest in sex

Low sex drive (also known as *low libido*) is more common than many men would like to believe. You may always have had low libido, or your sexual desire may have gone down gradually – or quickly – over time. In the normal course of events, after a peak in the teens and early twenties libido normally reduces slowly over the years – although quite a bit of variation exists between men. For some men as well as their partners, low libido may not be a problem. Others may worry or notice that it affects their relationship, thinking that partners don't find them attractive anymore.

If you suffer from low libido, go through the following list to see whether any of these potential causes may apply to you:

- ✔ **Alcohol:** Consuming larger amounts of alcohol can severely impact on your sex drive. Although small amounts of alcoholic drinks may help increase your sexual desire, drinking more than the recommended limit is often a 'turn-off', so try to reduce your alcohol intake or, ideally, stop drinking for a while: things usually return to normal quickly. If you find stopping difficult or you want to know more about alcohol-related problems, read Chapter 23, and consider discussing further management options with your GP.

- ✔ **Depression and anxiety:** Feeling low or anxious is bound to affect your sex life. When you don't feel well – particularly if you don't feel good about yourself – you're less likely to feel enthusiastic about sex. You can do a lot to help if you feel this way – checking out Chapter 21 is a good start, where you can discover how to spot the signs of depression and anxiety, and what you can do to improve your situation. If you're still concerned and things don't improve, visit your GP for further assessment and treatment.

- ✔ **Lack of hormones:** Your sex drive is affected by levels of the hormone *testosterone* in your blood. Although a fairly rare cause of loss of libido, your GP can diagnose a lack of hormones easily with a simple blood test, and treatment is fairly straightforward.

    Testosterone deficiency can also cause these other symptoms, although they don't necessarily mean that you're suffering from lack of hormones:

    • You feel tired all the time.

    • You have problems with erections.

- You put on weight for no reason.

- You feel low in yourself and have little energy.

- You find concentrating difficult.

- You get hot flushes or sweat increasingly.

- You lose body hair and your skin changes in some way.

✔ **Medication:** Taking tablets regularly for a medical condition may well have an impact on your sex drive. Common culprits are blood pressure lowering drugs, antidepressants, water tablets (known as *diuretics*) and drugs used for the treatment of epilepsy or anxiety. Often this problem is mild, but if you find that you lose interest in sex after taking a particular pill and the problem doesn't get better with time – or is severe – check the drug information leaflet or speak to your pharmacist or GP. They may be able to suggest an alternative type of medication for you.

✔ **'Natural causes':** If you've always had a low sex drive or you lost interest in sex gradually over time, this situation may just be normal for you and it doesn't have to mean that you can't enjoy sex anymore. Speak to your GP or consider arranging an appointment with a sex counsellor.

✔ **Relationship problems:** Unhappiness in a relationship and any issues causing trouble between you and your partner may well affect your desire to have sex. Losing interest in sex to a certain extent is also normal when the novelty effect of being in a new relationship wears off.

✔ **Sexual difficulties:** Any form of sexual problem can reduce your desire for sex. Examples include erection problems and premature ejaculation (check out the earlier sections, 'Tackling problems with erections' and 'Dealing with premature ejaculation', respectively) or your partner suffering from a dry vagina due to the menopause (turn to Chapter 18 for more details on problems that your partner may be experiencing).

✔ **Sexual orientation:** If you find that you don't feel attracted to women anymore but get aroused by men, your sexual orientation may have changed or you may have only just recognised this fact. You've nothing to worry about if you're happy with this development, but you – and perhaps other people around you – may find adjusting to your new situation difficult. Speak to your GP for advice on getting help and support.

✔ **Tiredness and stress:** If you're stressed at work or at home, have too much on your mind or don't get enough sleep, your libido is likely to be affected (turn to Chapter 21 for more on the problems that stress can cause). Chat to your partner and see whether you can both take action to get you back on track again: you may need to take some time off work, do something nice together, reduce some of your activities or make other changes to your lifestyle. If you're still concerned or things don't get better, consult your GP.

If you lose interest in sex for a while with no signs of improvement and you can't figure out the reason, consider speaking to your GP about the problem and to obtain advice on locally available sources of help and support. Also, the charity Relate has lots of useful information on its website (`www.relate.org.uk`): you can find out about telephone or online counselling and where to find a sex counsellor.

Spotting sexually transmitted infections

A number of infections transmitted through sexual intercourse (commonly referred to as *sexually transmitted infections*, or *STIs)* are mainly due to viruses or bacteria that may be present in semen, vaginal fluid or blood. Many people choose a variety of different activities to have a fulfilling sex life, some of which carry a higher risk of transmitting STIs than others.

Busting some myths about STIs

Many myths about STIs exist, so here I cover some of the activities that put you at higher risk – and those that don't:

 ✔ You can pass on STIs even if your penis doesn't fully enter your partner's vagina or you don't 'come' (called *ejaculate),* because your 'pre-come' (that is, your pre-ejaculate fluid) also contains the organisms that cause STIs.

 ✔ You and your partner are at risk of passing on STIs even if you only insert your penis slightly (sometimes referred to as *dipping).*

 ✔ You can also pass on STIs if you give or receive oral sex. If one of you has an STI, the risk of spreading this is even higher if either of you have any sores or cuts around the mouth, genitals or anus. You're probably at lower risk if you receive oral sex than

when you give it – this is because if you receive oral sex you don't come into contact with your partner's genital fluid (such as vaginal fluid or semen), although some risk of infection always remains.

 ✔ The risk of spreading STIs is higher in anal sex because the lining of the anus is thin, making it more vulnerable to damage, which opens up the route for infections.

 ✔ You can also pass on STIs through sharing sex toys.

 ✔ Although the chances of spreading STIs from inserting your fingers into your partner's vagina or anus is relatively small, the risk is there – particularly if either of you have any cuts on your hands.

Safe sex

The most important thing you can do to prevent STIs is to use condoms when you engage in sexual activities. Only use water-based lubricants (which you can get from your pharmacist), as oil-based ones can damage condoms, making them less effective. Also make sure you always wash sex toys (that is, any object that you use during sexual activities) between users, and use a new condom to cover them.

Some STIs are common in the UK, whereas others are quite rare. However, having unprotected sex with a new partner abroad can put you at much higher risk of contracting an STI.

Here's the low-down on some STIs that are worth knowing about:

- **Acquired immune-deficiency syndrome:** Safer sex can help prevent the spread of *human immunodeficiency virus*, or *HIV*, which can lead to the *acquired immune-deficiency syndrome*, or *AIDS*. You can find more information about HIV infection and AIDS in Chapter 7.

- **Chlamydia:** *Chlamydia* is a common infection that can cause *infertility* (which means you can't father children) if not treated, and so get checked over if you notice a clear or yellowish discharge from your penis. Treatment is simple (with antibiotics) and usually effective.

- **Genital warts:** Genital warts are common and caused by viruses that you can pass on through sexual contact. The virus may not necessarily lead to infection, however – in fact, many people don't develop any problems, or if they do the virus goes away on its own. Therefore, you may not know whether you've contracted the infection or not.

  Lesions may break out from about three weeks up to many months or even years after you've come into contact with the virus. Small fleshy bumps in your genital area or around your anus are typical. Antibiotics aren't effective with genital warts, so treatment aims to reduce the number of lesions by means of creams, toxic solutions, heat, freezing, surgery or laser, which is normally offered in specialist clinics only unless your GP has special expertise in this field.

- **Gonorrhoea:** A yellow to white or even greenish irritating discharge from your penis or anus is typical for *gonorrhoea*, which isn't particularly common. Your testicles and prostate gland may also become inflamed, causing pain inside your scrotum, deep behind the base of your penis and close to your anus. You may also get some pain or discomfort when you pass urine, and in rare cases – particularly if you had oral sex with an infected partner – you may get a throat or eye infection, too.

✔ **Herpes genitalis:** An itchy sensation on the shaft of your penis and a small crop of painful blisters may mean that you've contracted an infection with the *herpes virus*. You may also notice lesions on your buttocks or thighs. When the blisters burst after about a day or so, they tend to leave small red and moist little ulcers, which usually crust over after a day or two. You may also develop swollen and tender lymph glands in your groins, and you're likely to feel unwell in yourself. Unfortunately, although the blisters heal after a while, they're likely to recur.

You can't cure this infection, but antiviral drugs can help with keeping the infection in check. You can spread the infection while sores are present – so avoid having sex at that time.

✔ **Non-specific urethritis:** If you notice a thickish and usually clear discharge as well as pain, tingling or discomfort when you pass urine, you may have *non-specific urethritis* (or *NSU*) – an inflammation due to infection of your *urethra*. You may not in fact get any symptoms at all and may only find out that you have the infection when you're being checked because your partner has been diagnosed with it. Although the symptoms of NSU can settle without treatment over a few weeks or months, antibiotics are usually given.

✔ **Syphilis:** *Syphilis* isn't common in the UK, but the total number of cases has risen in the past 10 to 15 years. Local outbreaks of syphilis do occur. Syphilis has different stages, and recognising symptoms and signs of the disease can be tricky. The condition may take three months to show after you've had sexual contact with an infected person.

The first thing you normally notice is one or more painless sores, usually not earlier than three weeks after you've had contact with the disease. This sore is very infectious and may take a few weeks to heal. Unless you receive treatment, you then usually develop a rash all over your body, which typically involves the palms of your hands and the soles of your feet. Fleshy wart-like lesions around your anus are also common.

Other symptoms of syphilis at this stage include the following:

- You feel unwell – similar to a flu-like illness.

- You're tired all the time.

- You notice swollen lymph glands, such as in your groins, neck or armpits.

- You may be losing hair.

- You notice white patches inside your mouth (called *snail track ulcers*).

This stage is also very infectious, and you can still pass on the infection through sexual contact. If you get treatment, though, you can still be cured. However, leave the condition too long and you may develop problems with your heart and nervous system many years later. Blood samples and testing fluids from a sore can help with making the diagnosis, and if the diagnosis is confirmed you need to receive antibiotics, usually by injection into a muscle.

For more information on the later stages of syphilis check out the NHS Choices website at `www.nhs.uk/Conditions/Syphilis/Pages/Introduction.aspx`.

Sexually transmitted infection isn't a topic that many men are keen to talk about. If you suspect that you suffer from such an infection, getting checked over is very important. Until you've been tested and treated, you should ideally avoid sexual activities that put your partner(s) at risk, or tell your partners about the problem so that they're aware of the risk – and always use condoms.

Make an appointment directly with a clinic specialised in diagnosing and treating STIs – you can usually find one easily by looking under 'sexual health' in your local phone book. Alternatively call the Family Planning Association Helpline on 0845 1228690 or your GP Surgery to enquire about finding a clinic close to you. These clinics can also help with what's called *contact tracing*, so that partners you've been with may be offered checks and don't pass on any infections unknowingly.

You can find out more about STIs on the NHS Choices website at `www.nhs.uk/Livewell/STIs/Pages/STIs-hub.aspx`, which gives you the complete low-down and has a wealth of information and resources.

Appointments at the sexual health clinic tends to involve talking about your symptoms, a brief physical examination of your genitals, a blood test and usually a *swab* – taking a small sample of fluids or discharge from the tube that runs from your bladder into your penis (known as *urethra*), from any ulcers or from infected-looking skin. Don't worry – this process doesn't usually hurt, although it may be a bit uncomfortable for a moment. Most men can handle this. . . ! The majority of sexually transmitted infections require treatment with antibiotics.

Identifying obstacles to having children

If you and your partner have been trying for a baby for over 12 months without success, you may start to worry that the problem lies with you, particularly if you've had medical problems in your genital area in the past.

Check this list to decide whether any of these common factors may be affecting your fertility:

- **Alcohol:** Drinking large amounts of alcohol regularly not only makes you lose interest in sex and have difficulties with erections, but also directly reduces your sperm production. Try to reduce your alcohol intake (check out Chapter 23 on the dangers of alcohol).

- **Illness:** Long-term medical conditions as well as their treatment can occasionally affect your sperm production. If medicines are a possibility, check the drug information pack and speak to your GP.

- **Increased temperature in your scrotum:** You produce more and better sperm at a temperature that's below that of your body – which is why your testicles dangle between your legs, to stay cooler. For this reason, always wearing very tight underpants or frequently enjoying hot baths or saunas may potentially affect your fertility.

- **Problems with your testicles:** If you had mumps after the age of 12 and you later notice swelling or pain in your testicles, the illness may have affected your sperm count. Also, if you've had a testicular torsion (for more details look at the 'Coping with scrotal and testicular problems' section earlier in this chapter) that wasn't treated early enough, the affected testicle may have lost its ability to produce sperm.

- **Sexually transmitted infections:** Untreated sexually transmitted infections such as chlamydia can cause problems with fertility in both men and women (flip to the preceding section for more info). See your GP if you're concerned.

Various other factors can affect your sperm count and fertility in general, and so sperm testing is a quick and easy way of testing yours – see your GP to arrange this for you. You're usually asked to produce a sperm sample by masturbation, so that the laboratory can examine it for any abnormalities.

Taking the following steps can also increase the chances of your sperm being in good shape:

- Avoid wearing overly tight underpants.

- Go easy on alcohol and avoid other (illicit) drugs.

- Keep physically fit and active.

- Make sure that you include healthy foods such as fruit and vegetables as part of your regular diet.

Your sperm take about three months to grow and mature, so any changes that you make to your lifestyle now take three months to have any noticeable effect. If you and your partner have been trying for a baby for over a year and nothing happens – or other problems are causing difficulty for you (for example, erection problems and loss of libido) – consult your GP to find out why and to examine the treatment options. Chapter 18 contains loads more information on infertility from the woman's side.

Having 'the snip'

Whereas women have a choice of various contraceptive methods, the options are fairly limited for men. Condoms are the most easily available male contraceptive. Admittedly, they can be fiddly to use, and some men – and women – don't like the feel of them, but they don't have any long-term implications, are straightforward to put on with a bit of practice (consider practising on a not too ripe and unpeeled banana) and help prevent sexually transmitted infections.

If you're after a more permanent form of contraception – perhaps you already have children and you and your partner are sure that you don't want any more – having a *vasectomy* may be an option for you. Vasectomy surgery is fairly straightforward: a quick operation in which a couple of tubes in your scrotum are disconnected so that you can still ejaculate, but without any sperm being present anymore. However, only consider this option when you and your partner have thought about the implications – which means that you need to see this operation as *irreversible*. Although a reversal of a vasectomy is possible, that operation is much more difficult, not always successful – and not usually funded by the UK National Health Service.

The vasectomy operation is usually performed under local anaesthetic, which means that you're fully conscious but don't feel any pain – perhaps only a little bit of pulling. You may have a bit of pain afterwards, but in most cases this discomfort settles quickly, after a few days at most. Mild bleeding, bruising or infection are rare and usually short-lived mild complications. After a vasectomy, you're not sterile straight away – the remaining sperm take a couple of months to disappear. For further information, consult your GP or check out the Patient UK website at www.patient.co.uk, which has a useful patient information leaflet, with helpful illustrations.

Chapter 20

Dealing with Health Problems in Later Life

. . . .

In This Chapter

▶ Performing a 'later-life health check'

▶ Preventing common chronic diseases and falls

▶ Approaching mind and memory problems

▶ Knowing more about vision and hearing concerns

. . . .

Sorry to be the bearer of bad tidings, but you're getting older each day, as am I. In fact, the UK population as a whole is ageing. As in many countries, life expectancy has risen from around 50 years at the beginning of the last century to 75 years in men and 80 years in women. This increase means that a greater proportion of the population is older aged, but what is 'older age', exactly?

People in the later stages of their lives may go through these general stages:

1. **Entering old age:** The first years of older age come when you've had your career or been raising children but are still independent. You lead an active lifestyle and hope to continue doing so for years to come. In terms of your health, you hope to keep active for as long as possible and prevent diseases such as heart attack and stroke.

2. **Being in the transition phase:** In the transition phase, you're somewhere in-between leading an active, healthy lifestyle and starting to become frail. You may have begun to develop new health problems and are likely to be around 70–80 years old.

3. **Becoming frail:** At this latest stage in your life, you may have a number of health or social problems – or both. You're likely to be over 80 years old (though you may be much younger), and you aim to maintain your quality of life for as long as possible.

Not everyone goes through these stages – many people maintain their physical and mental fitness well into their 80s or 90s without signs of slowing down. However, being aware of these later stages of life helps you appreciate that you're at increased risk of developing certain health problems, such as:

- ✔ Arthritis.

- ✔ Bereavement reactions (such as depression and loneliness) and end-of-life concerns (worries about terminal illness, going into care or dying).

- ✔ Continence problems.

- ✔ Falls.

- ✔ Heart disease and stroke-related problems.

- ✔ High blood pressure and diabetes (conditions that increase the risk of suffering a heart attack or stroke).

- ✔ Issues around housing, disability, finances and social problems, which in turn can lead to health problems such as falls, depression and anxiety.

- ✔ Medication issues.

- ✔ Memory issues and dementia.

- ✔ Smoking-related illnesses (particularly heart and lung problems).

In this chapter I look at common conditions in later life, such as these, and how to prevent certain diseases. Of course, many medical conditions aren't limited to people in later life, and so if you can't find information on a specific topic in this chapter make sure that you look elsewhere in the book.

Considering General Health Concerns in Older Age

Preventing diseases to maintain your quality of life for as long as possible is important even if you're completely fit and well when going through the later stages of life. For example, taking up offers of flu vaccinations, getting support with stopping smoking, having your blood pressure checked at regular intervals and taking part in breast cancer screening (if you're a woman) are all worthwhile steps to take in keeping diseases at bay.

Trying to prevent falls is also extremely important, because this problem becomes more common in older age and can have devastating consequences, particularly when falls lead to fractures or serious head injury: about 14,000 people die every year in the United Kingdom just because of the result of a hip fracture!

This section looks at some of the more important medical problems in later life and helps you to keep yourself in good shape.

Getting support in older age

The vast majority of older people manage to live independently with or without various levels of support. The charity AgeUK provides information and advice on getting support and enjoying later life – check out the website (www.ageuk.org) – and remember that your GP surgery is always available for help and advice (also see Chapter 25 for other useful helplines and websites). Your GP needs to take on a more central role for you as you get older: co-ordinating various services for you, providing and monitoring your care, and – last but not least – being an advocate for you and your family.

Conducting a later-life MOT check

If you belong to an older age group and develop new medical symptoms or find coping with life more difficult, identifying potential underlying causes can help you to address the problem. Go through the following list, which is a bit like an MOT test for a car, to see whether any of these issues apply to you:

- **Alcohol:** Check how much alcohol you drink and whether you may be drinking too much (see Chapter 23 for more on alcohol problems).

- **General living:** Consider whether you have any problems with your housing (such as inadequate flooring or a steep staircase without a hand rail) or finances (such as mounting debts so that you can't pay your bills or afford healthy food) that impair your quality of life or pose a danger to your health.

- **Loneliness:** Think about whether you feel lonely or socially isolated – and whether you'd like to change this.

- **Medication:** Look at your regular medication if you take any. Check when you had your last medication review by a health professional and whether you have any problems such as side effects.

- **Mobility:** Consider your current level of mobility, and whether you or people close to you think that you're at an increased risk of falling over.

- **New health problems:** Review if you have current or new problems relating to your physical and mental health, which haven't yet been addressed.

- **Relationships:** Think about whether you have any problems relating to other people (in terms of arguments or resentment), such as your partner or your children, and whether this is something that you'd like to change or receive help with.

- **Self-care:** Consider whether you find looking after yourself (such as washing, getting dressed, shopping or cooking) difficult.

✔ **Senses:** Identify any problems with your eyesight, hearing or how you communicate with other people, and whether you think any of these could potentially be improved.

If any of these situations apply to you, contact your GP surgery for further assessment and information. A lot of help and support is available from a whole team of health and other professionals as well as various charities that specialise in supporting people as they get older. So please don't hesitate to ask – sometimes getting just this little bit of extra support (honestly, it often doesn't need much) can make a huge difference to your quality of life.

Preventing disease: Spotting early signs

Being able to recognise and identify the early signs of common diseases means that you can react to them more quickly. This section looks at some of the more common diseases in later life.

Heart attacks and strokes

Heart attacks and strokes are common and can cause a lot of suffering in later life, both for yourself as well as people close to you. To find out how to recognise a heart attack or stroke, flip to Chapter 5.

Diabetes mellitus

As you get older, you're at risk of developing a condition called *diabetes mellitus* – a long-term disorder in which the level of blood sugar (or *glucose*) in your blood is raised, which can lead to a number of acute and long-term health problems.

Getting to grips with glucose

Glucose is important for your body: you need it for energy. Your body obtains glucose by extracting it from the carbohydrates contained in starch and sugary foods, digesting and transforming them into glucose. Your body can get to the glucose within the carbohydrates from certain foods, such as sweets, fruit juice or jams, very quickly. But foods such as potatoes, rice or bread release their glucose more slowly, because your digestive system needs more time to break these foods up.

A gland near your stomach called the *pancreas* produces the hormone *insulin*, which then moves the glucose out of your bloodstream and into the various cells of your body (imagine insulin to be like a key unlocking a door), where it then acts as the main source of energy. As the insulin lets the glucose in, your blood level of glucose drops.

Diabetes comes in two main forms:

- **Type 1 diabetes:** *Type 1 diabetes* (also known as *insulin-dependent diabetes mellitus*, or *IDDM*) is a condition that destroys the insulin-producing cells in your pancreas. You need to replace the lack of insulin with insulin injections. You can't avoid this type of diabetes, which usually affects children and young adults and tends to develop quickly over a few weeks, or even within days.

- **Type 2 diabetes:** In *type 2 diabetes* (also known as *non-insulin dependent diabetes mellitus*, or *NIDDM*), your body doesn't produce sufficient amounts of insulin or can't properly use the insulin that's available (which can be due to what's called *insulin resistance*). This type of diabetes is very common – the UK has more than two million sufferers, and many people aren't aware that they have this condition – and often affects overweight people over the age of 45. Treatment may initially include diet and exercise (which are also both good for preventing diabetes in the first place), and perhaps medication as well. Sometimes you may need to take insulin in addition to tablets.

You may not show any symptoms at all with diabetes, but consider the possibility that you may have the condition if you notice the following symptoms, which usually develop gradually over time:

- You feel tired all the time.
- You feel thirsty and drink more than you used to.
- You've gradually lost weight without reason.
- You feel more hungry than usual.
- You go to the toilet all the time to pass urine – especially at night.
- You develop itching around your genitals (called *thrush*: check out Chapters 18 and 19).
- You discover that any wounds heal slower than they used to.
- You suffer from blurred vision.

These symptoms don't necessarily mean that you have diabetes, but they need to encourage you to see your GP, who can easily check for diabetes with a simple blood test. If you're found to have diabetes, your symptoms go quickly after you receive treatment.

Diabetes can give you a number of sudden as well as long-term health problems. But if you've been diagnosed with diabetes and stick to your recommended treatment, you've got a good chance of avoiding these problems in the future.

Eye tests are free if you have diabetes and you should make annual appointments to have one. Eye tests are also free if you're over the age of 60 and in other circumstances – check out the NHS Choices website www.nhs.uk for further details.

If you can't keep food down. . .

If you've been diagnosed as diabetic and for some reason you're vomiting so much that you can't keep any food or drink down, consult your GP or practice nurse who can advise you what to do.

If your blood sugar rises too high. . .

Even if you know that you have diabetes and take your treatment as prescribed, your blood sugar can still rise too high (called *hyperglycaemia*). Hyperglycaemia usually develops over a few days, during which you drink more and pass urine more frequently. The following reasons may be to blame:

- ✔ You don't take enough insulin or your other medication needs altering.
- ✔ You don't get enough exercise.
- ✔ You eat too much of the wrong kind of food.
- ✔ You suffer from an acute illness or an infection (such as the 'flu' or a chest infection), which are common causes for the blood sugar to go up.
- ✔ You're stressed.
- ✔ You've put on weight.

Consult your GP or practice nurse (many practice nurses are specially trained in the management of diabetes) for advice if you can't manage to get your blood sugar levels under control yourself, or if you're unsure what to do. With hyperglycaemia, you eventually lose more fluid than you take in, so immediately seeking medical help is really important.

If you have hyperglycaemia for a long time you can develop the following complications:

- ✔ Eyesight problems, such as blurred or reduced vision (flip to 'Watching the Senses' later in this chapter).
- ✔ Heart disease, such as angina or heart attack (see Chapter 5).
- ✔ Kidney problems (of which you may be unaware).
- ✔ Nerve damage, such as reduced sensation.
- ✔ Poor circulation in your legs and other areas (see Chapter 13).

If your blood sugar goes down too much. . .

If you're on treatment for diabetes, a possibility always exists that your blood sugar may go down too much, which is called a *hypoglycaemic attack*, or *hypo* in short.

You're more likely to develop a hypo in these circumstances:

- ✔ You're taking too much insulin or too high a dose of your other diabetes medication.
- ✔ You aren't eating enough.
- ✔ You're exercising more than usual but haven't eaten enough to compensate.
- ✔ You're drinking more alcohol than normal (see Chapter 23 for problems with alcohol).
- ✔ You're under stress (see Chapter 21 for more on stress-related problems).
- ✔ You're sweating more due to hot weather or working in a hot environment.

Here's how to recognise a hypo, which can develop quickly within a few minutes or over a few hours:

- ✔ You may feel hungry, sweaty, dizzy or faint.
- ✔ You may feel cold, tired, confused or irritable – or show odd behaviour (which you may not recognise yourself but you may realise this from how other people react to you).
- ✔ You may well notice a pounding heartbeat.
- ✔ You may pass out or have a fit.

If you suspect that you're suffering a hypo, eat or drink something sugary immediately, such as a sugary drink (but not a diet drink!), sweets or a sugar tablet. If you notice these symptoms in someone else, consider putting some sugar-containing jam into the inside of that person's cheek, particularly if she's drowsy or about to faint. Symptoms usually improve after five to ten minutes at the most: if not, give some more sugar. If everything fails or the person's losing consciousness or having fits, call '999'.

If you want further information on diabetes, speak to your practice nurse or contact the Diabetes UK careline on 0845 1202960 or check out its website at www.diabetes.org.uk, which has lots of further resources. In addition, *Diabetes For Dummies* by Sarah Jarvis and Alan Rubin gives lots of additional background and a whole lot of practical tips.

High blood pressure

Raised blood pressure, or *hypertension*, increases the risk of heart attack, stroke and other potentially serious conditions. For 90 per cent of people with hypertension, no underlying cause can be found, but sometimes chronic alcohol misuse or medical problems such as kidney or heart disease may be to blame. In the short-term, anxiety, exercise, caffeine, smoking or stress can make your blood pressure go up, but this effect is usually short-lasting.

Because high blood pressure usually doesn't cause any symptoms, checks in later life are important. Indeed, whenever you see your practice nurse or GP, they're likely to check whether you've had a recent blood pressure measurement. A number of readings over a period of time are usually necessary to confirm a diagnosis of high blood pressure.

Generally speaking, the higher your blood pressure, the higher your risk of developing problems in the future. If your blood pressure is borderline, your GP may recommend lifestyle measures such as losing weight or increasing exercise to try and bring your blood pressure down. Reducing your alcohol intake, stopping smoking and reducing your salt and caffeine intake are all likely to help. If your blood pressure is very high or doesn't improve with these measures, your GP can prescribe various forms of blood pressure lowering medication.

Raised cholesterol

As with high blood pressure, raised cholesterol increases the risk of blocking up your blood vessels. Also similarly, you unfortunately can't feel when your cholesterol is too high.

Because of the lack of symptoms, having a cholesterol check is a good idea if you're at an increased risk of heart attack or stroke (also known as *cardiovascular risk*). Important risk factors include:

- ✔ You're aged 40 or more: the risk of cardiovascular disease rises with age.
- ✔ You're any age, and raised cholesterol or other related conditions (called *lipid disorders*) run in your family.
- ✔ You have a strong family history of early heart disease or stroke.

If you haven't already been invited, contact your GP surgery to arrange a simple blood test. For further information about hypertension check out the Patient UK website (www.patient.co.uk) or NHS Choices (www.nhs.uk).

Stumbling over: Falls

Many people underestimate the risks to health from falling when they're older; the consequences can be potentially disastrous:

✔ You may become disabled; falls are the leading cause of death due to injury in people over 75 years of age.

✔ You have a 10 per cent chance of suffering a fracture (commonly the wrist or hip): one person in every five who falls needs medical attention.

✔ If you live alone and can't get up after a fall (which may happen at night, for example, when you have to go to the toilet), you can suffer a reduction in body temperature (called *hypothermia*), pressure sores, chest infection or loss of body fluid (known as *dehydration*) if you're unable to call someone to help you get up. This could have potentially serious consequences for your health.

✔ You may seriously lose your confidence and you (and any carers) may worry about you having further falls. You may then become afraid to go out and lose your fitness and perhaps your independence.

For these reasons, preventing falls is high on the UK National Health Service agenda. You can do your bit by being aware of the factors in yourself and your environment that increase your risk of falling, and by doing something about them. That way, you can stay 'up and running' for as long as possible.

Be aware of the following circumstances that increase your risk of falling:

✔ You've had multiple falls in the past.

✔ You have problems with your gait or your balance.

✔ You suffer from poor vision, or your specs need changing.

✔ You have problems remembering things or understanding others.

✔ You feel low in yourself and lack confidence.

✔ You already receive a high level of care.

✔ You're not as mobile as you used to be because of physical ailments (such as a urine or chest infection, angina, chest problems and so on).

✔ You suffer from weakness or arthritis in your legs.

✔ You have problems with your feet.

✔ You've had a stroke in the past or suffer from Parkinson's disease.

✔ You take medication that can make you drowsy or unstable on your feet (such as blood pressure lowering medication).

✔ You drink alcohol.

✔ You're at risk from your environment – for example, poor lighting, lack of hand rails, slippery floors, loose carpets, steep stairs, cluttered rooms, inadequate footwear, ice on the pavement in winter and so on.

Unless you can identify and adequately deal with any of these risk factors, consult your GP who may arrange a more formal *falls assessment*. You may be surprised what can be done to reduce your risk of falling and to make your house a safer place – often with little effort. If you have a fall, and particularly if you sustain an injury, seek medical advice immediately.

Allaying Nerve and Mind Concerns

Problems with thinking and memory become more common as you get older, which sometimes may be due to an underlying cause that can be treated. Such problems develop in later life because you tend to have fewer 'reserves' compared to when you're younger. For example, urine or chest infections are relatively common causes for confusion in older people – with things getting quickly back to normal when treatment with antibiotics kicks in.

Remembering memory problems and dementia (including Alzheimer's)

Most people occasionally can't put a name to someone's face or forget where they've put the house keys, and that's quite normal. Such lapses can be due to tiredness, lack of concentration or just because you have so many other things on your mind. But when this type of lapse happens more and more often or you can't remember things that you experienced recently (for example, what was on TV last night or details of a recent conversation), but your longer-term memory is unaffected, you may wonder whether you're starting to lose your powers of thinking (known as *dementia*), or getting a form of dementia called *Alzheimer's disease*. Having a bad memory throughout your life, however, is unlikely to be due to dementia.

Any of the following conditions can cause dementia and affect brain function:

- ✔ **Alzheimer's disease:** Named after the doctor who first described this condition, *Alzheimer's disease* is the most common cause of dementia. This condition leads to some shrinking of the brain and a reduction of certain chemicals that your brain needs to think and function properly.

- ✔ **Lewy-body dementia:** *Lewy-body dementia* is caused by abnormal protein deposits inside your brain (called *Lewy bodies*). Experts are unsure how this condition develops, but these deposits certainly lead to problems with brain function.

- ✔ **Vascular dementia:** If the blood vessels supplying your brain clog up and don't supply your brain sufficiently with nutrients such as oxygen, you're suffering from *vascular dementia* – the most common form of dementia. Smokers are at a greater risk of dementia. In a stroke (see

Chapter 5), a blood vessel supplying your brain blocks up completely so that no blood can get through, leading to damage or the death of the tissues that this vessel supplies. Vascular dementia is the result of a succession of small strokes, and so your mental abilities become affected. The risk factors for cardiovascular disease also apply to vascular dementia (Chapter 5 contains a list of these risk factors).

✔ **Other causes:** Many other potential causes exist for dementia, but these ones tend to be quite rare. One example is alcohol-related dementia, which you can prevent or stop from getting worse by drinking alcohol sensibly (check out Chapter 23 for alcohol-related information). Remember that depression and other physical conditions, such as an underactive thyroid gland, may also sometimes be responsible for memory problems or other temporary reduction in brain function (such as problems with concentration), and can also be treated.

If you're suffering from dementia, you may in addition to loss of memory notice one or more of the following symptoms:

✔ **Change in personality:** You may become more moody, feel low all the time or get irritated easily. You may also sometimes or regularly say things that are a bit out of character for you.

✔ **Concentration:** You may find sticking with mental tasks such as reading, doing crosswords or knitting harder.

✔ **Confusion and disorientation:** You may find coping with new surroundings or remembering new people difficult, which can be very confusing. You may feel much more comfortable if you can stick to your routines and be in familiar surroundings. You may also find that keeping track of the time is difficult, and may at times not know what day or what time of day it is.

✔ **Not looking after yourself:** Because of dementia you may not look after yourself as well as you used to. Forgetting to change your clothes or wash yourself are quite common.

✔ **Reduction in intellect:** Even if you've always thought of yourself as being quite clever, you may find that acquiring new skills or grasping new ideas becomes tricky.

✔ **Various other signs:** Other features of dementia include losing weight, falling, mood changes (low or excessively cheerful) and later speech problems, as well as physical conditions such as incontinence, reduced mobility and becoming generally frail.

If you suffer from thinking or memory problems, and any of the following scenarios apply to you, seek medical advice straight away:

✔ You've lost some of your memory because of a fall.

✔ You've suffered a recent head injury.

✔ You have a history of cancer.

✔ Your symptoms are getting rapidly worse.

✔ You're disabled and memory problems put your independence at risk.

✔ You suddenly become confused or muddled.

✔ You have other symptoms such as a fever, regular night sweats or have lost weight for no obvious reason.

Unless you have a specific underlying treatable cause, dementia can't be cured. However, consulting your GP is important: she can arrange tests and a more formal assessment at a memory clinic and discuss with you the different management options. Some treatments can slow the progress of dementia, and managing risk factors such as high blood pressure, diabetes and raised cholesterol can help. One of the most important things is to ensure that you get support, advice and care – and lots of it is usually available.

The information in this section should also help you recognise symptoms of dementia in other people. For further information on dementia and Alzheimer's disease, contact the Alzheimer's Society Dementia Helpline on 0845 3000336 or check out the website at www.alzheimers.org.uk. For further advice, see Chapter 25 for a list of useful helplines and websites.

Clearing the air regarding acute confusion

If you're suddenly unable to think clearly, you need to consider whether this problem may be due to an underlying medical cause, such as those in the list in this section. If in doubt, seek medical advice without delay so that you can get treatment quickly if appropriate.

Compare your symptoms with the following descriptions:

✔ **Acute infection:** Urinary symptoms such as burning or stinging on passing urine, perhaps together with a fever, suggest a urine infection (or *cystitis*). If you have a cough, feel unwell, have a fever and find breathing more difficult, you may have a chest infection (called *pneumonia*). Seek medical help as soon as possible, because you may need antibiotics.

✔ **Diabetic emergencies:** If you suffer from diabetes mellitus, you may become confused due to changes in your blood sugar level. Your blood sugar can be too low or too high – read the 'Diabetes mellitus' section earlier in this chapter for how to recognise important symptoms.

✔ **Head injury:** If you've recently injured your head and suddenly or gradually become confused, your symptoms can be due to a bleed inside your skull. You're likely to have a headache as well and may vomit. Seek medical help immediately.

✔ **Medication side effects:** Starting new medication or medicinal side effects can lead to acute confusion, and so always bear this possibility in mind. Types of drugs that may be responsible include painkillers (particularly the *opiate* type) or drugs used for depression or anxiety. Always consider side effects from over-the-counter medication as well. Remember that over-the-counter medication can be toxic if you take it in higher than recommended doses and may react with your regular prescribed medication. Consult your pharmacist or GP if you're unsure.

✔ **Stroke:** You may suddenly become confused when you suffer a stroke. The confusion usually comes on very suddenly, and important accompanying signs are one-sided limb weakness, facial weakness, speech problems and perhaps sudden loss of vision in one eye. For further information about how to recognise a stroke, check out Chapter 5.

✔ **Withdrawal symptoms:** If you've recently stopped medication or drinking alcohol (particularly if you've been drinking over the recommended limits previously), you may suffer from acute confusion because of a withdrawal effect. Medication that can cause withdrawal symptoms when stopped suddenly include sedatives (such as diazepam or some sleeping tablets), antidepressants or opiate-type painkillers.

Plenty of other medical conditions can cause acute confusion, and in most cases seeking medical help straight away is best, instead of trying to figure out the underlying cause. If you're passing out, feel very unwell, you deteriorate quickly or don't know what's going on but are very worried, call your GP or '999' immediately.

Tremor and suspected Parkinson's disease

Movement disorders become more common as people get older. When a part of your body starts to move or shake in ways that you can't control, or if your voice becomes more shaky, you may wonder what might be going on. Many people think that if they develop problems with uncontrollable movements, they must have a condition called *Parkinson's disease* – which may or may not sound familiar to you. In this section I tell you what such symptoms may mean, how to tell them apart and what you should do about them.

Tremor

A *tremor* is when any parts of your body shake uncontrollably. You may experience a tremor as a shaking or trembling sensation in your hands, feet or even your head. You may find it just annoying or embarrassing, but particularly if the tremor gets worse over time, it can start to impact on your daily activities. Many people seek medical advice only when the tremor affects their work or hobbies such as painting or needlework – activities for which your hands and fingers need to be able to make fine movements.

Various forms of tremor exist, so see if your symptoms compare with the descriptions in the following list:

- **Alcoholic tremor:** Drinking alcohol over the recommended limits regularly can cause you to develop a tremor over time (Chapter 23 contains information on the dangers of excessive drinking).

- **Essential tremor:** A gradually worsening tremor that mainly affects both your arms and hands may be *benign essential tremor*, which can run in families. Typically, this type of tremor may improve when you drink small amounts of alcohol.

- **Medication-related tremor:** Certain prescribed drugs (such as some antidepressants) may cause tremor. Check the drug information sheet or speak to your pharmacist or GP if you're concerned.

- **Physiological tremor:** People tend to have a mild tremor (called *physiological tremor*), barely noticeable because it's so 'fine'. This form is quite normal. You may start to notice physiological tremor when:

  • You feel tired.

  • You feel anxious.

  • You've been drinking lots of caffeine-containing drinks such as tea, coffee or cola.

- **Thyroid-related tremor:** An overactive thyroid gland (known as *hyperthyroidism*) may occasionally cause a fine tremor of your hands. You can make this type of tremor more obvious by placing an A4 sheet of paper on the backsides of your outstretched hands – the paper accentuates the tremor and makes it more obvious.

  Consult your GP particularly if you also have any of these symptoms:

  • You feel tense or 'on edge', or more tired.

  • You suffer from frequent loose stools or diarrhoea.

  • You develop bulging eyes.

  • You notice that your muscles have become weaker.

  • You get palpitations and notice your heartbeat more.

  • You sweat more than usual.

  • You lose weight for no apparent reason.

- **Tremor of Parkinson's disease:** This condition may cause a tremor that looks like 'pill-rolling' between the fingers and thumb and usually affects only one side of the body initially. Look at the following section for how to spot other signs of Parkinson's disease.

Because tremor is a feature of Parkinson's disease, many people who develop tremor worry that they've developed this disease – which may not be the case.

✔ **Withdrawal tremor:** Alcohol withdrawal and withdrawal from other drugs such as anti-anxiety medication, sleeping tablets and recreational drugs can all cause tremor.

Occasionally, other underlying conditions affecting the brain or nerves, or poisoning may cause tremor. Sometimes, more than one cause for tremor may be involved. Consult your GP for further assessment, to confirm the diagnosis and discuss the treatment options.

Parkinson's disease

This condition is named after Dr James Parkinson, who was the first to describe it. In essence, if you suffer from *Parkinson's disease*, your brain struggles to move certain muscles in a co-ordinated way. Parkinson's disease most commonly affects people over the age of 50, but can start at a younger age. The condition is caused by damage to the part of the brain that produces *dopamine,* a chemical substance that helps co-ordinate and control body movements. Experts are still trying to find out why this damage happens.

The following symptoms are typical of this condition:

✔ **Balance problems:** Problems with balance and subsequent falls are common in Parkinson's disease.

✔ **Depression:** You may suffer from low mood: Chapter 21 tells you more about symptoms of and treatment options for depression.

✔ **Dizziness:** You may feel increasingly dizzy when you get up from sitting or lying down.

✔ **Reduced movements:** You may find that starting and maintaining repetitive movements is difficult, and that your muscles feel tense and stiff. Walking becomes more tricky, and your gait may start to look as if you're shuffling. You may also find that your handwriting becomes smaller. Other people may notice that you lose some of your facial expressions. You may also find rising from a chair or turning in bed difficult, and doing up or undoing buttons tends to become harder.

✔ **Sleep problems:** Sleep problems and vivid dreams can become very distressing.

✔ **Swallowing:** You may start to dribble and find swallowing difficult.

✔ **Tremor:** Tremor is often the first symptom. You may notice this problem usually in one hand or arm initially, and the tremor may look as if you're rolling a pill between your fingers and thumb. Over time, the tremor may spread to other limbs.

Dementia may occur with Parkinson's disease but isn't directly caused by it. For symptoms of dementia, take a look at 'Remembering memory problems and dementia (including Alzheimer's)' earlier in this chapter.

Ask to see your doctor for further assessment or review of the condition when you spot any symptoms, particularly if you also notice the following:

✔ You fall once or more times.

✔ You suffer from symptoms of depression (see Chapter 21).

✔ You become socially isolated.

✔ You're severely disabled by the condition.

✔ You don't respond to treatment (when you've already been diagnosed).

Watching the Senses

Problems with the senses become more common in later life. In this section I give you an overview of potential causes and actions that you can take to help you deal with the problem. Chapter 9 also has more on eye problems.

Common eye problems in later life

Eye problems are common in older age and can seriously affect your quality of life. Many eye conditions are treatable, and some require urgent action. Here are some of the more common eye conditions:

✔ **Age-related cataracts:** A *cataract* is a clouding of the lens in the front bit of your eye. The causes are unknown. However, certain factors like smoking, overexposing your eyes to sunlight, taking steroid drugs for a long time, a history of cataracts in your family or poor diet may all play a role. When you develop cataracts, you may notice a 'glare' in bright light or when you drive at night, and you may have difficulty distinguishing objects in low light.

✔ **Age-related macular degeneration:** This condition affects an area in the back of your eye called the *macula.* You're at higher risk of developing it if, among other factors, you smoke, drink more than four units of alcohol a day or have been exposed to lots of sunlight in your life. You may find that straight edges such as bookshelves or door frames look distorted, or that your vision is generally more blurred. You may also develop blind spots.

✔ **Chronic glaucoma:** In this condition you have an increased pressure in one or both of your eyes – often caused by fluid within your eye not draining away freely. You may not notice this problem at first, but if left for too long, glaucoma may permanently affect your vision (which is why the condition is known as 'the thief of sight').

✔ **Diabetes:** Too much sugar in your blood (see 'Diabetes mellitus' earlier in this chapter) can lead to chronic eye problems, with damage to the back of your eye (called *diabetic retinopathy*) being an important one.

✔ **Dry eyes:** In *dry eye syndrome* (or *keratoconjunctivitis sicca*), your tears drain away or evaporate too fast. You may notice grittiness, tearing of your eyes and redness. We don't know what causes dry eyes, but ageing, hormonal changes, illnesses and medicines are all thought to play a role.

If you suffer from eye problems, consulting your optician or GP is usually best. Seek medical advice immediately if you notice any of these symptoms:

✔ You suddenly lose your vision fully or partially.

✔ You have a headache in addition to any visual symptoms.

✔ You can't think straight in connection with your eye problem.

✔ You have a painful eye at the same time as loss of vision.

These symptoms may indicate acute eye problems such as infection, inflammation or blocked blood vessels, which can lead to temporary or permanent loss of your vision unless you quickly receive treatment.

Many people wrongly believe that losing their vision is a normal part of ageing and that nothing can be done – but that's not true: many eye conditions can be successfully treated. And good vision is important for continuing to be able to drive, read or take part in certain leisure activities, which makes seeking medical advice all the more important.

(Not) hearing trouble

The first signs of worsening hearing may become apparent to you while taking part in group conversations or talking on the phone. Reduced hearing can impair your quality of life (and that of other people close to you!) considerably. Getting your ears checked early on is worthwhile when you suspect hearing problems, because a number of treatment options are available to you. Don't suffer in silence!

Hearing problems can be split into two general groups:

✔ **Problems with sound conduction:** This type of hearing loss is caused when sound isn't being transmitted properly from your outer to your inner ear. Common causes are infection, blockage of the ear canal due to wax, hardened bones in your ear, ear damage or a perforated eardrum.

✔ **Problems with sound sensation:** Your hearing is reduced because sound signals aren't being transmitted properly from the inner ear to your brain. Common causes include age-related hearing loss (called *presbyacusis* – a natural decline in your hearing), damage to your ear due to loud noise (perhaps work-related or from playing in a rock band in your youth!), certain medicines and other causes. (*Ménière's disease*, for example, is a rare condition where you may notice symptoms of hearing loss, dizziness and ringing in your ear – see Chapter 6.)

Get your hearing tested or see your GP if you have any of these symptoms:

✔ You ask people regularly to repeat themselves.

✔ You find that following conversations is difficult, particularly when you're in a group.

✔ You have trouble hearing in noisy places.

✔ You have to turn the TV or radio volume up loud.

✔ You have difficulty hearing the doorbell.

A number of aids are available when you have hearing problems:

✔ Devices to inform you when your smoke detector or alarm clock go off.

✔ Equipment to help you watch TV or listen to the radio.

✔ Devices that let you know when your telephone or doorbell rings.

Chapter 9 contains more on hearing problems. Also, check out the Royal National Institute for Deaf people website at www.rnid.org.uk for more information on hearing aids and other equipment.

Part V
Approaching Mental Health Problems and Addictive Behaviour

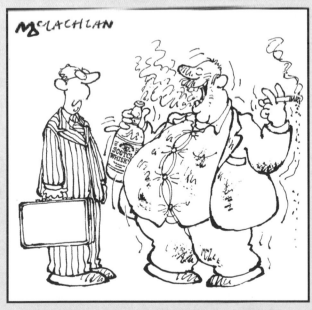

'I used to worry about my smoking
and alcohol intake so I doubled it
and now I don't worry at all.'

In this part . . .

Mental health problems such as depression, stress and anxiety are surprisingly common. Dealing with them can sometimes be hard because they're less 'concrete' than physical symptoms, and even accepting mental health problems can be difficult because they still sometimes carry a stigma. To help you identify and deal with these types of problems, Part V debunks some of the myths that surround these conditions and gives you some straight-talking guidance on how to tackle them.

Alcohol and drugs have the potential to cause significant health problems – physical as well as mental. This part provides some strategies to help you get a grip if you or someone close to you suffers from an alcohol or drug problem.

Chapter 21

Tackling Depression, Stress and Anxiety

. . . .

In This Chapter

▶ Becoming confident in recognising symptoms of depression

▶ Finding out more about self-harm

▶ Recognising the signs of stress and anxiety

. . . .

*F*eeling low or anxious is part of normal life. Your mood can be great one minute, but then day-to-day problems or life events such as work or relationship difficulties get in the way and your spirits go down or you feel nervous and stressed.

When you're emotionally and psychologically well (in other words, you're in a good state of mental health), you're in a great position to be getting on with your life, and so you feel better and bounce back quickly. But if the way you feel, think or behave gets so affected that you can't function properly, you may be suffering from depression, stress or anxiety. These mental health problems are common, but many people still don't like to talk about or even acknowledge them, and feelings of guilt, embarrassment or shame are not uncommon.

Symptoms of depression, stress and anxiety come in different forms and you may not be able to spot them easily, particularly when they're only mild. They may also overlap, and distinguishing clearly between them can be difficult. So, in this chapter I lay out the key information about the symptoms, what they mean, how to recognise when things are getting a bit more serious and when to seek help sooner rather than later. I also dispel some of the myths that surround these conditions and mental health problems in general.

Spotting Depression

Symptoms of depression are incredibly common – over two million people in the UK are depressed at any one time. Many of these people don't actually know that they suffer from this illness, and research shows that many people who are aware that they have it feel too embarrassed about it to see their GP. So if you suffer from symptoms of depression, do remember that you're not alone! A stigma remains attached to a diagnosis of depression, which is a real shame, because very effective treatments are available.

Dispelling common myths about depression

Many myths surround the term depression and its diagnosis and the time has come to set them straight:

✔ **Myth:** Depression is rare. **Fact:** Depression is common – in fact it's incredibly common and can affect anyone.

✔ **Myth:** Depression isn't an illness. **Fact:** Depression is a – sometimes serious – medical illness that may require treatment. GPs are very used to treating depression.

✔ **Myth:** You should be able to get out of depression yourself. **Fact:** Depression is an illness like asthma or diabetes and hasn't got anything to do with whether you're a so-called strong character or not. Typically, you can't just bounce back, although saying that, depression may sometimes get better by itself: it may just take a long time.

✔ **Myth:** Depression happens only when something bad happens in your life. **Fact:** You may develop depression for no apparent reason whatsoever.

✔ **Myth:** Talking about depression is pointless. **Fact:** Talking therapies can be very helpful and effective.

✔ **Myth:** Antidepressants are addictive and alter your personality. **Fact:** Antidepressants aren't addictive, and they don't change your personality. They may, however, help you to get back to your usual self. Some – often minor – side effects are common, particularly at the start of treatment, but these often settle after a week or two.

Identifying symptoms of depression

Spotting depression isn't always easy. In this section I explain how you can recognise the main symptoms of depression.

Finding out whether you may be depressed

To find out whether you may be depressed, try answering the following questions:

- ✔ Over the past four weeks, have you regularly or more often than not felt 'low', 'down' or 'hopeless'?

- ✔ Over the last month, have you often been bothered by having little interest or pleasure in doing things that you normally enjoy doing?

If your answer is 'no' to these questions, you're unlikely to be depressed. However, if you answered 'yes' to one or both of them, you may suffer from depression.

When you suffer from depression, you may not just feel low; a number of other symptoms can also affect you:

- ✔ **Appetite:** You may lose your appetite or develop a tendency for overeating.

- ✔ **Concentration:** You may have difficulty concentrating on things such as listening to the radio, watching television, reading the newspaper or books, or talking to other people.

- ✔ **Energy:** You may feel tired all the time, have little energy and not be bothered to do things, or do them only with a lot of effort on your part.

- ✔ **Interest:** You may lose interest in hobbies and sex, and find that nothing really gives you pleasure anymore.

- ✔ **Movement:** You or other people may notice that you're moving or speaking much slower than you used to. Or, you may be more fidgety or restless, moving around much more than usual.

- ✔ **Self-worth:** You may feel that you've let yourself or other people down and feel bad about yourself. You may see yourself as a failure.

- ✔ **Sleep:** You may find getting to sleep difficult, or you wake up once or more times in the middle of the night or too early in the morning. Alternatively, you may find that you sleep too much, and struggle to get up.

✔ **Thoughts of self-harm:** You may have thoughts that you'd be better off dead, that the world would be better off without you or that life is just not worth living anymore. Or, you may think that you want to hurt yourself in some other way. Such thoughts can be very distressing, which is why I cover them in more detail in the next section.

If you recognise any of the above symptoms in yourself – particularly if they've been going on for a couple of weeks or longer, or they're severe – consult your GP without delay. Various treatments, including talking therapies and medication, are available to you and can be very effective in getting you back on track.

Common reasons for feeling low

If you feel low, this doesn't necessarily mean that you suffer from depression. Here are some other common causes of low mood – which may at times turn into a 'full' depression:

✔ **Bereavement and major life events:** A time of mourning is a natural reaction to the death of someone close, and you're bound to feel low for a while, often for weeks, months or even years. Sometimes, other life events such as getting divorced or losing your job can lead to a period of feeling low. Seek medical advice when the death of a close person is affecting you more than you'd expect or when you find that getting back on with your day-to-day life is difficult.

✔ **Hormonal reasons:** Feeling low is common during pregnancy and after giving birth (called the *baby blues* when the feeling lasts for a few days only and *postnatal depression* when problems go on for longer and are more severe). You're also more likely to suffer from mood changes during the *menopause* (you can find more information in Chapter 18). See your midwife, health visitor or GP for further assessment.

Sometimes, an underactive thyroid gland – which can affect both sexes – may cause you to feel low and depressed, but you're likely to have additional symptoms such as feeling cold all the time, constipation, lack of energy and persistent tiredness as well (for more info turn to Chapter 6).

✔ **Illness:** Many infectious diseases and chronic conditions such as diabetes, heart disease and osteo- or rheumatoid arthritis can be accompanied by symptoms of depression. If your depressive symptoms last for longer than a couple of weeks or they're very severe, consult your GP.

✔ **Medication:** Certain drugs such as the oral contraceptive pill and blood pressure lowering medication can sometimes make you feel depressed. Check the information sheets that come with any medication that you take for possible effects on your mood, and consult your pharmacist or GP if you're concerned.

✔ **Premenstrual tension:** If you're a woman and you find that you tend to become irritable, unhappy, aggressive and low in spirit on the days leading up to your periods, you're likely to be suffering from *premenstrual syndrome*. This condition may be so bad that you also experience physical symptoms such as headaches or feeling bloated. Visit your GP if premenstrual syndrome regularly interferes with your life.

✔ **Seasonal affective disorder (SAD):** Some people regularly feel down and depressed during the winter months. When these symptoms are severe and impact on your daily life, you may be suffering from SAD, also known as the *winter blues*. Consult your GP if symptoms affect your day-to-day life or you're concerned.

✔ **Stress:** Feeling overworked or under pressure at home or work can bring on stress and low mood, particularly when this situation has been going on for a while. Check out the section on 'Feeling On Edge: Stress, Anxiety and Panic' later in this chapter.

If your depression alternates with bouts of mania – when you feel very 'high' – you may have a condition called *bipolar disorder*. Turn to Chapter 22 for more information on this illness.

Taking the first step towards getting help if you suffer from symptoms of depression can take a bit of courage, but I assure you that you'll be glad you did so. You've got a very good chance of getting better after receiving appropriate treatment, and your GP should be the first port of call. Don't feel that you're bothering the doctor; most GPs see between two and six patients with depression every day and are well used to managing this condition.

For further information, visit the Depression Alliance website at www.depressionalliance.org.

Looking at self-harming behaviour

Self-harming behaviour can take several forms, from self-cutting with a sharp object or self-burning with a cigarette to attempted suicide. Such behaviour can be an impulsive response to an argument or drinking alcohol, or a response to emotional distress. People who self-harm often say that it gives them a feeling of 'release' and makes them feel better. The extreme of attempted suicide often follows a longer period during which a person may have been experiencing suicidal thoughts for weeks or even months. For issues around self-harm in teenagers turn to Chapter 17.

If you have thoughts of harming yourself, you may recognise any number of the following feelings:

- You don't like yourself.

- You're deeply embarrassed about something.

- You feel very ashamed for some reason.

- You feel socially isolated or lonely.

- You feel helpless, or you're in a situation from which you can't see a way out.

- You're angry with yourself or other people.

- You feel deeply frustrated for some reason.

- You may have particular worries, for example about your or other people's health, your finances, or about the future in general.

If you experience such thoughts of self-harm, the following factors increase the risk that you're in danger of hurting yourself:

- **Bereavement:** Losing a loved one is always a difficult situation, particularly when you or someone close to you loses a partner or child.

- **Chronic illness:** If you suffer from chronic pain or illness and have dark thoughts, particularly if your illness is getting worse or has a poor prognosis, you may be at higher risk of suicide.

- **Depression:** Symptoms of severe depression, such as thoughts of guilt, hopelessness or low mood can make self-harm more likely (for more info on this aspect, read the 'Identifying symptoms of depression' section earlier in this chapter).

- **Hearing voices:** Hearing voices commanding and encouraging self-harming behaviour puts you at a higher risk of hurting yourself. For more details on intrusive thoughts, check out Chapter 22.

- **Illegal drugs:** Use of illegal drugs increases the risk of self-harm.

- **Planning:** If you find yourself planning self-harm or suicide, you're at a higher risk of carrying your plans through. Generally speaking, the more detailed and prepared your plan is, the higher your risk.

- **Previous attempts:** You're at increased risk of self-harm if you've self-harmed in the past.

If you feel that your life is no longer worth living, or you contemplate suicide, take your feelings very seriously. Speak to your GP immediately if you notice any of the warning signs. Alternatively, you can phone the Samaritans for help and advice 24 hours a day on 0845 7909090; or visit the website at www. samaritans.org for further information.

Thoughts of self-harm are common and are often due to depression – an illness that can be treated. Don't hesitate to seek professional help if you have these thoughts – you're not the only one, and you've nothing to be ashamed of. Your GP is always a good first port of call – and everything you discuss or talk about will be treated confidentially.

If you're dealing with self-harming behaviour in other people, remember that even if a thought or act on their part seems trivial, the intent may still be serious.

Feeling on Edge: Stress, Anxiety and Panic

Feelings of tension and stress are common and may go hand in hand with physical symptoms such as sweating, a racing heart or feeling unwell. Most people get stressed at times in certain situations – admittedly some people do so more than others – and usually this feeling doesn't last for long. However, if symptoms of stress seem to be taking over your life, or if you feel increasingly anxious or even panicky, you may benefit from seeking professional help.

This section helps you to recognise the warning signs of stress and anxiety.

Identifying stress

Stress is pressure or worry caused by physical or emotional problems. Not all stress is bad for you. For example, thinking of an upcoming deadline can make you work harder, having to pick up the kids from school at a set time may prompt you to get the shopping done beforehand and having a baby may get you excited. A certain amount of stress can therefore be good for you – it can be stimulating and actually improve your quality of life.

However, people react differently as regards tolerating stress; some people seem to thrive on it, whereas others find that dealing with any change or events outside their daily routine is difficult. When stress rises above a certain level – perhaps when you're going through a major life event such as getting married, getting divorced, moving house or changing jobs, or when you're finding increasing stress more difficult to deal with – you may develop actual symptoms of stress and suffer as a result.

Common causes of stress in the UK are as follows:

- **Exams:** Many people find that coping with the pressure of exams, or having to speak or perform in public, is very stressful.

- **Family issues:** You may have problems with your children, difficulties in a relationship or struggles in your role as a carer.

- **Legal disputes:** Court appearances in particular can be very stressful.

- **Money:** Financial difficulties can cause a lot of stress.

- **Work:** You may experience work problems such as bullying, employment disputes or other problems with your colleagues or boss.

Recognising stress can be difficult, particularly if it comes on gradually. But when you're stressed you may notice any of the following symptoms:

- You suffer from mood swings and feel low a lot of the time.

- You feel anxious or irritable (being 'snappy').

- You feel your self-esteem dropping.

- You find concentrating and remembering difficult.

- You feel tired and lethargic.

- You find getting to sleep difficult because you can't switch off; alternatively, you wake regularly in the middle of the night.

- You get headaches and other physical problems such as palpitations, a 'knot' in your stomach, other unexplained aches and pains, or increased sweating.

- You drink more alcohol, coffee or tea than you normally do.

- You eat more or much less than you usually do.

If you suffer from a chronic condition such as asthma, migraine or eczema, these illnesses may get worse when you're stressed.

Some of these symptoms overlap with those of depression that I cover in the earlier section 'Identifying symptoms of depression' – and too much stress can therefore lead to depression. If you find that you can't function properly due to stress, particularly if you don't get better and your symptoms last for longer than a couple of weeks, see your GP for further assessment.

Many people suffer from too much stress at times, which is nothing to be ashamed of. Don't hesitate to seek professional help if you feel too stressed and this seems to affect your day-to-day life and your health in general – it can make all the difference.

Stress-busting strategies

Sometimes, for whatever reason, life just 'gets in the way' and you feel increasingly tense. The good news is that you can take steps to keep stress at bay:

✔ Make sure that you get enough sleep and avoid taking sleeping tablets if possible.

✔ Avoid coffee, tea, alcohol and cigarettes.

✔ Look after your health: eat regularly and healthily, and be sure to spend time with your family and friends.

✔ Remember that exercise is great for stress relief!

✔ Try to pinpoint the cause of your stress and sort it out by, for example, talking to your line manager at work, arranging additional child care or booking an appointment with a debt or marriage counsellor.

✔ Treat yourself by booking in for a nice sauna or massage, going to the cinema or doing something else that you enjoy doing but haven't made time for lately.

✔ Improve your time management: make lists and prioritise tasks in order of importance. Try to get out of commitments or appointments that can wait or are unimportant. Look at your 'to do' list and strike out anything that you can safely drop without any major consequences.

For further help and advice, contact the Stress Management Society on 0844 3578629 or visit the website at www.stress.org.uk.

Understanding anxiety

Feeling anxious can be quite normal, as long as any feelings of apprehension or tension go away again by themselves or aren't severe enough to impact on your life. Anxiety often accompanies depression, and as with depression and stress most people feel anxious at times, particularly when confronted with a stressful situation. You can also experience symptoms of anxiety for no apparent reason, and particularly when worries seem to take over your life you may suffer from what's known as *generalised anxiety disorder*. This can be difficult to distinguish from depression and stress.

Anxiety isn't always easy to recognise, and so consider these indicators:

✔ You feel nervous or on edge.

✔ You find relaxing and controlling your worries difficult.

✔ You tend to worry a lot, perhaps much more than you or other people feel is 'normal', and tend to think the worst.

✔ You're so fidgety that you find sitting still difficult at times.

✔ You suffer from mood swings or get easily wound up.

✔ Your worrying affects your day-to-day life significantly – including your social life and work.

✔ You often think that something bad's going to happen.

✔ You find your worries upsetting and stressful.

✔ You suffer nightmares or from increased sensitivity to noise.

Physical symptoms commonly develop when you suffer from anxiety, and so you may also notice the following:

✔ Your hands are shaking and you may notice strange sensations such as tingling or numbness.

✔ You easily get a dry mouth or find swallowing difficult.

✔ You get headaches or feel dizzy.

✔ You experience chest discomfort or palpitations.

✔ You pass urine or open your bowels frequently.

If you feel that you may be suffering from anxiety – particularly if you've had symptoms of anxiety for a few months or longer – visit your GP for further assessment and to discuss the treatment options. If appropriate, your GP may want to exclude other possible causes that can also lead to symptoms of anxiety, such as:

✔ Developing an overactive thyroid gland (called *hyperthyroidism*).

✔ Drinking too much coffee or tea.

✔ Experiencing low blood sugar (known as *hypoglycaemia*).

✔ Withdrawing from drugs or alcohol.

Anxiety is incredibly common, but many people with symptoms of anxiety struggle to summon up the courage and seek professional help because they're anxious or because they're ashamed or embarrassed about the way they feel and think. Remember that your GP is well trained in dealing with anxiety, and that lots of other people also have these symptoms.

Grappling with phobias

A form of anxiety that occurs only when you're in a certain situation is called a *phobia*. If you suffer from a phobia, you typically try to avoid the situation that provokes your symptoms and you may become anxious even just thinking about getting into that situation.

Some examples of phobias are as follows, starting with simple phobia and followed by the more complex ones:

- **Simple phobia:** You're inappropriately anxious when faced with an object such as a spider or mouse, or in certain situations such as flying or being in enclosed spaces. Simple phobias commonly start in the early years of life following a stressful situation or some frightening life event, although experts don't always know why this type of phobia occurs.

- **Agoraphobia:** You feel panicky or may even faint when you're part of a crowd, out of the house or in a situation from which escape is difficult. To avoid these situations, you may avoid going out altogether, which can sometimes lead to depression and other mental health problems. We don't know exactly why agoraphobia occurs, but it's thought that life experiences, genetic reasons and changes of chemicals in the brain may all play a role.

- **Social phobia:** You have a strong and persistent fear of being negatively seen by others, and so you try to avoid social situations such as talking to groups, speaking on the telephone or going out with friends. In contrast to just being shy, social phobia can be quite disabling. Previous anxious or intense experiences in certain social situations may cause social phobias – particularly if you've always been shy since childhood and haven't been able to fully develop your social confidence.

To avoid a phobia getting out of hand, consult your GP to discuss the many forms of treatment and therapy that are available. If you're in a situation and start to feel anxious, try to relax and take control of your breathing. Open and stretch your hands, which can help release tension – our natural reaction to stress and anxiety is to close our hands or make a fist.

To find out more, you can contact *Triumph Over Phobia (TOP)* on 0845 6009601 or visit their website at www.topuk.org. Turn to the next section on 'Handling panic attacks' for info on dealing with more severe symptoms that you may experience when you suffer from phobia.

Handling panic attacks

Panic attacks are when you suddenly experience an intense feeling of apprehension or impending disaster. You're likely to become anxious very quickly – often without warning and for no apparent reason. These attacks affect a lot of people and can be very frightening. Nobody really knows why panic attacks occur, but experts think that traumatic life experiences like the death of a close family member, unpleasant childhood experiences or changes in the chemicals within your brain, for example, may play a role.

If you suffer from panic attacks, you may recognise some of the following symptoms, at least four of which typically show during an attack:

- ✔ You suffer from a fast heart rate or palpitations.
- ✔ You feel short of breath or that you're choking.
- ✔ You notice chest pain or discomfort.
- ✔ You feel dizzy, unsteady on your feet or faint.
- ✔ You feel sick or have stomach pain.
- ✔ You feel flushed or suddenly cold.
- ✔ You feel shaky and tremble.
- ✔ You're afraid of doing something that you can't control or that may seem crazy to other people.
- ✔ You feel like you're not yourself.
- ✔ You may feel as if you're about to die.

During a panic attack, try to tell yourself that you're not coming to any harm, and that the symptoms you experience are due to anxiety. Remind yourself that attacks will pass, and 'ride it out'. Try not to leave the situation that is causing you to have a panic attack and 'confront' your fear. By staying in the situation you give yourself the opportunity to discover that nothing serious is going to happen to you.

If you feel that you may suffer from panic attacks and that these attacks impact on your life, consult your GP. She can then exclude any potential underlying physical causes and discuss the different management options with you.

Useful sources of more information are No More Panic (www.nomorepanic.co.uk) and Anxiety Care at www.anxietycare.co.org.uk.

Chapter 22

Considering Unusual Thoughts, Feelings and Behaviour

In This Chapter

▶ Working through problems with feelings and thinking

▶ Handling extreme ups and downs

▶ Dealing with obsessive, compulsive or other extraordinary behaviour

*A*long with everybody else, you have ups and downs in your daily life and experience a range of emotions over time. Everyone is different, and some people feel or experience things more intensely than others. Most people, however, know which feelings and thoughts are normal for them.

A change in your normal self – such as developing obsessive thoughts or behaviours, feeling that you're 'in two minds' or starting to experience the world around you in a way that seems strange, threatening or unsettling for you – can be quite frightening. You may wonder whether having these symptoms is okay, or whether you need to seek help from a health professional.

This chapter aims to give you some idea of what certain thoughts, feelings and behaviours may mean, whether they may indicate an illness that can be regarded as a *mental health disorder* (for example, *psychosis* or *compulsive behaviour)* and when seeking medical advice is appropriate. (If you feel low, anxious or stressed, also take a look at Chapter 21. If you think that the way you feel or think may be influenced by drinking too much alcohol or using drugs, check out Chapter 23.)

Feeling ashamed or embarrassed when you develop thoughts that are unusual for you is natural, and it may put you off seeking professional help. If you feel that any of the problems mentioned in this section apply to you and these interfere with your life, though, don't hesitate to contact your GP or the other sources of support I mention – they've heard and seen it all before. And remember that you're not the only one, so don't 'bottle it up' for too long if you're worried.

Feeling 'Different'

In this section, I help you decide whether to seek advice if you – or someone you know – start to worry that any of your feelings, thoughts or behaviours have become abnormal.

Dealing with unusual feelings and thoughts

Changes to the way humans feel or think are often caused by common mental health conditions and problems, such as the following:

- **Alcohol and drugs:** Drinking too much alcohol or using drugs are common causes for problems with thinking, feeling and behaviour. (Read more about this subject in Chapter 23.)

- **Anxiety:** *Anxiety* (when worries seem to take over your life) and *panic attacks* (when you suddenly experience an intense feeling of apprehension or impending disaster) can cause a whole range of unusual feelings and thoughts. (Chapter 21 has more on anxiety and panic attacks.)

- **Depression:** If you suffer from depression you may feel low in mood, worthless or guilty, often with no obvious reason. You may be convinced that people hate you, or feel that your life isn't worth living. Depression is a treatable illness, so see your GP for further assessment. (You can discover more about depression in Chapter 21.)

Other mental health disorders such as *schizophrenia*, which you can read about in the following section 'Sussing out schizophrenia', can also be the root of unusual thoughts. Medical causes such as acute infections or conditions affecting your brain can also be to blame.

Making sense of mental health symptoms can be quite difficult, even for experienced doctors and other health professionals. Therefore, do consult your GP if you notice any of the following symptoms, which may suggest that you need professional help:

- **Abnormal beliefs/delusions** are where you hold onto unshakeable – and usually wrong – beliefs despite evidence to the contrary, which other people may find unexpected and unusual for you.

- **Abnormal perceptions:** When you wrongly interpret what's happening around you, you experience an *illusion*. When you see something that isn't really there, you experience a *hallucination*. Or, you may not feel 'real', as if someone else is playing yourself – a bit like an actor. Similarly, things around you may feel unreal or dreamlike.

✔ **Abnormal thoughts:** Your ideas may leap around like a yoyo, or your thoughts may suddenly get completely interrupted, with your mind going blank. You may also feel that your thoughts don't belong to yourself, but have been planted into your mind by someone else, or that someone is taking your thoughts away.

Delusions and hallucinations are sometimes also called *psychotic symptoms* (or *symptoms of psychosis*), which suggest that you can't really distinguish between what's real and what you imagine.

Countless more examples of unusual feelings and thoughts exist, including disturbed and confused thoughts as well as lack of self-awareness and insight. Any such beliefs, perceptions or thoughts should prompt you to see your GP for further assessment. Likewise, concerns about other thoughts, perhaps around your sexuality, or becoming unusually aggressive or tense – particularly when this change is affecting your life or that of those around you – mean that you need to consult your GP to find out what's going on.

Sussing out schizophrenia

Schizophrenia is a fairly common and chronic serious mental health condition. If you suffer from schizophrenia, you show symptoms of psychosis and may hold abnormal beliefs (called *delusions*), see or hear things that aren't there (known as *hallucinations*), have abnormal thoughts of someone persecuting you or feel that your thoughts don't belong to yourself. Typical of schizophrenia is that you're unable to distinguish between what's real and what's in your imagination, which can be quite frightening.

Nobody knows exactly why some people develop schizophrenia, but experts believe that a mixture of environmental and genetic factors may be responsible. Schizophrenia may occur together with other mental health problems such as depression and anxiety, and drug and alcohol misuse is not uncommon. Refer to Chapters 21 and 23 for further information on these issues.

A common belief holds that when you have schizophrenia, you must have a so-called split personality – which isn't true – and that you're violent towards others. Again, this belief is a myth – most people with schizophrenia aren't violent towards others and are in fact much more vulnerable to violence from other people themselves.

Forget the myths about schizophrenia, and use this list to help you recognise the actual symptoms:

✔ **Decision making:** You may find that making decisions is difficult, or that you make decisions that seem impulsive or foolish to others. Your decisions may have endangered you or other people in some way.

- ✔ **Delusions:** You may hold an irrational belief that, for example, an elaborate conspiracy against you exists. You may fear that someone is out to harm you and may interpret normal occurrences in an unusual way. Again, you may not notice this symptom, but other people may do and bring it to your attention.

- ✔ **Drive:** If you suffer from schizophrenia, you may lack drive and ambition, and find engaging with the world around you to be difficult. Other people may tell you that you seem apathetic. Your friends and family may feel that you've become emotionally flat and lack motivation. You may not bother looking after yourself and cease wanting to socialise with other people.

- ✔ **Hearing voices:** A typical symptom of schizophrenia is 'hearing' voices, often as if two people are talking about you. You may feel that the voices are giving a running commentary of what you're doing, or that the voices are arguing with each other. However, the experience may feel normal to you.

- ✔ **Influence from others:** You may feel that other people or organisations are influencing and controlling your thoughts and behaviour, perhaps by 'broadcasting' messages to you, or have a feeling that other people can read or hear your thoughts.

- ✔ **Language and speech:** Friends or family may tell you that your use of language seems odd and that you're using words that no one else understands. You may also talk much less than you used to.

- ✔ **Self-esteem and the way you feel about yourself:** Your self-esteem may be low, and you may feel that 'something funny is going on' in the way you perceive the world or other people around you. You may not realise that this feeling is a problem, but other people may worry about you.

Noticing any of these symptoms in yourself doesn't automatically mean that you suffer from schizophrenia. Other issues can produce similar symptoms; for example, medical causes such as infections, hormone disorders, other physical conditions and dementia can mimic schizophrenia. In addition, intoxication due to alcohol or drug misuse (cannabis or stimulating drugs called amphetamines are typical examples) or a drug overdose can produce the same symptoms.

If you think that your symptoms may be due to drug use or overdose, call your GP urgently or go straight to the nearest Accident & Emergency (A&E) department. Call '999' in an emergency.

If drugs aren't a likely cause, do still see your GP to get checked out, particularly when you find that coping with and/or looking after your own affairs is hard. Many people who suffer from schizophrenia often talk to their GP late or not at all, particularly when their symptoms are mild, and so they miss out on receiving appropriate and often effective treatment.

For further information about schizophrenia or other mental health disorders, contact Mind (the National Association For Mental Health) on 0845 7660163 or visit the website at www.mind.org.uk. The charity Rethink also helps people with mental illness as well as their relatives and carers; you can contact the charity on 0845 4560455 or visit the website at www.rethink.org.

Coping With Boundless Energy and Depression: Mania and Bipolar Disorder

Being elated and full of grandiose ideas and energy can be a great feeling, but may also be a sign of *mania* or the less severe form, *hypomania* – which is mania without any delusions or hallucinations. The main problem with suffering from mania or hypomania is that you can lose touch with reality. You may not realise that you're doing so, but to other people you may be behaving oddly or even bizarrely. No-one knows exactly what causes mania, but experts think that a combination of physical, environmental and social factors may play a role.

When mania or hypomania alternates with episodes of depression (check out Chapter 21 for more details), it's called *bipolar disorder*. Bipolar disorder is a serious mental health condition that can severely impact on people's lives. The ups and downs of bipolar disorder are quite different from what people experience in their daily lives, in that the episodes of depression and mania can each last for a few weeks. During the depressive phases, your thoughts are more negative, your mood and energy levels are low – particularly in the morning – and you no longer enjoy your daily activities. You may also start to feel guilty or develop low self-esteem for no apparent reason.

Check the following list to see if you recognise any of these symptoms in yourself:

- ✔ **Activity:** You may be very active – both mentally and physically – and feel out of control or even 'unstoppable'. You may also have an increased or (more commonly) erratic appetite and have grandiose or self-important ideas. Although you may not recognise all these symptoms in yourself, other people may tell you about them. Your sleep pattern may be all over the place, and not surprisingly you may feel exhausted.

- ✔ **Finances:** Recklessness with money is common during manic phases, and may affect you and your family considerably. Debt problems aren't unusual.

- ✔ **Hallucinations:** Hearing voices that aren't really there may also occur in mania.

✓ **Ideas and delusions:** During manic phases, you may feel that your ideas are of great importance or brilliance, or that you have extraordinary abilities, powers or privileges – without much evidence to support your delusions.

✓ **Mood:** You may feel extremely happy or be irritable and angry. Each of these feelings may last for several weeks at a time.

✓ **Physical health:** Without treatment, your physical health may also be affected in that you may eventually lack sleep, feel tired and lose weight.

✓ **Risk taking:** You may become less risk-averse and engage in behaviour that may put your health at risk. For example, you may have an increased sexual drive and become sexually disinhibited, exposing you to a higher risk of sexually transmitted infections.

If your symptoms are severe, you may even lose the will to live and stop looking after yourself. See your GP for further assessment and advice. For more information, contact The BiPolar Organisation on 0845 6340540 or visit the website at www.mdf.org.uk.

Looking at Unusual Behaviour

Your thoughts and feelings directly influence the way in which you behave. Unusual, strange, bizarre or in any other way extraordinary behaviour can be due to an underlying mental health problem. Some behaviour disorders such as *obsessive compulsive disorder* (*OCD*) are very common, and can create real difficulties for yourself, as well as for co-workers, friends and family.

Experiencing obsessions and compulsive behaviour

Images, urges or thoughts that keep coming into your mind (for example, a fear of being locked in, or having to check something over and over again) are called *obsessions*. Obsessions are more than just your normal worries in day-to-day life – they tend to be unpleasant for you and may make you feel anxious. Even if you try to ignore your thoughts or suppress them, you may not be able to get rid of them, with the end result that your obsessions can start to rule your life. Some people develop strategies to work around their obsessions, but life can become difficult when these attempts fail.

Here are some examples of common obsessions:

✓ An exaggerated or unpleasant fear of making a mistake.

✓ A fear of getting contaminated with germs.

- An extreme need for exactness or symmetry.

- An excessive worry that you'll come to harm.

- A powerful fear of behaving unacceptably.

- A strong sexual or religious urge that you feel is unpleasant.

Obsessions such as these ones can lead to actions that you feel you need to repeat constantly – a condition called *compulsive behaviour*. Compulsive behaviour is usually directly linked to obsessions – you're trying to respond to the anxiety or distress that your obsessions cause.

Obsessions may lead to compulsive behaviour such as the following:

- Having to carry out certain rituals on most days.

- Needing to perform certain acts or having to behave in fixed repetitive ways most of the time.

- Cleaning things or washing your hands very frequently, perhaps every few minutes.

- Having to order and arrange things in a certain way.

- Checking again and again that you've switched off the lights or your oven (you may regularly get up again to do so after you've gone to bed), or when you calculate sums you go over your results over and over again . . . just to make sure.

- Hoarding items to what other people would consider to be an excessive extent, although you yourself may not perceive this behaviour as a problem.

- Carrying out mental acts such as repeating words silently, counting or ruminating.

When obsessions and compulsions impact on your life, they become jointly known as *obsessive compulsive disorder*, or *OCD*. OCD can be very mild (in fact, many people sometimes show OCD-like behaviour some of the time, and this can be entirely normal) or so severe that you're quite disabled and distressed.

OCD can start at any age, but most people develop this condition in childhood or adolescence. The exact causes of OCD aren't known, but experts believe that genetic factors, adverse life events, abnormalities within a group of nerves in the brain (called the *basal ganglia*) and changes of some chemicals in the brain play a role.

> # Getting vocal about Tourette's
>
> Many people think that everyone with Tourette's syndrome shouts and screams obscenities and swear words (called *coprolalia*). However, this is uncommon – only about one in ten people with Tourette's show this particular symptom. Instead, nine out of ten Tourette's sufferers develop a neurological disorder such as OCD or *attention deficit hyperactivity disorder (ADHD)* – flip to Chapter 16 for more on this. You can find out more about Tourette's syndrome by calling the Tourette's Action helpline on 0845 4581252 or visiting the website at www. tourettes-action.org.uk.

People often don't realise that they have OCD, because they're unaware of the typical symptoms. The key feature of OCD is that you feel your obsessions don't fit in with your view of yourself, and that they're unpleasant for you. Go through the following checklist to see if any of these additional symptoms also apply to you:

- ✔ You wash or clean yourself or your possessions a lot.

- ✔ You have thoughts that keep bothering you or that you'd like to get rid of – but can't.

- ✔ You take a long time to finish daily activities such as cleaning, washing, calculating and checking that all the lights are off, because you have to do them repeatedly and check them afterwards.

- ✔ You're troubled by your behaviour and these problems are affecting your life negatively.

Seeking help sooner rather than later is particularly important if you also suffer from the following symptoms:

- ✔ You feel depressed and/or have thoughts of harming yourself (also check out Chapter 21).

- ✔ You drink alcohol over the recommended limits (turn to Chapter 23 for more details).

- ✔ You feel socially isolated and don't go out much, because you try to avoid situations where obsessive thoughts or compulsions may occur.

- ✔ You find that your symptoms are severely disabling and that they considerably interfere with your life, perhaps to the extent that your family life suffers or you're at risk of losing your job.

If any of these points sound familiar, you may be suffering from OCD. Many sufferers choose not to get help because they feel too embarrassed to tell their doctor. However, seeing your GP for an early diagnosis is important because effective treatment can reduce your symptoms and your suffering considerably. Various forms of help are available to you. For further assistance, you can also contact the charity Mind on 0845 7660163 or visit its website at www.mind.org.uk.

If you do suffer from OCD, you're also more likely to have other mental health issues, such as:

- ✔ Problems with anxiety or panic (read Chapter 21).
- ✔ Symptoms of depression (check out Chapter 21).
- ✔ Unusual thoughts or behaviour (discussed throughout this chapter).
- ✔ *Tourette's syndrome*, which is an inherited condition that usually starts in childhood. Characteristic symptoms for Tourette's are as follows:
  - *Tics*, which are sudden and repetitive involuntary muscle movements which in Tourette's often affect the head and face. Vocal tics include uttering words or making sounds like coughing or throat-clearing.
  - Being unable to control your sounds or certain movements.

Suspecting autism and Asperger syndrome

Autism is a form of developmental disability that interferes with the way people communicate with, and relate to, other people and the world around them. *Asperger syndrome* is a particular form of autism.

People with autism and Asperger syndrome have difficulties in the following three areas:

- ✔ Social communication.
- ✔ Social interaction.
- ✔ Social imagination.

Although all people with autism have difficulties in similar areas, their condition impacts on their lives in different ways. Experts think that both environmental and genetic factors may lead to changes in the way the brain develops in people with these conditions, but no-one knows for sure.

Experts are fairly certain that autism hasn't got anything to do with the way you're brought up or your particular social circumstances – and be reassured, the condition is certainly not your fault or that of your family! You're born with the condition – and you can't catch it from other people or from childhood immunisations such as the MMR vaccine.

Saying 'no!' to acting under compulsion

If you suffer from obsessive thoughts or have to carry out compulsive acts, try these simple tricks to help get around the problem:

✔ Don't let gloomy thoughts get the better of you. Write them down, and for each thought try to find a positive argument against it. Imagine that you're another person advising yourself.

✔ Focus and concentrate on the positive things – not the bad things – in your life.

✔ Give yourself praise or a reward of some sort each time you manage to avoid carrying out a compulsive act.

✔ Try to reduce your compulsive behaviour slowly instead of attempting a complete behaviour change in one go. This approach causes less anxiety and is more likely to succeed.

Autism

Autism is a condition in which you have problems with social interaction, and find communicating or interacting with other people difficult. If you have autism, you find that making sense of the world around you is difficult, which in turn can create a feeling of anxiety.

Autism stays with people for life but can affect them in a variety of different ways, which is why professionals tend to refer to it by the term *autism spectrum disorder*. Many people with autism can lead an almost normal life, whereas others may struggle and need a lot of help and support because of their learning difficulties.

If you suffer from autism you're likely to experience the following problems in the areas of social communication, interaction and imagination:

✔ You find communicating with other people difficult.

✔ You struggle to interact with other people socially. Doing so just doesn't come naturally. You may find social rules – such as how close to stand to people or what are acceptable topics to talk about in certain situations – hard to understand.

✔ You may find that you're misunderstood a lot of the time and struggle to get jokes or understand sarcasm.

✔ You don't easily understand other people's body language and have problems appreciating the significance of tone of voice or facial expressions.

✔ You have a hard time expressing your emotions or feelings.

> ✔ You struggle to imagine what other people may be thinking or to understand abstract ideas.
>
> ✔ You may find predicting 'what will happen next' difficult.

If you have autism, you may also display these other characteristics:

> ✔ You may like routine and have a fixed daily schedule or way of doing things.
>
> ✔ You may be very creative – lots of people with autism are talented and skilled writers, musicians or artists.
>
> ✔ You may show increased or reduced sensitivity to certain senses – taste, smell, sound, touch or sight.
>
> ✔ You may develop a very strong interest in a certain subject or hobby – reaching a level of 'obsession' which other people find unusual.

Many more possible characteristics exist in addition to these examples. If you feel that you're showing symptoms of autism spectrum disorder or if you notice these in your child, particularly if these symptoms impact on your daily life, speak to your GP who can arrange further assessment and support.

For more information on autism, call the National Autistic Society Helpline on 0845 0704004 or visit www.autism.org.uk. You can find more information specifically about autism in children in Chapter 16.

Asperger syndrome

Asperger syndrome is a form of autism. People with Asperger syndrome have fewer problems engaging in conversation, are often of average – or above average – intelligence and are without the learning difficulties that many people with autism suffer from (look at the previous section on 'Autism' for info on typical symptoms). However, people with Asperger syndrome may have specific but often less disabling learning difficulties such as *dyspraxia* (difficulties with thinking out, planning out and executing planned movements or tasks) or *dyslexia* (which may include problems with reading, spelling, writing, speaking or listening), as well as other conditions such as attention deficit hyperactivity disorder (ADHD) and epilepsy.

A key feature of Asperger syndrome, however, is that you tend to be preoccupied with complex issues. For example, people with Asperger typically hold jobs in engineering, computing, mathematics or academia because their concrete thinking is often much better developed than their abstract thinking. You may also find that other people think of you as eccentric, because you're more likely to take up activities such as trainspotting or collecting.

With Asperger syndrome you may have quite complex emotional or relationship needs, and so if you show symptoms, consult your GP who may offer to refer you to a specialist for further assessment and arrange help and support for you.

With the right support and encouragement, you're likely to lead a full and independent life. You can improve your quality of life in many ways, and various therapies and interventions are available such as behavioural therapy and dietary changes.

Unfortunately, if you have Asperger syndrome you may find accessing and maintaining employment difficult despite perhaps having a great deal of skill and knowledge. To help, and to find out more about Asperger syndrome and the support available to you, visit the National Autistic Society website www.autism.org.uk/asperger . In addition, you can contact the OAASIS (Office for Advice, Assistance, Support and Information on Special needs) helpline on 0800 1973907 or through the website at www.oaasis.co.uk.

Chapter 23

Addressing Addictive Behaviour and Substance Misuse

In This Chapter

▶ Finding out about alcohol misuse and associated problems

▶ Recognising the signs of drug misuse

▶ Approaching other addictive behaviours

*R*obert Palmer famously sang about being 'Addicted to Love', but he could just as easily have sung about any of the other addictions to substances or behaviours that can be dangerous to your health. As well as the personal problems that can result, the misuse of alcohol and drugs, in particular, is a huge issue worldwide, which creates massive health and social problems, such as family breakdowns and crime.

If you're concerned that you, or someone close to you, have problems of being or becoming addicted to a particular substance or type of behaviour, use this chapter for information on how to spot the danger signs and when to get professional help.

Spotting Symptoms and Signs of Alcohol Misuse

Many people drink alcohol socially and in moderation. Nothing's wrong with that. However, drinking alcohol regularly and in larger amounts than your body can cope with puts you in danger of suffering long-term physical and mental damage, and of eventually becoming dependent on alcohol. Drinking alcohol to excess can affect your judgement and body control and make you less averse to risks. You can even become aggressive and violent. Such problems can severely impact on your life: difficulties with relationships or at work are very common as a result of alcohol misuse, and many road traffic accidents, injuries and domestic rows are alcohol-related, too.

Hitting the bottle: Alcohol misuse

You misuse alcohol when you drink it in greater amounts and more frequently than your body can cope with. The recommended limits for men are 21 units of alcohol per week, and no more than four units in a day. For women, the figures are 14 units of alcohol per week, and no more than three units in a day (with no alcohol intake at all for pregnant women).

Depending on your drinking habits, you can easily exceed these limits if you don't keep tabs on your intake. For example, going for after-work drinks on three days a week and having three pints of beer each time means that you're already taking in at least 18 to 20 units of alcohol, which is close to the recommended limits. Drinking three pints (which is at least six units of alcohol) in one session is over the safe limit for drinks on a single day. Drinking more than two 750-millilitre bottles of wine containing 12 per cent of alcohol a week means that you're already close to 18 units – more than the recommended limit for women. If you drink for fun or as a response to problems such as stress, anxiety or feeling depressed (check out Chapter 21 for more info on these), your drinking can easily become a serious problem.

Drinking sensibly: Doing the maths

Keeping tabs on how much alcohol you're drinking – and how much is safe to drink – enables you to know when to stop. To measure your alcohol intake, think of your drinks in terms of *units of alcohol*, with one unit being 10 millilitres of pure alcohol (or 8 grams if you measure this by weight). You can find more information and an online calculator at www.drinkaware. co.uk.

The following quantities of drink each contain one unit of alcohol:

✔ **Beer:** Half a pint of standard-strength (containing 3–4 per cent of alcohol by volume) lager, beer or cider.

✔ **Spirits:** A small pub measure (25 millilitres) of spirits containing 40 per cent of alcohol by volume.

✔ **Fortified wine:** A standard pub measure (50 millilitres) of sherry or port containing 20 per cent alcohol by volume.

The following drinks contain about one and a half units of alcohol:

✔ **Wine:** A small glass of standard-strength wine (125 millilitres) containing 12 per cent of alcohol by volume.

✔ **Spirits:** A standard pub measure (35 millilitres) of spirits containing 40 per cent of alcohol by volume.

Remember to check the label or ask the barperson for the strength of your drink – many beers and wines are stronger than the standard-strength ones. If you're good at maths (and even if you're not) you can easily calculate the number of units of alcohol in a drink by remembering:

The number of units in 1 litre of alcoholic drink = the percentage of alcohol by volume.

Okay, that was a bit of a mouthful, so here are some examples of how it works:

✔ One litre of strong beer with 6 per cent of alcohol by volume contains 6 units. So, if you're drinking a pint, which is the same as 568 millilitres (or just a bit more than half a litre), your intake is just over three units. Easy!

✔ One litre of wine with 12 per cent of alcohol by volume contains 12 units. So, by drinking 250 millilitres, or a quarter of a litre (one large glass or two small ones), you're taking in three units of alcohol. From this figure, you can also work out that a standard bottle of wine (750 millilitres) with 12 per cent of alcohol by volume contains 9 units of alcohol.

Everyone is different, but research shows that for most people the following amounts of alcohol don't cause problems to their health. These reflect, amongst other things, the differences between sexes when it comes to absorbing and metabolising alcohol:

✔ **Men:** 21 units of alcohol per week, and no more than four units in a day.

✔ **Women:** 14 units of alcohol per week, and no more than three units in a day. If you're pregnant, you shouldn't drink any alcohol to avoid harming your baby.

Health professionals sometimes refer to four broad categories of drinking, with increasing risk to your health and safety from one level to the next. Read through to decide whether you may fit into any of these types:

✔ **Social drinker:** You drink small amounts of alcohol at a time, and not all the time, up to the recommended limits.

Social drinking is unlikely to harm your health, but drinking even small amounts of alcohol can affect your driving and your ability to operate tools or machinery, and can still react with any medication that you take.

✔ **Heavy drinker:** You drink above the recommended limits (refer to the information in the sidebar 'Drinking sensibly: doing the maths').

Your drinking puts your health at risk and increases your chance of developing damage to your liver (known as *cirrhosis of the liver*) and another important organ in your abdomen called the *pancreas*. You're also more likely to develop sexual problems, cancer, high blood pressure or problems with your heart.

✔ **Problem drinker:** You continue to drink alcohol even though you've already damaged your health or run into difficulties with your family and other people (such as your colleagues or wider society). Problem drinking includes binge drinking, or where you have to take time off work or behave in a socially unacceptable way because of alcohol.

To be a problem drinker you don't necessarily need to get drunk; just drinking small amounts of alcohol can cause health problems, particularly if you already suffer from liver damage. If you're a problem drinker, you can probably still stop drinking if you want to.

✔ **Alcohol-dependent:** You drink every day and have to drink to avoid unpleasant withdrawal effects, and you're likely to have a strong desire for or be addicted to alcohol. You're unable to control your drinking.

Any attempt to stop drinking brings on withdrawal symptoms such as a craving for alcohol, nausea and vomiting, sweating, shaking and generally feeling unwell. You're also at an increased danger of suffering a fit. (Also check out the later section 'Avoiding delirium tremens'.)

You can identify a possible alcohol problem if any or all the following signs apply to you:

✔ You drink regularly and over the recommended limits.

✔ You may have six or more drinks on any one occasion.

✔ You sometimes fail to do what other people expect of you because of drinking.

✔ You drink alcohol first thing in the morning to help you get going.

✔ You sometimes feel guilty or remorseful after drinking.

✔ You often drink alone.

✔ You occasionally can't remember what happened the night before because of your drinking.

✔ You or someone else has been injured because of your drinking.

✔ You cause concern among friends, relatives or health professionals about your drinking or receive suggestions that you drink less.

✔ You feel annoyed if people say that you drink too much.

If, after comparing your own situation with these signs, you think that you may have an alcohol problem and you have difficulty reducing your alcohol intake or stopping drinking, check out the Drinkaware website (www. drinkaware.co.uk) for more information and consult your GP for further help and advice. Your GP is likely to give you a thorough medical check-over and may recommend various treatments.

Understanding alcohol-related illness

Many people underestimate the potential harm that alcohol misuse can cause, particularly when they're unaware of the safe limits of consumption.

Drinking too much alcohol over a prolonged period of time can directly lead to a number of serious health problems:

✔ **Alcoholic liver disease:** *Alcoholic liver disease* is an overarching term for conditions such as *alcoholic hepatitis* (inflammation of the liver), *fatty liver* and *cirrhosis of the liver* (scarring of the liver), as well as liver cancer, which are common and important consequences of drinking too much alcohol for too long.

✔ **Blood problems:** Alcohol can have direct toxic effects on your blood. Bruising easily is a sign that something may be wrong with your blood.

✔ **Brain damage:** Too much alcohol can damage your brain in many ways; acute alcohol intoxication and longstanding alcohol misuse, as well as acute alcohol withdrawal, may affect your brain function. Your personality can change as well – and probably not for the better.

✔ **General health problems:** You're more likely to feel tired all the time, lose your 'drive', feel unwell and develop poor sleeping patterns.

✔ **Heart-related problems:** You're more likely to develop high blood pressure and be at increased risk of suffering a heart attack or stroke. You may also suffer from *alcoholic myopathy*, where your heart muscle becomes weaker due to alcohol.

✔ **Hormonal problems:** Obesity and diabetes are more common in people with alcohol problems. Remember that alcohol contains a lot of calories.

✔ **Injuries:** Many deaths are directly caused by injuries sustained as a result of drinking too much alcohol.

✔ **Mental health problems:** Depression, anxiety, loss of confidence and confusion are common effects. As a result, you're more likely to abstain from work, lose your job, become socially isolated, run into marriage problems, drift into poverty or lose your home.

✔ **Mouth, gullet and tummy problems:** You're at higher risk of developing cancer of the mouth, throat and gullet. If you feel sick and have a burning sensation in your upper stomach, you're likely to be suffering from *alcoholic gastritis* (inflammation of the stomach lining). If you already have cirrhosis of the liver, you may develop *oesophageal varices*, or swollen blood vessels, in your lower gullet which, if they leak, can lead to severe and life-threatening bleeding.

✔ **Nerve problems:** You're likely to lack essential vitamins and develop 'nervous' symptoms such as a fuzzy feeling in your limbs, eye problems or losing the sensation in your skin.

✔ **Sexual problems:** Although small amounts of alcohol can be stimulating, your sex drive is likely to go down when you drink too much. If you're a man, you may become *impotent* (where you're unable to have erections) and eventually your testicles shrink so that you're *infertile* (unable to father children). If you're a pregnant woman, too much alcohol can negatively affect your growing unborn baby.

✔ **Skin lesions:** You may develop itching of the skin, which can be severe and unpleasant. As a result, you scratch a lot and may develop unsightly skin lesions. You're also more likely to bruise easily, and any wounds and skin infections tend to heal slowly. An affected liver can cause your skin and the whites of your eyes to become yellow (called *jaundice*). Skin lesions such as prominent small blood vessels (called *spider naevi*) and a rash on the palm of your hands (also knows as *palmar erythema*) can occur when liver disease is in more advanced stages.

As you can see, the list is long, which is why health professionals and the NHS are so keen for people to know the risks of drinking too much alcohol, and to bring down excessive alcohol consumption. Check out the Drinkaware website at www.drinkaware.co.uk for more information about the complications of excessive alcohol consumption.

Beating the bottle: Tackling your problem

Contact your doctor as soon as possible if you notice the following symptoms:

✔ You have ongoing stomach problems such as pain or feeling sick.

✔ Your health is affected in any of the areas covered in the preceding list.

✔ You find that your alcohol drinking adversely impacts on your life.

Consult your GP urgently or call '999' in an emergency if you experience any of the following symptoms:

✔ You develop severe withdrawal symptoms such as hallucinations, restlessness, agitation and persistent vomiting (you can find more on this aspect in the following section 'Avoiding delirium tremens').

✔ You vomit blood or find that your stools change to a black, tarry colour.

✔ You suddenly become confused, can't walk properly or find that your eyes make jerking movements. (These symptoms may be due to a problem in connection with a vitamin deficiency called *Wernicke-Korsakoff Syndrome* – a medical emergency.)

✔ You suddenly develop severe, constant abdominal pain. (This problem may be due to a stomach ulcer or inflammation of your *pancreas* – a large gland behind your stomach secreting digestive juices and a hormone called *insulin* – particularly if you also vomit.)

Avoiding delirium tremens

Attempting to rectify your alcohol problem by abruptly stopping drinking can bring on withdrawal symptoms, and even a severe reaction called *delirium tremens*, or *DTs*.

DTs can be dangerous and even life-threatening, and so be aware of the warning symptoms, which include the following:

✔ You get agitated and confused.

✔ You get 'the shakes'.

✔ You may see or hear things that aren't there (known as *hallucinations*).

✔ You may have a fit.

✔ You may become dehydrated.

If you experience these, contact your GP urgently or call '999' in an emergency.

Although stopping drinking is the right move when you're alcohol dependent, weaning yourself off drink gradually to safer levels of alcohol consumption is the way to proceed (see the sidebar 'Cutting down on the booze').

Cutting down on the booze

If you drink too much alcohol and want to cut down, try taking up these suggestions:

✔ Drink slowly.

✔ Alternate alcoholic drinks with soft drinks or water.

✔ Switch to drinks with a lower alcohol content and avoid the stronger varieties.

✔ Avoid situations and social activities in which you know you drink too much.

✔ Whenever you buy other people a drink, get a non-alcoholic one for yourself.

✔ Don't be afraid to say 'no' or 'not now' to anyone who urges you to drink.

Contact your GP for help with reducing or stopping your alcohol intake, which may involve taking medication or taking part in a *community detoxification* programme, usually arranged by local alcohol services.

Getting additional help

You can get further information about alcohol and its related problems from the NHS and from a number of websites, self-help organisations and charities, such as the following:

- ✔ **Alcoholics Anonymous:** Phone the helpline on 0845 7697555 or visit `www.alcoholics-anonymous.org.uk`.

- ✔ **Drinkline – National Alcohol Helpline:** Phone the helpline on 0800 9178282.

- ✔ **Know Your Units Campaign:** Visit the campaign's website at `www.units.nhs.uk`.

- ✔ **NHS Choices:** Visit `www.nhs.uk/conditions/alcohol-misuse/Pages/Introduction.aspx` for information on diagnosis, risks and treatment of alcohol misuse – and more.

- ✔ **Patient UK:** Visit `www.patient.co.uk` for a number of excellent alcohol-related patient information leaflets.

- ✔ **The Department of Health**: Visit the alcohol misuse website at `www.dh.gov.uk/en/Publichealth/Healthimprovement/Alcoholmisuse/index.htm`.

For support for your family contact:

- ✔ **ADFAM:** Call 020 7553 7640 or visit `www.adfam.org.uk` to access the support they offer for families.

- ✔ **AL-Anon Family Groups:** Call 020 7403 0888 or visit `www.al-anonuk.org.uk`.

- ✔ **National Association for Children of Alcoholics:** Call the Helpline on 0800 3583456 or visit `www.nacoa.org.uk`.

Many people with alcohol problems do successfully manage to stop drinking. Doing so can be very hard, and you may need several attempts to eventually become 'dry', but the pain will be worth it – both for you and for people close to you. I've met many people whose lives suddenly 'fell into place' again when they managed to get their alcohol problem under control. If other people can do it, so can you!

Identifying Drug Problems

Drugs are chemical substances that can change your emotions, mood, behaviour and state of consciousness because of their effect on your brain and nervous system. Drug *misuse* is when you regularly take one or more drugs to bring on such states of mind. The biggest danger of misusing drugs is that you can become *addicted*, which can happen in two forms:

- **Physical addiction:** Stopping using a drug leads you to suffer withdrawal symptoms such as feeling sick or vomiting, and agitation.

- **Psychological addiction:** You have a psychological addiction when you feel a need or you have a compulsion to use a drug regularly. When you stop taking the drug, you may not suffer physical symptoms as such, but you can become depressed, anxious and irritable.

In the UK, most drugs are illegal, with the exception of caffeine, alcohol and cigarettes. This doesn't mean that these three drugs are harmless, though: in England, drinking alcohol and smoking kill more people each year than all illegal drugs combined. Also, prescribed medication such as certain sleeping pills or strong painkillers can lead to misuse when the clinical need to take them has passed because of the effects they can have on your mood. Possessing certain prescription-only medication such as morphine or methadone without prescription is also illegal.

As well as the risk of becoming addicted, drug use can seriously affect your health by causing a host of physical and psychological medical conditions, which lead to an estimated 2,000 deaths each year in England and Wales.

Spotting substance misuse

If you misuse substances, you may recognise the effects that various drugs have on your physical and mental state. You can distinguish between three major groups:

- **Stimulants:** Drugs like cocaine give people energy and make them more alert.

- **Depressants (or *sedatives*):** Heroin, for example, makes people feel relaxed.

- **Hallucinogens:** Drugs like LSD make people feel, hear or see things that aren't there or aren't real.

In the UK, drugs are classified under the terms of the Misuse of Drugs Act as Classes A (for example, heroin), B (such as cannabis) or C (including tranquillisers). Class A is the most dangerous and class C the least dangerous – although class C drugs can still cause serious health problems.

Certain drug sub-classes have specific effects:

✔ **Amphetamines (class B)** lead to heightened alertness, concentration and confidence. Adverse effects include dehydration, difficulty concentrating, jaw clenching, irregular heartbeat, severe mental health problems and in very rare cases sudden death due to burst blood vessels.

✔ **Cocaine (class A)** brings on positive feelings and elated mood, but can also lead to severe mental health symptoms such as anxiety and paranoia, dizziness and muscle twitching. Violent behaviour and aggression are common. Cocaine may also cause heart problems such as *cardiomyopathy* (weakness of the heart muscles) and irregular heartbeat. A nasal discharge due to direct damage of the lining is also common.

✔ **Ecstasy (class A)** leads to positive mood, feelings of intimacy and increased energy. Adverse effects are similar to those of amphetamines.

✔ **Opiates (class A)**, such as heroin, produce calming sensations, elated mood and a feeling of increased wellbeing. Adverse effects include skin infections, collapse, heart and other organ damage, drug dependence, reduced breathing effort and death.

Many other drugs are also used in the UK. For a fuller list of drugs and their adverse effects check out the NHS Choices website at www.nhs.uk or the 'A–Z of Drugs' on the FRANK website www.talktofrank.com.

You may also notice the following signs if you use illicit drugs:

✔ You occasionally or regularly behave in an inappropriate way, such as being uncharacteristically rude to people or walking out of situations unexpectedly.

✔ Your family and social life may be affected, perhaps by having relationship problems or not getting on with your friends anymore.

✔ You're more likely to run into problems with employment and your finances (for example, you find it difficult to cope with your workload or run into financial difficulties because of your drug taking).

✔ You may be involved in illegal or criminal activities to finance your drug habit.

If you or someone close to you suffers from a drug problem, contact your GP for assessment and suggestions for sources of help and support, particularly those available locally. You can also contact these organisations for advice:

✔ **DrugScope:** This organisation provides lots of information about drug use and how to get treatment. Visit the website at www.drugscope.org.uk.

> ✔ **Release:** For legal advice about a drug-related issue contact Release on 0845 4500215 or visit the www.release.org.uk website.
>
> ✔ **Talk to FRANK:** This government-run information, advice and referral service is available on 0800 776600 or via the website – www.talkto frank.com.

Identifying drug-related problems

Using illicit drugs puts you at increased risk of medical and social complications. As a rule, the higher the dose of a drug you take, the higher your risk of suffering serious medical problems.

If you develop medical complications, compare your symptoms with those in this list (which is a selection of examples – many others exist):

> ✔ **Hepatitis:** Drug use, and especially sharing needles, puts you at an increased risk of liver infection – hepatitis B and C in particular. With hepatitis, you're likely to feel tired all the time and may notice that your skin and the white parts of your eyes become yellow.
>
> ✔ **HIV:** Using drugs – again, particularly if you share needles – puts you at increased risk of getting infected with the HIV virus, which causes AIDS. For symptoms and signs of HIV infection, check out Chapter 7.
>
> ✔ **Mental health problems:** You're more likely to suffer from mental health problems such as depression, anxiety or other more serious disorders (turn to Chapters 21 and 22 for more information).
>
> ✔ **Social problems:** Homelessness and other social problems are more common in drug users.

Many people with drug problems are wary of health professionals, and of doctors in particular. However, your GP is aware of drug-related issues and can be a central figure as regards organising further help for you – and everything you say or discuss will be treated confidentially. The chances are that a specialist drug service operates in your area, with specially trained staff who are familiar with the situation that many drug users are in and who can offer you support and treatment as appropriate.

Dealing with drug problems

Consult your GP if any of the following situations apply to you – because you're at risk of damaging your health or even your life:

✔ You share needles or other drug-taking equipment.

✔ You use high or increasing amounts of drugs.

✔ You use cocktails of drugs or a number of different drugs.

✔ You have thoughts of harming yourself or of taking your own life.

✔ You think you may suffer from liver infection.

✔ You think you may have overdosed on a drug (check out Chapter 5 for details on how to deal with medical emergencies).

✔ You consider yourself to be at risk from HIV infection.

If you avoid drugs for a while and then start taking them again, you're at an increased risk of an overdose if you suddenly take the same amount that you used to.

Tackling Other Addictive Behaviours

Certain behaviours can become addictive. Contact the organisations I list below or see your GP for help if any of the following problems impact on your life, or cause you financial or social difficulties:

✔ **Benzodiazepine addiction:** Becoming addicted to prescription drugs such as benzodiazepines or sleeping tablets is easier than you think. If you feel as if you can't stop taking them, feel nervous just at the thought of having to do without them or if you need to take increasingly higher doses, speak to your GP. For further information and support contact BAT (Battle Against Tranquillisers) on 0117 9663629 or visit www.bataid.org. Patient UK provides a useful Patient Information Leaflet on its website at www.patient.co.uk.

✔ **Gambling:** If you have a compulsive urge to gamble, you can get help and support from Gamblers Anonymous – visit the website at www.gamblersanonymous.org.uk for further information.

✔ **Sex:** If you think that you may be suffering from *sex addiction* – where you can't control your sexual behaviour and this leads to detrimental consequences, such as keeping you from an honest and long-term relationship, or your behaviour leads you to deceive your partner – contact Relate on 0300 1001234 or visit the website at www.relate.org.uk.

✔ **Shopping:** Many people consider themselves to be shopaholics, but for some the urge to spend becomes hard to resist and the habit gets out of control. If this behaviour sounds like you, consult your GP, who may be able to refer you to local sources of help and advice. In this case, 'retail therapy' isn't necessarily good for you!

Part VI
The Part of Tens

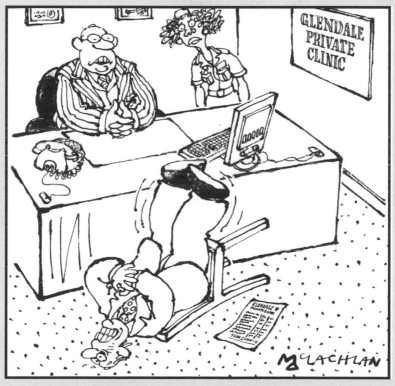

'He thought he was very ill but his thorough
medical examination showed he was in
perfect health–until we gave him our bill.'

In this part . . .

This part is all about picking out the most helpful tips and advice on providing first aid and dealing with medical emergencies.

Many people consult the Internet for health information but often don't know where to look or what to make of the bewildering number of websites available. If you want to find out more about your health symptoms or where to get further help and advice – particularly if you're unsure whether to seek medical advice or if you can't pluck up courage to do so because you feel embarrassed – I give you details of some trustworthy health-related websites that you can rely on.

Just in case you need any medical tests to investigate your symptoms further, I provide the low-down on blood tests, X-rays, and other procedures that you may need.

Chapter 24

Ten (okay, Nine) Things to Know About First Aid

In This Chapter

- Approaching emergencies
- Equipping yourself with knowledge and skills

This book is mainly about diagnosing and managing your own health symptoms. However, because we humans don't live isolated lives, I also cover health symptoms in your wider family (for example, Chapters 14 to 16 are all about your children's health) because for most people the lives and health of people close to them is just as precious as their own. For this reason, I've included this chapter on first aid for both yourself and in other people – regardless of the specific underlying cause.

Thankfully, serious medical emergencies are rare. Many people would rather not think about the possibility of an emergency occurring, but being able to provide first aid or give basic life support can potentially save your own or another person's life when an emergency does strike, as well as prevent further health problems. Many first aid techniques and skills aren't that tricky to pick up, and following a few simple rules can make all the difference.

Stocking Up With Essential Equipment

Keeping your home well stocked with essential first aid equipment means that you're well prepared for the majority of health problems that you may encounter. Put together a simple first aid kit that contains these items:

- Adhesive Tape.
- Bandages.
- Disposable gloves.
- Eye pads, sterile.

- Plasters, individually wrapped and in assorted sizes.

- Safety pins.

- Scissors.

- Sterile eye pads.

- Triangular bandages, preferably sterile and individually wrapped.

- Wipes, individually wrapped and moist.

- Wound dressings, medium size (approximately 12 centimetres x 12 centimetres/4.5 inches x 4.5 inches) and large (approximately 18 centimetres x 18 centimetres/7 inches x 7 inches), sterile.

Standard emergency first aid kits, where all the hard work of compiling the items is already done for you, are available online or from your pharmacist. Make sure you remember to check items for their 'use by' date and replace them when they're out of date.

Brushing Up on Your First Aid Skills

The guidance in this chapter is no substitute for thorough knowledge and skills in first aid. Acquiring first aid skills is best done by attending an approved training course, such as those run by the following:

- **St John Ambulance** (www.sja.org.uk; tel: 0870 0104950).

- **The British Red Cross** (www.redcross.org.uk; tel: 0844 8711111).

- **First Response Resuscitation & First Aid Training Ltd** (www.first response.org.uk; tel: 0117 9490944).

These courses are interesting and fun, and definitely worth the money. With the knowledge and skills that you gain you really can save someone's life – as well as your own – which is a pretty good reason to add taking a first aid course to your 'to-do' list, if you haven't attended one yet.

So that you remain prepared, also consider revising at regular intervals (say, at least every 6–12 months), so that your first aid knowledge and skills become second nature to you.

Staying Safe

The first thing to do in an emergency or accident situation is to check whether you or the casualty are in any further danger. Before you do anything else, look around and go through a mental checklist of anything that may pose an additional risk, such as road traffic, electricity, poison or water. Don't put your own life in any unnecessary danger and have a quick think about how you can make the situation immediately safer for everyone present – for example, switching off the electricity mains, moving dangerous objects out of the way, shouting warnings or asking someone to stop or divert any traffic in the event of a road traffic accident.

Assessing an Emergency

If you or someone else is injured or suddenly becomes unwell, you need to determine what may be wrong – which is a very important part of the treatment. Try to obtain information on what's actually happened, consider any symptoms (what you or the casualty experiences – such as pain, dizziness or feeling sick) and check for any obvious signs (things you can smell, hear, see or touch on you or the casualty such as swelling, noisy breathing or the smell of alcohol).

Ask yourself questions in the following areas:

- ✔ **Clues to causes**: Look for clues – for example, an empty medicine bottle may suggest an overdose or a cut lawnmower cable on a wet lawn would point towards an electric shock. Such information can be invaluable, particularly when someone becomes unresponsive.

- ✔ **Details of the incident:** Question yourself or the casualty (if possible), or other bystanders, to try and get a bit more information, especially when you didn't witness what happened.

- ✔ **Major risk to health:** Check for any life-threatening conditions, such as severe bleeding.

- ✔ **Pain:** Ask about any pain or other symptoms, such as numbness or a loss of feeling in a limb.

- ✔ **Personal information:** If you're attending an accident scene, ask the casualty's name and address, and check whether she has any pre-existing medical conditions.

Giving Life Support to an Unconscious Casualty

Giving life support (also known as *cardio-pulmonary resuscitation*, or *CPR*) can literally save lives. Check someone who appears to be unconscious by talking loudly or shouting to them: 'Are you all right?', 'Open your eyes!' or 'Can you hear me?'. Gently shake the person's shoulders at the same time. If you get a response, don't move her but call for help if required. While you wait for help to arrive, keep an eye on the casualty's responses and breathing.

If the person isn't breathing, call for help or call '999' immediately. While you wait for medical help to arrive, you can help to keep the injured or ill person alive by performing *rescue breaths* – where you breathe oxygen into the casualty (the air you breathe out still contains enough oxygen potentially to enable someone to survive). You then need to help the body to pump the oxygen around by doing *chest compressions* – where you repeatedly press down on the chest. Here are the steps to take:

1. **Check the airway:** Put one hand on the person's forehead and gently tilt the head back to open her mouth (see Figure 24-1). Check for anything that may block the airway (such as dentures that have come loose, or food) and, using only two fingers, lift the chin up. This simple procedure helps you to move the tongue away from the back of the mouth where it can obstruct the throat and lead to death if not corrected.

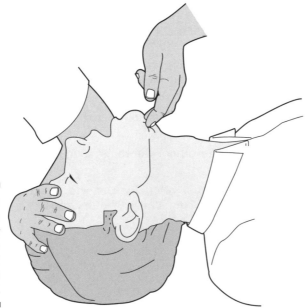

Figure 24-1:
Opening up the airway using the 'head tilt' and 'chin lift'.

2. **Check whether the person is breathing normally:** Look for chest movements, listen for breath sounds by placing your ear close to the person's nose and mouth and feel for any breaths against your cheek.

   A normal breathing rate is around 12–15 breaths per minute. If someone is breathing normally and you hear or feel at least 2–3 breaths over a period of 10 seconds or so, place her in the recovery position (check out the next section for details). If 10 seconds go by and you don't detect any breaths, go on to step 3.

3. **Call '999':** Call '999' or get someone else to do this for you.

4. **Perform 30 chest compressions:** If someone isn't breathing, find the centre of the chest near the lower end of the casualty's breast bone and place the heel of your hand about 5 centimetres (2 inches) up in the direction of the person's head. Press her chest down (see Figure 24-2) by 4–5 centimetres (1½–2 inches) at a rate of around 100 compressions per minute – a bit faster than 1 compression per second.

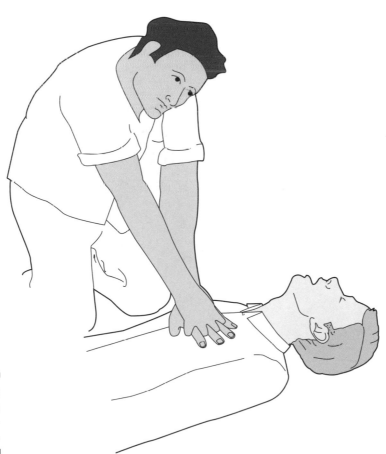

Figure 24-2: Performing chest compressions.

5. **Give two rescue breaths:** Assuming the airways are open, pinch the person's nose and place your mouth over her mouth (as shown in Figure 24-2). Attempt two rescue breaths (see Figure 24-3) by blowing gently for one second each. If this technique is successful, you will see the chest rise and fall.

6. **Go back to step 4 and perform 30 chest compressions.**

Continue alternating between steps 4 and 5 until help arrives or the person breathes normally again.

If someone's heart stops beating, she may still take sudden irregular gasps for breath in the first few minutes afterwards. Don't mistake this activity for normal breathing – still dial '999' and start CPR.

Performing basic life support on children is slightly different, but you can keep children's airways open by performing a head tilt and chin lift in a similar fashion as you would for an adult. For details look at the websites for St John Ambulance (www.sja.org.uk) or the British Red Cross (www.redcross.org.uk) for more information. Remember that these steps aren't a substitute for attending a full class and gaining instruction for giving CPR, but if you're unsure what to do, following the adult sequence of giving life support on a child who is unresponsive and not breathing is better than not doing anything.

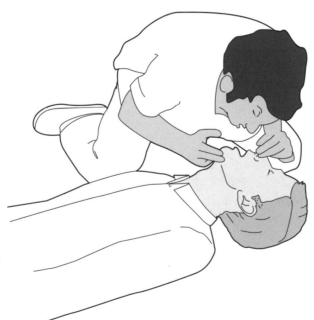

Figure 24-3:
Giving res-
cue breaths.

Placing Someone in the Recovery Position

To avoid the airway being compromised by the tongue touching the back of the throat or by vomit (should the person be sick), place an unconscious casualty who is breathing but has no other life-threatening conditions in the *recovery position* (as shown in Figure 24-4).

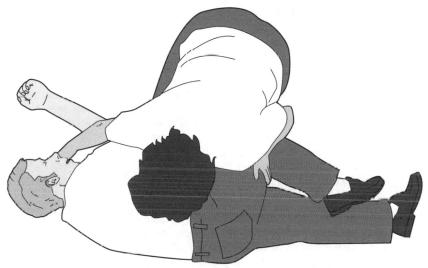

Figure 24-4: The recovery position.

To move someone into the recovery position, follow these steps:

1. **Turn the casualty onto her side.**

2. **Lift the chin forward to open up the airways and put the person's hand under the cheek if necessary.**

3. **Make sure that the casualty can't roll over onto either side and keep monitoring the airways and breathing.**

For children under the age of one year, use the *modified recovery position*. Here, you cradle the baby in your arms and tilt the head slightly downwards to prevent her from choking on the tongue or inhaling vomit. Check regularly (ideally continuously, but at least every 30 seconds) how the baby responds and whether she breathes.

Providing Simple First Aid for Bleeding

Bleeding can range in severity from a simple scratch to life-threatening loss of blood. Here's a quick low-down on dealing with some forms of bleeding:

- **Bleeding from minor cuts and grazes:** Wash and dry your hands, put on disposable gloves and then clean any of your dirty cuts or minor wounds under running water. Raise the affected area above the level of the heart if at all possible. Use a sterile dressing to cover the wound temporarily and clean the surrounding skin with water and soap. Instead of then patting the area dry, always take one swipe with a clean pad and then use a new one if possible. Finally, cover the wound completely with a sterile dressing or plaster.

- **Nosebleed:** A common reaction to nosebleeds is to tilt your head back, but avoid the temptation to do so – you may swallow blood and vomit as a result – and also placing a cold object on the base of your neck is unlikely to make any difference. Instead, sit down, lean forward and pinch the soft fleshy tip of your nose rather than the hard bit. Avoid coughing, sneezing and speaking, because doing so may set off the bleed again. If you feel weak, lie down on the floor and take up the recovery position (as I describe in the preceding section) until the bleeding stops and you feel better. Go to hospital if the bleeding doesn't stop or is very severe.

- **Severe bleeding:** Wearing disposable gloves, press onto the wound with a dressing pad, or with your fingers (to interrupt the bleeding and prevent further blood loss) until you have a sterile dressing to hand. If you can, raise and support the injured area, but be particularly gentle if you think you may have broken a bone. Lay down to aid circulation if a danger of *shock* exists (a dangerous loss of body fluid – refer to Chapter 5 for further info). Bandage the dressing pad firmly until you control the bleeding, but make sure that you don't make it so tight that you stop the blood circulating to your fingers or toes. If the bleeding continues and seeps through the bandage, apply a second layer of bandage. If this process still doesn't work, remove everything, start again and call '999' for an ambulance.

Knowing What Not to Do When Giving First Aid

Knowing what not to do is just as important as knowing what to do in an emergency situation. Take care and try to avoid these common mistakes when dealing with an emergency:

✔ **Don't put butter, ice or anything else apart from a clean dressing onto a large or deep burn:** Anything you put on a deep burn, other than a clean dressing, is of no use and would need to be removed in hospital – ouch! Using ice can even cause additional damage. Instead, put your burn under running water for at least 10 minutes and wrap it loosely in clean cling film or a clean non-fluffy cloth. Go to an Accident & Emergency (A&E) department if you suffer any burn that's larger than the cap of a milk bottle, because even small burns can be deep.

✔ **Don't take large objects out of wounds:** You may cause even more damage and set off a major bleed, ending up in a right old mess. Instead, build a 'bridge' over the object by applying pads to the skin surrounding it. Build up padding around it until this bridge is higher than the object. Finally, cover everything with a clean bandage and call '999'.

✔ **Don't put your finger in the mouth of a choking child:** You may induce vomiting or damage the child's throat.

✔ **Don't hang a choking child upside down by the feet:** Doing so can be very stressful for the child and you run the risk of accidentally causing a head injury if you drop the child or bang the head against another object.

✔ **Don't move if you suspect an injury to the spine:** Doing so may make things worse. In the worst-case scenario, you may even cause serious permanent damage.

Keeping Calm and Providing Comfort

Unsurprisingly, being faced with an emergency makes everyone's blood pressure go up, particularly when you're the casualty! Not panicking, and staying calm as you give or receive first aid in such situations isn't easy, but keeping your cool and being in control can prevent a situation getting worse.

Remaining calm, and being comforting and reassuring to a casualty has a more practical purpose than just being nice – it can help to prevent problems that may result from panicking (like wanting to get up in the case of a serious spinal injury where lying still is essential until help arrives, or in the event of a heart attack). Being calm also helps to keep the situation controlled and makes providing care easier for you and the medical professionals. If you're the casualty, you also reduce the impact of an emergency on your health by staying calm. Not panicking can make all the difference.

One way to make sure that you stay calm in an emergency is to prepare by keeping important telephone numbers, such as those for your GP surgery, dentist and pharmacist (also see Chapter 25 for a list of useful numbers), in an obvious place near your phone and stored on your mobile phone so you can find them easily in the heat of the moment.

Chapter 25

Ten Reliable Websites and Helplines

In This Chapter

▶ Finding health information you can trust online

▶ Discovering which websites to consult for particular problems

*T*hanks to the Internet, accessing medical information from the comfort of your own home has never been easier, and when you or a family member fall ill, the temptation is to have a look online for information. In theory, this idea isn't a bad one, because the high-quality information provided on certain websites can increase your knowledge about medical issues, which then helps you to make better decisions about your healthcare. This in turn enables you to enter into a more active partnership with health professionals. The downside is that a lot of poor advice is also on offer, with many websites containing material that's inaccurate, unfounded and sometimes plainly wrong. Unfortunately commercial or other interests sometimes get in the way, so not all of the medical information on the Internet is sufficiently reliable. The trick is to know where to look for information that you can rely on.

The ten websites I look at in this chapter are authoritative, reliable and good sources of information when you want to discover more about your symptoms or certain medical conditions. Most of these sites are reviewed and checked by experts, and you stand a good chance of finding further information on almost all your health problems on these websites alone – and if not, these sites give you the relevant links and tell you where else you can look.

The most important thing to remember is that the Internet is no substitute for sound medical advice from a health professional, particularly if you're not sure what's going on or you're potentially seriously ill.

NHS Websites and Helplines

England: NHS Choices (www.nhs.uk) and NHS Direct (www.nhsdirect.nhs.uk) (Tel: 0845 46 47).

Scotland: NHS Scotland – Scotland's Health on the Web (www.show.scot.nhs.uk) and NHS 24 (www.nhs24.com) (Tel: 08454 242424).

Wales: Health of Wales Information Service (www.wales.nhs.uk) and NHS Direct Wales (www.nhsdirect.wales.nhs.uk) (Tel: 0845 46 47).

Northern Ireland: Health and Social Care in Northern Ireland (www.hscni.net).

These websites are the gateway to the NHS, and they contain all the information you need for making choices about your health. Tons of useful health advice is available here – for example, about living well, medication issues and health risks – and you can discover more about hundreds of medical conditions, all explained in plain English. You can find and choose all the health services you need, read about the NHS and how it works, and get the low-down on major health stories.

The NHS Direct website in England and Wales and NHS 24 in Scotland also run helplines that are available 24 hours a day, 365 days a year, and are great places to turn to for help and reassurance when you have health worries. The websites provide a huge amount of advice and information, and you can even assess your medical symptoms with the health and symptom checker. You can access self-help advice on making your symptoms better before seeking medical help, and find straight-talking, informed and up-to-date information and advice about the latest health scares. You can get telephone advice on long-term medical conditions and receive pre- and postoperative support.

NHS Clinical Knowledge Summaries – Information for Patients

www.cks.nhs.uk/information_for_patients

The NHS Clinical Knowledge Summaries provide access to reliable and up-to-date patient information developed by NHS Direct and established major UK Charities such as The Arthritis Research Campaign, Epilepsy Research UK and the Family Planning Association. The website offers easy access to a vast range of patient information leaflets on various conditions, medications and complementary therapies, as well as health and social services.

Patient UK

www.patient.co.uk

Patient UK has a huge selection of patient information leaflets about medical conditions, symptoms, medicines and drugs, which many doctors give to their patients. You can find details of more than 1,800 UK patient support organisations and self-help groups plus selected Internet links to over 500 health-related online videos and to information aimed at carers.

Healthtalk Online and YouthHealthTalk

www.healthtalkonline.org and www.youthhealthtalk.org

These two websites give you access to real-life experiences that people and their carers have had of over 40 different illnesses and health conditions. Aimed at patients, their carers, family and friends as well as health professionals, these sites not only provide amazing insights into the patient perspective but also into the impact that an illness or medical condition has on the people around them. You can read about, listen to and watch people talking about their experiences and join their discussion forums.

The Royal College of General Practitioners

www.rcgp.org.uk/patient_information.aspx

The Royal College of General Practitioners is the professional membership body for family doctors in the UK and abroad; it aims to improve patient care, clinical standards and general practitioner training. The website has a useful section for patients where you can find information about medical conditions, health advice, links to support groups and tips on getting the most from your local surgery.

Patients Association

www.patients-association.com

The Patients Association (telephone helpline: 0845 6084455) is one of the UK's most established national healthcare charities, which helps patients by signposting advice and information about getting the best out of your healthcare, about medical problems and concerns, and much more. The Association is independent from the Department of Health or any other government body and campaigns to improve services across the country.

NetDoctor

www.netdoctor.co.uk

On this website you can join medical discussion forums, ask a large team of medical professionals questions online and access information about conditions, medicines, news stories, medical terms and support organisations. The authors who provide information on this website take care to follow the same standards as leading medical journals.

The Health Protection Agency

www.hpa.org.uk

This independent UK organisation aims to protect the public from threats to their health from infectious diseases and environmental hazards. On the website you can obtain advice and information about health hazards and emergencies caused by infectious disease, hazardous chemicals, poisons or radiation – all underpinned by evidence-based research.

Sixpartswater

www.sixpartswater.org

Sixpartswater is a new and visually appealing site that provides information about prevention and easy-to-follow knowledge about various medical conditions. This website also has a section called BodyWorks, which features great computer-generated animations of the human body. You can also download software applications from this site to help you gather your own personal health information on your home computer. Neat!

Cancer Research UK

www.cancerresearchuk.org

This charity website aims to help people understand cancer and gives information and advice about the choices each person can make about cancer diagnosis and treatment. The site also has lots of tips on how to spot cancer early, and information about cancer treatments, ways of adopting a healthier lifestyle to prevent cancer and statistics about the disease.

Chapter 26

Ten Medical Tests You May Need

In This Chapter

▶ Finding out what tests your doctor may arrange

▶ Discovering what certain tests involve

Medical professionals sometimes need to monitor disease or the effect of treatments, and confirm diagnoses by arranging further medical tests for you. Many people worry about what medical tests are for, whether they really need them, what the results may mean and whether the tests are painful. In this chapter I look at some common tests. (For more detailed information about these and other tests, check out the Patient UK website at www. patient.co.uk.)

Medical tests have limitations and your doctor chooses them carefully. You aren't sent for one without good reason. Generally, doctors send you for a test only when the result can potentially lead to a change in the management of your problem. For example, you don't normally need an X-ray for diagnosing a suspected rib fracture, because in managing the problem whether your rib is broken or not is irrelevant; the treatment (pain relief) is exactly the same.

Testing Your Blood

Blood tests can be useful for diagnosing and monitoring many medical conditions and can tell you whether some organs are functioning properly or if they're struggling because of some kind of damage. The thought of needles may put you off, but blood tests don't hurt much. You feel only a little sting, like pinching your skin gently between your fingernails. Here's a brief glance at a few types of blood test:

✔ **Blood sugar (or glucose):** Doctors use this test in diagnosing diabetes.

✔ **Full blood count (or FBC):** This test looks at various cells and platelets in your blood and is helpful in investigating anaemia, infection or bleeding problems (see Chapter 1 for more info on blood cells).

✔ **Kidney function (U&Es or C&Es):** This test looks at the salts in your blood and overall kidney function. Doctors commonly send you for this test to monitor diabetes and when you're prescribed certain medications.

✔ **Liver function (or LFTs):** Although called liver function, this series of tests is more about assessing liver damage.

✔ **Tests for inflammation or infection:** Plasma viscosity (or PV) or erythrocyte sedimentation rate (or ESR) tests rise in infection or inflammation such as arthritis.

✔ **Thyroid function (or TSH):** This test is useful when diagnosing and monitoring an underactive or overactive thyroid gland, which can cause symptoms such as tiredness and constantly feeling cold.

Getting to the Bare Bones With X-rays

X-rays are basically images produced on a photographic film by radiation that passes through objects or parts of the body, and are often used in medicine as a diagnostic tool. Because they're good for showing up bone and certain tissues – the denser the tissue, the whiter the appearance on the film – your doctor may send you for an X-ray to get a look at your bones and joints, your heart's size and shape or, on a chest X-ray, look for fluid collections or other masses in your lungs. Having an X-ray takes a few minutes, and they're completely painless, but the radiation can potentially damage certain tissues such as the testicles or ovaries, which is why they're used only when needed.

Testing Your Urine With a Sample

Doctors can test your urine for organisms that cause infection in a *mid-stream urine sample*, or MSU – all you need to do is pee into a little pot. This test can also indicate to medical professionals the best antibiotics to use in case you have a urine infection. This test isn't always necessary in simple and uncomplicated infections – a urine dipstick test can be useful to check for blood, sugar, protein and other various chemicals in your urine.

Tunnelling With CT and MRI Scans

Computerised Tomography (CT) and *Magnetic Resonance Imaging* (MRI) scans are generally safe and painless tests that efficiently show up organs and other structures inside your body. The scanners are tunnels that look like huge

Polo mints and, in the case of MRI, use strong magnetic fields rather than X-rays. You need to lie still during the procedure, which may last between 15 and 45 minutes and can be quite noisy. Some people can feel claustrophobic in these machines and, if necessary, you can receive medication to make you feel more relaxed. You don't have any after-effects from the scan.

Peering Inside With Ultrasound

Ultrasound tests are safe and painless, and good for looking at structures inside your body, and for seeing babies in pregnancy. Pictures are taken with a blunt probe (which is round and smooth); to get better pictures, a blob of jelly is used to provide good contact with your skin. Because the picture the doctor sees is updated quickly, ultrasound can show movement and assess the shape, size and consistency of unborn babies, and structures or organs such as your liver, kidney, gall bladder, ovaries, testes, breasts, bladder or blood vessels. Depending on the area under investigation, you may get instructions prior to the test, such as not to eat or drink, or to attend the test with a full bladder.

Looking at Bowels With a Barium Enema

A barium enema is a test for looking at your large bowel (or *colon*) lining, and is good for showing up things such as inflammation, pouches in your colon wall or tumours. The gut doesn't show up particularly well on standard X-ray pictures, and so a thick liquid containing a substance called *barium* is injected through your rectum into your gut – which can be uncomfortable. Because X-rays don't go through barium, they make your gut show up clearly on the X-ray film. This procedure is less common these days – endoscopy is often used instead – but it still has its place.

Approaching the Heart of the Matter With an Electrocardiogram

An *electrocardiogram* (ECG) is a harmless, painless test that takes a few minutes to look at your heart's electrical activity, without giving you an electric shock. ECGs can detect rhythm abnormalities and help your doctor to investigate chest pain, but they're also sometimes done routinely before operations. Electrodes are placed on your chest, and a reading is recorded over a few seconds. Special forms of ECGs include *exercise ECGs* (useful for assessing chest pain, and involves taking serial ECGs under increasing exercise) and *ambulatory ECGs* (when you wear a mobile ECG for 24 hours or more).

ECGs do have their limitations, and normal ECGs don't necessarily rule out underlying conditions, so sometimes further tests are necessary.

Viewing the Engine Room With an Echocardiogram

An *echocardiogram* (or ECHO) is a simple ultrasound test that doctors use to assess your heart's structure and function, to check whether a heart is working properly after a heart attack or whether the heart valves are doing their job properly (check out 'Peering Inside with Ultrasound' earlier in this chapter on how it's done). The test is painless, harmless and usually doesn't last longer than 15–30 minutes or so. Other special forms of ECHO are sometimes used, for example to check the flow of blood in your heart.

Delving Deep With Endoscopes

Doctors can use a flexible telescope called an *endoscope* to look inside your body. An endoscope has the thickness of an average little finger. At its tip is a light and a tiny video camera, which transmits images to a television screen, making riveting viewing! The operator can even pass instruments through a side tunnel within the endoscope, enabling her to take small tissue samples and perform other nifty little tricks. Going in from your mouth (*gastroscopy*) is useful for diagnosing symptoms such as heartburn or vomiting; going up from your back passage (*colonoscopy*) is useful for investigating a change in bowel habit or bleeding from the back passage. Having an endoscopy isn't the most pleasant experience, so you may be offered relaxing medication.

Feeling Itchy With Allergy Testing

Doctors sometimes use *skin prick testing* to find out what may be causing certain allergies. Potential *allergens* (substances that may be the cause of an allergy) are put on your skin in drops. The skin is then pricked and you wait for a reaction about 20–30 minutes later. If your skin becomes red and itchy or swells up, you've had a positive reaction, and doctors then discover more about what you may be allergic to. A different form of allergy testing called *patch testing* can also help to pinpoint the cause of an allergic skin reaction. In patch testing, certain substances are placed directly on your skin to identify skin allergies. Allergy testing is useful only when you don't really know what you're allergic to, and so that you can identify potential causes.

Index

• U •

• V •

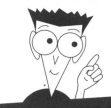

FOR DUMMIES®

Making Everything Easier! ™

UK editions

BUSINESS

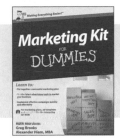

Marketing Kit
978-0-470-74490-1

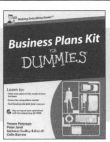

Business Plans Kit
978-0-470-74381-2

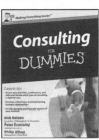

Consulting
978-0-470-71382-2

Anger Management For Dummies
978-0-470-68216-6

Boosting Self-Esteem For Dummies
978-0-470-74193-1

British Sign Language
For Dummies
978-0-470-69477-0

Business NLP For Dummies
978-0-470-69757-3

Cricket For Dummies
978-0-470-03454-5

CVs For Dummies, 2nd Edition
978-0-470-74491-8

Divorce For Dummies, 2nd Edition
978-0-470-74128-3

Emotional Freedom Technique
For Dummies
978-0-470-75876-2

Emotional Healing For Dummies
978-0-470-74764-3

English Grammar For Dummies
978-0-470-05752-0

Flirting For Dummies
978-0-470-74259-4

IBS For Dummies
978-0-470-51737-6

Improving Your Relationship For
Dummies
978-0-470-68472-6

Lean Six Sigma For Dummies
978-0-470-75626-3

Life Coaching For Dummies,
2nd Edition
978-0-470-66554-1

REFERENCE

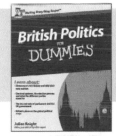

British Politics
978-0-470-68637-9

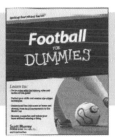

Football
978-0-470-68837-3

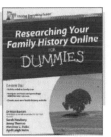

Researching Your Family History Online
978-0-470-74535-9

HOBBIES

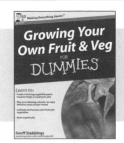

Growing Your Own Fruit & Veg
978-0-470-69960-7

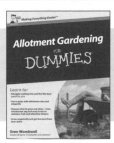

Allotment Gardening
978-0-470-68641-6

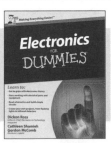

Electronics
978-0-470-68178-7

14652 (p1)

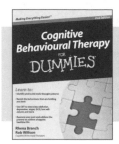
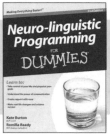
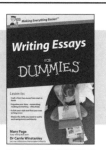

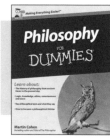
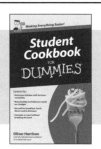
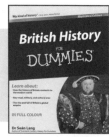
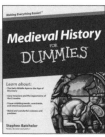
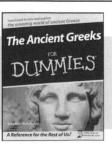

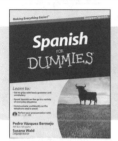
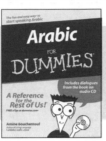
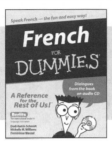
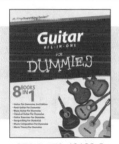
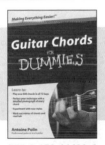
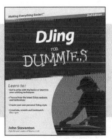
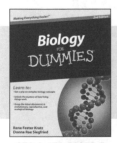
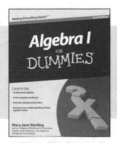
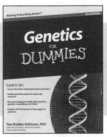

FOR DUMMIES®

Helping you expand your horizons and achieve your potential

COMPUTER BASICS

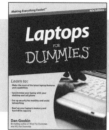

978-0-470-57829-2

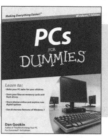

978-0-470-46542-4

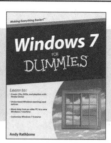

978-0-470-49743-2

DIGITAL PHOTOGRAPHY

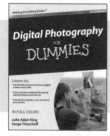

978-0-470-25074-7

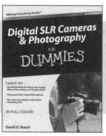

978-0-470-46606-3

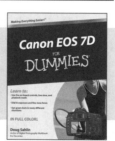

978-0-470-59591-6

MICROSOFT OFFICE 2010

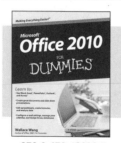

978-0-470-48998-7

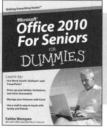

978-0-470-58302-9

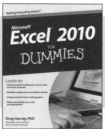

978-0-470-48953-6

Access 2007 For Dummies
978-0-470-04612-8

Adobe Creative Suite 5 Design
Premium All-in-One For Dummies
978-0-470-60746-6

AutoCAD 2011 For Dummies
978-0-470-59539-8

C++ For Dummies, 6th Edition
978-0-470-31726-6

Computers For Seniors For Dummies,
2nd Edition
978-0-470-53483-0

Dreamweaver CS5 For Dummies
978-0-470-61076-3

Excel 2007 All-In-One Desk Reference
For Dummies
978-0-470-03738-6

Green IT For Dummies
978-0-470-38688-0

Macs For Dummies, 10th Edition
978-0-470-27817-8

Mac OS X Snow Leopard For Dummies
978-0-470-43543-4

Networking All-in-One Desk Reference
For Dummies, 3rd Edition
978-0-470-17915-4

Photoshop CS5 For Dummies
978-0-470-61078-7

Photoshop Elements 8 For Dummies
978-0-470-52967-6

Search Engine Optimization
For Dummies, 3rd Edition
978-0-470-26270-2

The Internet For Dummies,
12th Edition
978-0-470-56095-2

Visual Studio 2008 All-In-One Desk
Reference For Dummies
978-0-470-19108-8

Web Analytics For Dummies
978-0-470-09824-0